AGING AND LEVELS
OF BIOLOGICAL
ORGANIZATION

CONTRIBUTORS

KIMBALL C. ATWOOD

C. H. BARROWS

JAMES E. BIRREN

AUSTIN M. BRUES, *Chairman*

HANS COTTIER

W. M. COURT-BROWN

TH. DOBZHANSKY

CHARLES F. EHRET

WALLACE O. FENN

FRANK FREMONT-SMITH

R. J. MICHAEL FRY

LISSY JARVIK

FRANZ J. KALLMAN

ANCEL KEYS

ALBERT I. LANSING

PATRICIA J. LINDOP

HENRY QUASTLER

FREEMAN H. QUIMBY

GEORGE A. SACHER

HENRY S. SIMMS

H. BURR STEINBACH

JOHN B. STORER

ALBERT TYLER

AGING AND LEVELS OF BIOLOGICAL ORGANIZATION

Edited by
AUSTIN M. BRUES
and GEORGE A. SACHER

THE UNIVERSITY OF CHICAGO PRESS

CHICAGO AND LONDON

PROCEEDINGS OF A CONFERENCE
AT PRINCETON, NEW JERSEY
December 2–5, 1962

Library of Congress Catalog Card Number: 65-17281

THE UNIVERSITY OF CHICAGO PRESS, CHICAGO & LONDON
The University of Toronto Press, Toronto 5, Canada

THIS VOLUME IS DEDICATED TO THE MEMORY OF

HENRY QUASTLER
1908–63

TO WHOM MANY OF THE PARTICIPANTS ARE
INDEBTED FOR HIS BROAD AND IMAGINATIVE
WISDOM AND FOR HIS UNFAILING GENEROSITY IN
SHARING IT WITH HIS FRIENDS AND COLLEAGUES

Preface

This conference was sponsored by the American Institute of Biological Sciences and supported by the National Heart Institute, National Institutes of Health.*

It was originally proposed that an interdisciplinary conference of this type be directed to the subject of radiation-induced aging. After some discussion among the organizers, however, it became clear that this somewhat limited topic had been covered rather thoroughly in other recent conferences and that it would be more fruitful from all points of view to broaden the scope. The participants, therefore, were asked to examine the problem of metazoan aging at all levels of organization, ranging from molecules and cells to ecosystems. Only one of the six sessions treated primarily problems of ionizing radiation; and that one centered on the basic and rather elusive question of the extent to which effects of radiation on life span actually represent acceleration of the natural processes of aging. Although several of the participants have been closely identified with radiation physiology and pathology, this should be taken to reflect only the special concern that investigators in these fields have had for problems of aging.

The conference was conducted along lines familiar to those who are acquainted with other conferences held under the interdisciplinary conference program of the American Institute of Biological Sciences. Each of the sessions was opened by a selected discussant. He was asked to present his recent work and current views in the context of the major questions in the field, and the participants were encouraged to present their own data and thoughts in the same context; a number of

*The conference was supported by grants from the National Institutes of Health (H 3650 and HTS 5326) and publication of the proceedings was supported by an additional grant (HEO 8532).

them, in so doing, bridged gaps between various levels of organization.

The discussions were all free and informal and were transcribed verbatim. Each participant reviewed the transcript and edited his remarks under the admonition of the editors to preserve the informal atmosphere of the meeting. The editors then undertook to prepare the final text, with a minimum of deletions and rearrangements.

We wish to acknowledge gratefully the assistance of Elizabeth Purcell and Catherine Calabretta in conducting the preparations for the conference and in much of the work of editing this volume, and of Elaine Bart and Donna Daniel of the Argonne National Laboratory in preparation of the final text.

Austin M. Brues
George A. Sacher

Division of Biological and Medical Research
Argonne National Laboratory
Argonne, Illinois

Contents

Genetics and Environment

PART I

<u>Dobzhansky</u>: I have been asked to give an introduction to the subject of genetics and environment.

I suppose no biological concept is as widely, persistently, and stubbornly misunderstood as the concept of heredity. To many people, the idea that biological inheritance can have something to do with human traits which are of any importance to individuals or to society is intensely repugnant.

I submit that this prejudice is due to two kinds of misunderstanding, which we may analyze as far as we can.

One of the misunderstandings is semantic: in English, and apparently in all other languages, the word "heredity," or "inheritance," means two completely different things. One is biological inheritance; the other is legal inheritance—inheritance of property.

I am told that there is only one language in which this is not true, and that is Malay, Indonesian. The Malay language has separate words for the two concepts. The fact that most other languages use the same word has led to countless difficulties and mix-ups. Indeed, when we speak about having inherited skin color, longevity, or intelligence from our parents, we do not mean the same thing at all as when we speak about having inherited a house or a diamond from them. When parents pass on skin pigmentation and intelligence, they presumably have kept their own skin and their own pigment, and, presumably, they have also kept their own intelligence intact.

Obviously, inheritance of biological properties means something very different from legal inheritance. This ambiguity has been realized for a long time. The earliest, very clear and very beautiful statement was made by Montaigne (26) in the sixteenth century. He was greatly worried about having inherited gallstones from his father, and he asked, very reasonably: "How could my father pass to me bladder

1

stones which he himself did not have at the time I was conceived?" (Laughter)

Now, of course, the difficulty is resolved relatively simply: we do not inherit bladder stones, or intelligence, or even skin color—we inherit genes.

The other difficulty is, perhaps, a little more subtle and has something to do with the history of genetics.

The reason Mendel succeeded where many others failed was that he worked on the inheritance in crosses between parents differing in discrete qualities. Many experimenters crossed plants and animals before Mendel, but they tried to work with the entire habitus of an organism and, of course, precise analysis of that proved to be impossible. What Mendel did was to study the inheritance of single, discrete, clear-cut qualities—yellow versus green, tall versus short—and follow the distribution of these qualities in the progeny. This was the basis of his success, and the classical geneticists quite reasonably followed Mendel.

Morgan (27) started to observe the mutants in Drosophila. He found two kinds of mutants: there were some of these beautiful, wonderful, clear-cut mutants with short wings, vestigial wings, and no wings at all, with vermilion, purple, and white eyes instead of the normal red. These were the mutants selected for experiments. Anybody who has worked with Drosophila, or any other material, knows that, apart from these "good" mutants, a tremendous number of what are known as "bad" mutants are found—mutants which differ from the normal fly only slightly—and especially those "bad" mutants which are subject to environmental modification. The differences are so variable that the flies cannot be classified into clear-cut classes. These "bad" mutants usually are dispatched down the drain, and that is the end of them.

Fremont-Smith: Along with the environmental factor.

Dobzhansky: Indeed. I would like to repeat: The fact that geneticists selected these unusual sorts of mutants, these unusual kinds of clear-cut, hereditary variants, was tactically well justified for the purpose they had in mind—to study the rules of hereditary transmission from parents to children, and to make chromosome maps. These are the kinds of traits, the "good" mutants, which are most desirable for genetic studies of the classical type. Of course, up to this day in microbial genetics or biochemical genetics, the types of hereditary variants selected are in most cases mutants which produce all-or-none effects. A "bug" grows or does not grow in the presence or absence of a certain antibiotic substance. If it grows merely a little more or a little less than the normal type, it is not a good type of variant to work with.

Of course, geneticists were always quite well aware of the existence of genetic variants of the less convenient kinds, such as those called the "quantitative traits." Moreover, geneticists were also quite well aware that these quantitative traits, such as variants with a little bigger or little smaller body, greater or lesser weight, a little more or little less pigmentation, are quite common. Those are the really important traits in agricultural practice. Such traits are what people who are working on animal- and plant-breeding are chiefly interested in. These are what they study and select when they try to improve the breeds of agricultural animals and plants.

Genetically, traits of this sort are difficult to work with. One does not get a beautiful 3:1 Mendelian segregation. As a matter of fact, in the early days of genetics there was a considerable amount of doubt and polemic as to whether these quantitative traits were subject to Mendel's laws at all.

There was a powerful school in genetics of those who believed in genetic dualism: gene heredity, Mendelian heredity, on one side, and some kind of hazy, non-Mendelian heredity dealing chiefly with quantitative traits on the other. This disagreement has been resolved; it is now generally accepted that almost all heredity is Mendelian heredity. There is no dualism in heredity; there are no two kinds of genes. Genes are all basically similar. It is their phenotypic effects which are different.

Fremont-Smith: Was the dualism due, in part, to the assumption that genes had all aspects of environment constant, and that there were variants in the environment which had not been recognized?

Dobzhansky: In experiments, obviously, we try to make our environment as uniform as possible. So the good mutants in Drosophila are those mutants which appear reasonably constantly within the range of environments which exists in the laboratory, where the temperature is controlled, where the food is as uniform as possible, and so on.

On the other hand, geneticists came to study, let's say, the yield of corn, or the growth rate in pigs, or the responses to climatic variations, to seasonal variations, to differences in food. All these factors act to obscure the clear-cut specimens' inheritance. What is really involved is not a dualism of hereditary elements, but a dualism of methods of study (8, 24).

The small quantitative changes are now habitually described as due to polygenic changes or to polygenic heredity. This is a most unfortunate term. Etymologically, "polygene" is clearly a nonsensical word: "polygene" means "many genes." A "many genes" is nonsense. But the term is well established in the literature; let's not fight it. We have to put up with it.

Fremont-Smith: Put quotes around it.

Dobzhansky: I'm afraid it is no longer used even with quotes.

Fremont-Smith: You don't think we could reintroduce them?

Dobzhansky: The modern usage of the word "polygene" was introduced by Mather (24), currently a professor in Birmingham, England.

The main difference between "good" genes and polygenes is a difference in technique used for their study. Instead of crossing strains and observing the segregation of discrete traits, we have to use statistical, mathematical techniques which are very difficult indeed and very uncomfortable to most geneticists who are, like myself, ignorant of mathematics. There are geneticists who study the quantitative characters, and geneticists who study the classical 3:1 Mendelian trait.

I submit that polygenic traits are very important, because the adaptively significant human and animal and plant traits are usually of that kind. This, again, is no accident. This is no perversity of nature.

A number of evolutionists, especially Schmalhausen in Russia, have argued, and I believe quite cogently, that natural selection will tend to establish an adaptively significant trait on a polygenic rather than on a monogenic basis; that there will be a greater plasticity in the process of evolutionary transformation if a trait is built, not on a single, major gene, but on a system of minor polygenes (9).

Incidentally, it is worth quoting Mather's definition of a polygene, a definition which does not imply any absolute distinctness. He spoke about polygenes as genes with phenotypic effects of a magnitude less than, or equal to, the usual environmental phenotypic variation.

Here, then, is a gene such that two alleles, or variant forms, produce a difference of phenotypic effect that is at most as large as what the environment can produce by way of phenotypic modification.

Whether a character is environmentally plastic or environmentally rigid is a matter not of accident but rather of natural selection establishing a developmental pattern most favorable to the organism.

By and large, the traits which are adaptively significant, in the sense that an organism must have them, are developmentally buffered in such a way that, if life goes on at all, they always appear in the process of development.

Fremont-Smith: Does "developmentally stable" imply we haven't yet found the environment that will cause a change?

Dobzhansky: Indeed. In principle, I think it can be safely said that any characteristic may be modified by environmental as well as by genetic variables. What I am talking about is simply that certain traits—for example, the presence of two eyes instead of one eye in vertebrate development—arise in almost every developing individual. The cyclopic monsters are rare. Another example is the suckling instinct, which is, as far as I know, present in every newborn baby.

Fremont-Smith: How about anencephaly?

Dobzhansky: The formation of the head in the embryo is, presumably, also one of the characteristics which are buffered against environmental disturbances.

On the other hand, there is a category of traits where an environmental plasticity is, presumably, adaptively desirable. The simplest example is skin color, skin pigmentation. My skin at present is fairly well bleached. However, I can develop a healthy, dark pigmentation if I spend a good summer somewhere in the bosom of nature.

Where the organism is exposed, in its natural habitat, to a variety of environments which can be coped with most easily by modifying some traits, we are likely to find a genetically established plasticity rather than a fixity of the developmental pattern. Let me emphasize this expression, genetically established plasticity. When a trait is environmentally plastic, easily modified by the environment, this environmental plasticity is genetically conditioned.

Probably the most remarkably plastic trait in man is his behavior. Here the developmental pattern is genetically made most responsive to environmental variations, so that the outcome of the development is most easily modified by the environment in which it takes place. And the outcome of the development is not something fixed; there is no final stage of development. Development continues from fertilization to death. The phenotypes which can develop during this time span, from fertilization to death, are, in some cases, rigidly fixed, where this is adaptively advantageous to the organism, and in other cases plastic and responsive to the environment where this is advantageous.

I think this is worth stressing because, particularly in

early genetic literature, attempts were made to distinguish two classes of traits, the environmental and the genetic traits. We get into trouble every time we attempt to classify the characters of any organism, be it Drosophila, Homo sapiens, or anything else, into these two categories. They are not two distinct categories. In every case there is in principle the possibility of both genetic and environmental modification; and the degree to which this modifiability can be achieved by the variety of environments normally encountered by an organism is, in turn, a genetically established characteristic.

Sacher: In human evolution, has there been a selection toward greater plasticity?

Dobzhansky: We are speaking about different kinds of plasticity. On the one hand, there may be a plasticity of the individual development. Given a certain genotype, the outcome of the development may depend on the environmental setting, and the plasticity may be greater or less.

On the other hand, there may be a variety of genotypes in the population. Such a population may respond to the environment in a different way. The incidence in the population of certain genotypes may increase in some environments and decrease in others.

Adaptation of the population, or of the species, to the environment, then, can be achieved in at least two ways. One possible way is developmental plasticity. Some genotypes can react to different environments by producing a variety of adaptive phenotypes. This is one kind of adaptive mechanism. The other kind is genetic diversification, existence of a variety of genotypes. A population of a sexually reproducing species is a mixture of a large number of genotypes. In a human population—in the entire species, in fact—the number of genotypes is equal to the number of individuals, identical twins being an exception. Assuming that none of us has an identical twin—I do not—each of our genotypes is unique. There has never been anybody with a genotype exactly like mine, and there never will be.

Fremont-Smith: We regret that, sir.

Dobzhansky: I'm not sure it is regrettable. (Laughter) I think it is just as well. Well, some populations are relatively uniform, genetically; others are highly polymorphic, or variable. This genetic population variability is also an adaptive mechanism whereby a species may adjust itself to the variety of the environment it faces.

These are the two equally effective methods of adaptation to the environment that most biological species, including

Homo sapiens, have utilized: individual plasticity—homeo-stasis—and genetic variety.

Birren: Medawar (25) used the word "precession" of fa-vorable characteristics and "recession" of unfavorable char-acteristics, implying, I believe, that a favorable trait is likely to advance in the age at which it will appear. Negative traits would thus appear later in life. Does this mean that most polygenetic characteristics would be characteristics of early life, whereas genetic characteristics of late life would be sin-gle-gene characteristics?

Dobzhansky: No. There is no particular reason, at least no reason that I know of, to make such a differentiation. Per-haps, on the average, the early development processes have oftener been buffered. The later processes may more often be plastic. I would be reluctant to go as far as you say Med-awar is inclined to go.

Birren: Are early-life characteristics more likely to be polygenic?

Dobzhansky: I don't know whether there is any indica-tion of that.

Ehret: We seem to be approaching one of the crucial questions for the aging process, namely, what is the physical basis for developmental plasticity? Very simply stated, there are at least these alternatives: that plasticity is based upon a variety of genes that may be switched off or on or, contrari-wise, that it is based upon genes with inherent plasticity of product-character output. The first alternative seems favored by evidence from a number of studies in microbial genetics. In _Paramecium_ the serotype transformations with tempera-ture (2) are such that the character of the surface proteins is related not only to the growth temperature but also and, pre-dictably, to the specific Mendelian genes of the nucleus, switched off or on according to the temperature. Most of our contemporary models, including those of Jacob and Monod (15) are of a similar sort: a variety of genes with switch mecha-nisms, rather than genes with inherent plasticity. For the stu-dent of aging, an interesting question that arises from the _Paramecium_ results is whether there is a differential ther-molability of the various serotype proteins that would lead to a differential wearing out of the very fabric of the cell.

Quastler: Is there any known adaptive advantage in switching serotypes?

Ehret: Only one that I know of: the serotype induced by

the antibiotic patulin can withstand higher concentrations of patulin than the other serotypes (1).

Dobzhansky: I think the point you brought up is by no means irrelevant to the problem. The existence of environmentally plastic traits and of environmentally fixed traits, is, of course, a matter of considerable importance for the theme of this conference. I would like, however, to warn that one should not get into the habit of thinking of these as two distinct and different categories of traits. Some confusion has been caused in the genetic literature by making the polygenes and the "oligogenes," the major genes, two different classes of genes. They are not. There exist all possible intermediate situations, from environmental rigidity to environmental plasticity. It is not that some traits are completely fixed and others are completely plastic; there is every possible degree of plasticity and fixity.

Furthermore, "fixity" means fixity within the range of the environments which the species normally encounters in its natural habitat. If we expose an organism to environmental variables which it does not encounter in its natural habitat—high energy radiation in large amounts, for example—the traits which are normally fixed may become plastic. This is sometimes described as "modification" versus "morphosis." Modifications are changes due to environmental factors, factors which occur in the habitat of the species more or less frequently. Morphoses are responses to agents to which the species has not become adapted in its evolution. Modifications are usually adaptively valuable. Morphoses are adaptively random and, consequently, very frequently not valuable but harmful.

The effect of poisons can be used as an example of morphosis. A poison is a poison because the organism cannot react adaptively to its effects.

Fremont-Smith: If we talk about the usual environment to which the organism is exposed, doesn't this tend to ignore evolution, which has provided a variety of environments in the past, sometimes with high radiation?

Dobzhansky: I think, Dr. Fremont-Smith, that is an excellent question. There you have, if you please, evidence of the imperfection of our world. Ours is not the best of all possible worlds. The evolutionary process makes the organism adapted best to the environment which has just lapsed. We are always backward in our adaptedness. In the case of man, that becomes, of course, a fundamental problem. Our genes have not made us adapted to the environment of the Nassau Inn, or of the twentieth century; we are, presumably, best adapted to the environment of some of our ancestors—perhaps a hundred or a thousand generations back. That is, however, a necessary consequence of adaptation by means of natural selection.

If evolution should make us adapted to the present or to the future environment, that would be nothing short of a miracle. The adaptedness is often, of necessity, imperfect in the retrospective sense that the adaptedness achieved is adaptedness to the environment of the past.

Storer: Could we go back to one point that confused me a little? As I understand your argument, the genotype showing the greatest plasticity, allowing the greatest phenotypic variability, is the best adapted. Is that, roughly, your point?

Dobzhansky: If is not quite so simple, Dr. Storer, I'm afraid. The genotype which would make the development plastic with respect to all possible environmental agencies would not be very good. I mentioned learning ability. You will agree that a genotypic fixity of a kind which would permit a fellow to learn only one thing, to become, shall we say, a very excellent barber, and nothing else, would not be adaptive in many environments. Suppose an individual can learn only barbering, or only gardening, or only the priestcraft. This type of fixity would be disadvantageous. Conditions change; cultural environments change extremely rapidly. Genetic fixity would be disadvantageous. The plasticity which permits one to become a barber or a gardener or a priest or a scientist is adaptively far more valuable.

On the other hand, the presence of, for example, resistance to cold, which I seem unfortunately to lack, is probably a genotypic trait that is desirable in every individual. So I would not say that either fixity or plasticity is always, per se, desirable. It depends on the environment.

Ehret: When we talk about genetic plasticity, we don't mean non-constancy of genes within the individual; in fact, we expect gene constancy. Of course, as the raw material of evolution for the population, a certain amount of non-constancy, or error in the gene replication process, is a healthy thing. But what we are concerned with in aging is the physical basis of developmental plasticity for the individual. Perhaps Dr. Dobzhansky can help clarify this.

Dobzhansky: Developmental plasticity is the ability of a genotype to react to various environments by evolving different phenotypes which are adaptively suitable to those environments. That is developmental plasticity, or phenotypic plasticity, if you wish.

Now, genotypic plasticity is a property of a population. If a population is genetically uniform, it contains only one genotype. It may very well be adapted to the environment as it exists at a given moment, in a given place. As the environment changes, the species may find itself at a disadvantage; it has no genetic plasticity.

If, on the other hand, a population contains a great variety of genotypes, then it may also be genetically plastic. It can respond to environmental change by adaptive genetic change.

Sex, that ancient and venerable institution, is, of course, a biological adaptation which confers genetic plasticity on the species because it is able to manufacture ever new genotypes.

Sacher: A well-adapted fruit fly population has members, all of which have good survival in a given environment and, therefore, a minimum of variability of this presumably vital characteristic. Is that not the case?

Dobzhansky: No. I could talk about this for an hour, since it happens to be my particular line of research. Some Drosophila fly populations are genetically more or less uniform, others are more or less polymorphic, non-uniform. Species which are ecologically most versatile, most successful, are, as a rule, those which are genetically most variable in the sense I have tried to define. When we speak about environment, we are likely to think of it as being a unit—the species faces the environment. That is obviously an oversimplification. Any species faces a variety of environments. Even a blood parasite living, presumably, in the most uniform environment, never lives in an environment which is absolutely constant.

For a species which faces a variety of environments— and, again, Homo sapiens is undoubtedly one such—genetic variety may be adaptive. In fact, genetic variety may confer on a population the ability to exploit a great variety of ecological niches which would be inaccessible to a population consisting of only a single genotype or only a few genotypes. Let's not forget that there is never an environment; there are always environments—many of them.

Kallmann: Is it possible to define such vague terms as genetic plasticity and relative fixity of a trait, and how can they be distinguished? I wonder, for instance, how much of a variation in genetic plasticity might be necessary to account for the difference between the abilities to survive as a barber and as a gardener. I would like to understand why this difference can be regarded as an indication of genetic plasticity.

Dobzhansky: Dr. Kallmann, imagine a genotype so specialized that its carrier could be brought up only as a member of a certain occupation or profession. This situation would be adaptively less favorable than a genotype which would permit its carrier to be trained for a variety of occupations. Consider different social systems: on the one hand, in India there are castes and subcastes which are, or were, genetically closed systems. The castes were specialized for different occupations. A member of each Indian caste generally went into a definite profession. That is one way of organizing a human society. It consists of a variety of types, each specialized for a given profession.

On the other hand there is a situation where an individual can be trained for any kind of profession. That would be plasticity. This kind of genetic adaptation, which permits such a plasticity, will usually be advantageous, will it not?

Kallmann: I can visualize one well-defined situation, in which a person with the ability to survive as a gardener might have no chance of surviving as a barber. In a society where shaves and haircuts are in conflict with cultural or political rules, no member would be able to survive as a barber. I doubt, however, that this inability can be accounted for in terms of genetic plasticity.

Ehret: I think that if we use human populations and argue by analogy we have some difficulty; what concerns us is aging of the individual.

Fixity of watchmaking as a profession is good as long as watches are sold, and may be advantageous to a small country for a while. But in this conference we are concerned not so much with the aging of populations or groups of individuals (in the sense in which Toynbee would analyze society); we are concerned with the aging of the individual. As a method, reasoning by analogy may lead to interesting relations that parallel reality mathematically, but the underlying physical causes and structures are entirely different. This realization is the very essence of the levels-of-organization approach (12).

Just as there are physical reasons for the deterioration or "aging" of a social order, so there are also physical reasons for organism, tissue, cell, and perhaps even molecular aging. Of course we normally don't speak of "molecular aging." At the lower levels of organization we speak of "changes." We say: "This is the reaction sequence." Other transitions in time are more complex, and to certain categories of these we apply the term "aging." An understanding of aging in living systems will come from an understanding of the physical aspects of gene action, and consequential sequelae up the levels-of-organization ladder. As soon as we start talking about human populations, barbering, and watch-making, we confuse the issue by introducing an extra-genic code that includes tools, libraries, and tradition, even drugs and the practice of medicine—all highly interesting and un-doubtedly contributing to average human longevity, but not basic to the aging process common to all living systems.

Kallmann: I have raised this issue only in view of some recent statements made on television in relation to the evo-lutionary theory. In one of those round-table discussions dealing with mental illness, a well-known scientist stated: "Inasmuch as schizophrenics are able to survive, and schizo-phrenia is rather common in all populations, this mental dis-ease must confer some biological advantage upon its carri-ers." Is there any reliable evidence supporting this hypoth-esis?

Dobzhansky: I'm afraid I can't take responsibility for what is said on television.

Ehret: Perhaps sickle-cell anemia in Mediterranean areas might be an example to use.

Dobzhansky: That is what I would suggest. Possibly that statement was a garbled version of a perfectly sound idea which I am sure is familiar to you, namely, that heterozygous carriers of sickle-cell anemia have a gene which is unfavor-able in a homozygous condition, and that they may have an ad-vantage. I trust you are not shocked by that.

Kallmann: No, I am not really shocked. I am merely con-cerned about the possible consequences which such categor-ical statements may have in terms of the reproduction of schizophrenics. I am reluctant to jump from normal, plastic traits showing many graded differences within a certain range of ordinary responses, to clearly pathological conditions pre-sumed to be adaptively advantageous under certain circum-stances. In my opinion, such analogies are rather hazardous.

Dobzhansky: We have discussed this topic with Dr. Kall-mann several times. I believe that normal and pathological conditions are not two distinct classes and that we not only can but, indeed, should jump from one to the other. I know Dr. Kallmann does not agree.

Keys: Isn't one difficulty here that there is a good deal of talk about "advantage," without saying advantage for what?

Dobzhansky: That is a crucial point. What is natural selection doing? It is selection for reproductive proficiency. Reproductive proficiency, however, is not the only quality we admire in our fellow men and women. Consequently, the biological process of natural selection may not be a satisfactory one from the human standpoint. However, when we speak about biological adaptedness, we may distinguish between "adaptedness" and "adaptation." Adaptation is a process of becoming adapted; adaptedness is a state of being adapted. Adaptedness is the ability to survive and reproduce in a given environment. Biological adaptedness need not necessarily be identical with what we, as people, regard as desirable or admirable.

Fremont-Smith: Because we are a thousand generations further on now, in terms of what you said.

Dobzhansky: In terms of population explosion, which has made us rather skeptical about the virtues of reproductive efficiency.

Birren: May I go back to the contrasts between early and late life? I should add that my questions are more for getting information than exposing a point of view.

You say that there is selection for reproductive proficiency; yet for men this would mean, by and large, that natural selection doesn't operate for characteristics which appear after the age of 50.

We know that Alzheimer's disease, and a few other diseases, commonly appear for the first time after the age of reproduction. I am trying to question the likelihood of these late-life characteristics having a different kind of genetic basis from early-life characteristics. One might expect to find some difference in these characteristics since those of late life are less likely to be subjected to natural selection or the force of selection.

Dobzhansky: This matter was treated for the first time, I believe, by Haldane (13); it has been discussed many times since. Since natural selection, in the biological sense, is concerned with reproductive efficiency, it will not directly regulate, modify, or maintain characteristics of postreproductive age. It may do so, indirectly, on the population level.

Haldane pointed out that if the presence of old people in a tribe constitutes a burden, if having to maintain them is disadvantageous to the tribe, natural selection may act to speed up their demise. If, on the other hand, postreproductive individuals, because of their wisdom, or whatever it may be, confer an advantage on the group, then natural selection may act to improve the conditions of old age. The same thing is true for all kinds of conditions which interfere with repro-

14 AGING AND LEVELS OF BIOLOGICAL ORGANIZATION

duction. They may conceivably be selectively advantageous, if they confer some advantage on the group.

I think the most interesting paper on that was published a few years ago (14) by G. Evelyn Hutchinson of Yale. I am sure Dr. Kallmann knows about this paper. He used the term paraphilia for genetic variants which are reproductively ineffective, but which may still be favored by natural selection because of their indirect effects.

Kallmann: Hutchinson (14) suggested that the most probable mode of operation of the genetic determinants of homosexual behavior in man might be "on the rates of development of neuropsychological mechanisms involved in identification processes and other aspects of object relationship in infancy" and, as such, may have important pleiotropic effects. In his opinion, the tendency to substitute reproductively non-significant sexual goals for a mate of the opposite sex is sufficiently widespread in human populations, results in sufficiently lowered fertility, and is under enough genetic control to affect the distribution of human genotypes. Hence, certain aspects of sexual selection in man "may involve mechanisms neutralizing castration fear, and so may ultimately influence such maturation rates." The given type of display was called "cryptandric."

Sacher: This assumes a great deal of importance because, in Medawar's view (25)—and I think it is a view attractive to many biologists—natural selection does not operate after the end of reproductive life, and this leads to a model of aging that Medawar aptly described as running out of program. According to this position, aging is an adventitious process rather than a programed process under genetic control throughout the life of the individual. This "running-out-of-program" model is easy to fall into if one's attention is restricted to consideration of the mammal. But I believe that the zoologist or geneticist who works with other material would realize there are actual, specific mechanisms of life termination which are under quite definite genetic control.

Dobzhansky: This has been discussed in recent years, particularly by Comfort (7) in England, and by Williams (37) in this country. There, again, we ought to distinguish between these two kinds of selection: interindividual—intrapopulation—selection and interpopulational selection.

Intrapopulation selection will, as these scientists have shown, favor the organism at an age when its reproductive efficiency is highest. Interpopulational selection, however, may be a more versatile mechanism, favoring conditions disadvantageous to individuals, if they confer an advantage on the group.

Perhaps the most obvious example of this latter mechanism is the balanced polymorphism situation. Dr. Ehret mentioned the sickle-cell trait. There, the adaptedness of the population is compensated for by unadaptedness of some of the component individuals who die of sickle-cell anemia. That is the clearest example of natural selection being able to do two different things. This is obviously a pathological, in fact, a lethal condition favored by natural selection, because of the increase in fitness of the heterozygote. I take it this is what Dr. Kallmann's television speaker was talking about.

Kallmann: While the life span as a whole is assumed to be an evolutionary product of natural selection, it has been postulated that there is no selection following the effective reproductive period. According to this theory, there is no selection against senescent decrepitude or Alzheimer's disease or similar pathological conditions occurring in the senile or presenile periods.

On the other hand, if schizophrenia tends to become more and more common and we are really adapted only to environments which prevailed a thousand years ago, might it not be possible that the best state of affairs for all of us would be a completely schizophrenic form of society?

Dobzhansky: That doesn't quite follow, does it?

Kallmann: Why doesn't it follow?

Fremont-Smith: The environment has changed since a thousand years ago.

Kallmann: Let us assume that our environment would change in such a way as to become more and more propitious to the adaptation of schizophrenics.

Dobzhansky: The gene for schizophrenia may, by natural selection, be maintained indefinitely in a state of equilibrium at one frequency, and the normal, non-schizophrenic condition at another frequency. We will not all be schizophrenic, I hope.

Kallmann: How about a thousand years from now?

Dobzhansky: The equilibrium will be constant, provided the selective advantages and disadvantages are constant. The selection will never establish either the schizophrenic gene or the non-schizophrenic gene. It will establish an equilibrium at a value which is a function of the two selection coefficients. It is possible to calculate that the average adaptive value of an individual in the population will be maximal when the equilibrium is reached.

Natural selection maximizes the mean adaptive value of the population. There is no danger of everybody being schizophrenic.

Keys: It seems to me this is all obviously and completely unrealistic. These selective advantages and disadvantages do not stay constant.

Tyler: In sickle-cell anemia, the selective agent, the malarial organism itself, may change.

Dobzhansky: It is a very nice mathematical exercise because it shows that the population in which adaptedness is due to this mechanism of balanced polymorphism will be, genetically, most plastic, that is, able to respond most rapidly to changes in the environment. Environments will change the magnitudes of S_1 and S_2. So long as the maximum fitness, 1, is the property of the heterozygote, both genotypes will be preserved in the population. The relative frequency will be a matter of the environmental situation.

Brues: In addition to the equilibrium values for these things, I think some of us are interested in the matter of how long it takes for a change to take place in natural selection.

A good case to consider might be the one Dr. Tyler brought up. Now that we don't need to have malaria, how long will it be before there is an appreciable shift in the sickle-cell trait in the Mediterranean region? Is that a matter of ten generations or a great many more?

Dobzhansky: Selective changes are generally slow. In human terms, they are quite slow. In the case of sickle-cell anemia, it has been calculated that the changes are rapid enough so that, for American Negroes, who presumably had a high frequency of the sickle-cell gene when they were brought from Africa to an environment where malaria was less of a danger, the time lapse has been sufficient to cause a perceptible decrease of the frequence of the gene. I do not remember the figures, but some people believe they can demonstrate a drop in the frequency of the sickle-cell gene.

Keys: That is only a matter of a few generations in evolutionary span; therefore, the implication is that not having the sickle-cell trait offers a positive advantage that can be acted upon, in an evolutionary sense, in this short period of time. Does this seem reasonable?

Dobzhansky: Presumably it will take quite a long time

until the very last sickle-cell gene has been eliminated.

Sacher: How quickly did industrial melanism develop in moths and other species?

Dobzhansky: That is an excellent example. It took less than a century. But there, of course, selection was quite intense.

Jarvik: I would like to try and relate this fitness which Dr. Dobzhansky is talking about, and which I think is a purely reproductive fitness, to human aging.

If we think of an increase in life span as largely due to the elimination of specific diseases in the younger age groups, then factors operating prior to reproduction or during reproduction could readily explain genetic differences. But, if we want to postulate genetic effects occurring in later life, one of the most useful concepts is that of pleiotropism. We may postulate that there are genes with functions which are important to the organism at earlier ages and which, incidentally, prolong life. There are people here who know far more about this subject than I do. Thus, I recall one study by Roderick and Storer (33) showing a positive correlation between litter size in mice and the life span of the dams. Going a little further afield, some of our own data have shown a correlation between intelligence and life span (19, 21).

Dobzhansky: I hope, for goodness' sake, that higher intelligence increases in the life span, not the other way around. (Laughter)

Jarvik: It is reassuring; the correlation is a positive one. Later on, perhaps we could discuss some ideas of how genetic mechanisms, other than on a purely genic level, could operate in aging.

Lansing: I am puzzled, through my own inadequacy, about what we are driving at in the several references to the notion that natural selection is relatively ineffective in the postreproductive individual.

This first assumes that there is a fixed reproductive period, quite apart from the aging system. I think, as Medawar (25) uses the notion, that this is a means of establishing a genetic basis for senescence. It assumes there is a fixed reproductive period.

If we are talking specifically and only of the human species, in which the female has a three-decade reproductive period, that is well and good. If we are thinking about senescence through all populations, then I must see the evidence that in most species in which aging does occur, there is a fixed reproductive period. As far as I know, there are very few species in which there is a limited reproductive period, other than man and perhaps a few other higher forms.

I don't know the fixed reproductive period in the rat. In our laboratory, the rats of advanced age are still very busy reproducing, but we have senescence in rats. Our 7- and 8-year-old rabbits are still very busy reproducing. In the rotifer, eggs are laid throughout the major portion of the span.

Though this is a pretty notion, one has to limit it only to those populations in which we are dealing with a fixed reproductive period.

Keys: There is another consideration beyond that. In the first place, of course, with regard to man, the limitation is a good deal more concrete in the one sex than the other. I recall a day with an old gentleman in Russian Georgia whose younger brother, aged 96 (so they said), had to help his wife (his eighth) and his youngest son, aged 22, wash dishes because the older men were the center of the stage. Extreme longevity can be a force in natural selection. If we consider the situation in many societies where advancing age means acquiring wealth or prestige and thus giving a preferred status to the offspring, then one can see how, beyond the reproductive age, the mere ability to live on gives advantages to the children and the grandchildren. The offspring are favored to acquire and support wives and, therefore, to produce more offspring. This kind of factor operates in most societies.

Sacher: One particular instance of programed aging which has impressed me is connected with the life termination in certain moths. An English zoologist named Blest (3, 4) studied the family of Saturniid moths in which there are cryptic (protectively-colored) as well as aposematic (bad-tasting and vividly-colored) moths. The obvious teleological conclusion is that the cryptic ones should die out very soon after reproduction and the aposematics stay around for quite a long time to give their possible predator a good taste of them. Apparently this is the case.

The next point he investigated was this: What is the mechanism of life termination? There seems to be a specific mechanism having to do with the release of an inhibitor which keeps the moths from resuming flight. When it decays, they fly themselves to death. By actual measurement, the aposematics have a greater persistence of this specific, presumably enzymatic, mechanism that retarded the self-destructive process.

Dobzhansky: I think Dr. Jarvik mentioned a very important concept which we should not overlook here, namely, the pleiotropic effects of genes. It would be altogether wrong to consider that a gene controls aging and does nothing else.

A gene which makes the aging process more rapid or less rapid may have other effects; in fact, it almost certainly does have other effects during the reproductive period. Such a gene will be selected according to what it does, not in postreproductive, but in reproductive stages.

We do not postulate specific genes which make life longer or shorter. It is a matter of genes acting during the entire life span of the organism, and being selected, for or against, according to the benefits or disadvantages they confer on the organism with respect to its reproductive efficiency. There is no contradiction here at all. A contradiction will arise only if we say there are genes specialized to work on a given stage, in a given part of the life cycle, which is not necessary at all. That is true of major genes, and of polygenes, to the same extent.

Court-Brown: Are all these arguments based on the process of natural selection? Assuming that, do they all assume that there is random, unassortive mating?

Dobzhansky: Not necessarily. Mating that is random, or assortive mating, would produce genetic effects, but they would not necessarily change the selective values. In this case, for example, random mating would lead to predictable frequencies of the S_1S_1, S_1S_2, and S_2S_2 genotypes. Assortive matings of like with like would cause a drop in the relative incidence of the heterozygote S_1S_2. Assortive matings of unlikes would increase the frequency of heterozygotes. That is about all (8, 10).

Court-Brown: When geneticists tried to predict what might be the effect of, let us say, a dose of radiation in a given population, that was based on the assumption of random mating within the population?

Dobzhansky: I don't think so.

Storer: If I understand Dr. Dobzhansky's remarks correctly, selection for or against senescence at the population level should be possible. Is that correct?

Dobzhansky: Yes. That is not my original idea, by any means. There is a considerable literature about it. I believe I quoted Haldane (13), but I am not even sure that he was the first to propound the theory.

Storer: Since I am a novice in the area, could you explain briefly the genetic mechanism by which this could occur?

<u>Dobzhansky</u>: Suppose there are a series of endogamous tribes which are more or less isolated genetically. Two kinds of situations may exist. In the first, the postreproductive individuals in the community are an economic drag on the community or, in general, are harmful to the community in some way. In the second situation, the postreproductive individuals are advantageous to the community as leaders, teachers, and so on.

In the first case, natural selection would favor genes that would decrease the number of postreproductive individuals. In the second case, it would favor genotypes that would increase the number of such individuals. Quite an analogous situation and, again, Haldane's original thesis. He considered genes for altruism and genes for criminal behavior. If altruism is defined as a quality whereby an individual acts for the benefit of the community but for his own disadvantage, and criminal behavior as the opposite, an individual harming the community for his own advantage, Haldane argued that in small endogamous populations, there may be a selection of genes for altruistic behavior and elimination of genes for criminal behavior; and, alas, in a large panmictic population, the other way round.

I would like, again, to emphasize Dr. Jarvik's point: There are no genes which regulate longevity and do nothing else; no genes which produce altruistic versus criminal behavior, and do nothing else. The selective value of a gene is a function of the over-all balance of its effects.

So, if we know that a given gene produces a certain effect, we cannot jump to the conclusion that it will be favored or disfavored by natural selection.

<u>Storer</u>: Going back to these theoretical tribes you spoke of, how would these genes for elimination of the old members of society ever become fixed in that population?

<u>Dobzhansky</u>: They may increase in frequency because tribes which have such genes, according to Haldane, will have an advantage in the intertribal competition. If oldsters are a disadvantage to the interest of the community, a tribe which has genes which kill off older people will prosper, become more numerous, displace other tribes in which such genes are absent.

<u>Storer</u>: So this has to be a completely chance occurrence?

<u>Dobzhansky</u>: No. Granting Haldane's (13) assumptions, namely, that the presence of oldsters is disadvantageous, then tribes which contain genes which finish them off sooner will

almost necessarily have an advantage, and the tribes which do not contain these genes will be at a disadvantage. After passage of a certain number of generations, mankind would then contain a higher frequency of genes for shorter longevity.

Storer: The tribe's having the genes that finish off the oldsters would, initially, be simply a chance occurrence. Would there be no mechanism for increasing the frequency of these genes?

Dobzhansky: Suppose we have a mutation rate which produces such genes; then every tribe would stand a certain chance of acquiring such a gene by mutation. Mutation is a chance phenomenon, in a sense, but since every mutation has a certain probability of appearing, this chance is calculable and predictable to that extent—predictable in probability terms. The mechanism for increasing the incidence will be the selection of tribes or colonies which contain these genes.

Birren: Suppose the late-life change was related to size and strength, for example. Here the question is the logic of the relationship between the early- and late-life characteristic. It might be difficult to eliminate it because the desirable late-life characteristics might be malassociated here.

Dobzhansky: This, then, is a matter of manifold effect which could make selection possible without requiring small endogamous tribes or colonies. A gene which might have an advantageous effect in youth, increasing the reproductive efficiency of the young groups and, also, producing early death, might be selected as such in a tribe of any size.

Fremont-Smith: But the opposite could take place. It could have advantages necessary for the reproductive period as well as a longevity factor.

Dobzhansky: Then the situation is not exceptional. Indeed, it is the most universal. The selective value, the adaptive value of a genotype, is a result of summation of all its advantages and disadvantages over the range of environment which the population faces in its normal habitats.

A gene which is advantageous in some respects may be disadvantageous in others. A beautiful example of that is a tropical bird, the man-of-war bird, which has short legs and consequently cannot raise itself into the air from a flat place. It has to have a jumping-off place. But it happens to be a supremely efficient flier, a supremely efficient hunter. It is a very common tropical bird (8).

How did natural selection permit such an absurd animal to survive? Why should natural selection have permitted such legs to develop? If we consider bad legs in isolation from everything else, that becomes an impossibility.

What natural selection was doing in these birds was selecting an efficient organism which happens to have a biological defect in its legs—legs of clay, if you please.

Fremont-Smith: There is a mouse with a lethal tail gene that operates during embryonic life. Could there be lethal genes which would operate at the end of a long life period, and could this have something to do with the longevity of species—that they carried a gene which terminated life in a certain range?

Dobzhansky: This mouse with lethal genes concerned with tails was studied particularly by my colleague, Dr. L. C. Dunn (11). It is an example of a still different phenomenon, the possible importance of which is at present hard to assess. It is the phenomenon sometimes called "meiotic drive." A male which is heterozygous for this gene fails to produce one-half of the sperm carrying this gene and the other half free from this gene, as according to Mendel's law it should; it produces up to 95% of the sperm that carries the gene which, in homozygous condition, is lethal, and that confers on this gene a tremendous selective advantage.

Dr. Dunn has now analyzed some mouse populations in various parts of the United States and—I believe I quote him correctly—with one or two exceptions, every mouse population carries this gene. This gene acquires a selective advantage by subverting the reproductive processes in a way which is disadvantageous to the species but which, nevertheless, confers on the gene a selective advantage—a peculiar situation. How widespread such situations are, nobody knows.

Fremont-Smith: My question was, could there be an analogous kind of gene which would operate at the end of a long life, but terminate life? Could the termination of life in a species be by the fact that it carries a gene that operates late?

Dobzhansky: I take it you refer to Huntington's chorea, which is a straightforward dominant gene, isn't it?

Fremont-Smith: But I suppose there could be one that operated in a way which didn't knock out a particular system but, perhaps, knocked out the correlative factor, so that an individual gradually died, let's say, at 90.

Dobzhansky: A lethal gene which manifests itself in post-reproductive individuals?

Fremont-Smith: That is right.

Dobzhansky: Technically, that would not be called "lethal" in a genetic sense. A lethal gene kills 100% of individuals before they reach reproductive age.

Fremont-Smith: Then we have to have a new kind of lethality, don't we? What would you call it, and is there any evidence for this kind of a late-acting lethal gene?

Dobzhansky: There are a lot of people in the field who love to invent new terms. They probably have a good Greek dictionary; I don't. So a new term may well be proposed for this purpose.

Tyler: I would like to mention, in this connection, the Pacific salmon as an example of the operation of a kind of lethal gene that manifests itself suddenly, immediately following reproduction. It is like the case Mr. Sacher described in the moth. As is well known, after the Pacific salmon spawns, it very soon dies.

The basis for this seems to be reasonably well worked out, by O. H. Robertson, Emeritus Professor of Medicine at the University of Chicago, who is now at Stanford (31, 32). This is perhaps an example of very rapid senescence, since the Pacific salmon dies very soon after a very vigorous period. It dies, apparently from Cushing's syndrome, hyperadrenocorticism. During the spawning migration, the pituitary undoubtedly becomes very active, secreting much gonadotrophic hormone, along with plenty of the adrenocorticotrophic hormone. This is all to the good during the migration period, up to spawning. On spawning, a large mass of tissue is lost. As a result of this loss, and I am adding a little bit perhaps to Robertson's story, there would be a relative excess of pituitary hormones in the body. The excess of gonadotrophin probably does no harm, since there is not much gonad on which it can work, but the excess of adrenocorticotrophic hormone would cause an excess stimulation of the adrenals and result in Cushing's syndrome. So the simple cure would be a partial adrenalectomy.

Fremont-Smith: Do they survive then?

Tyler: I have seen no reports of successful experiments. However, the reverse has been done, giving trout hydrocortisone, and thus imitating the symptoms that the Pacific salmon exhibits after spawning; namely, the osmotic upset, blood sugar symptoms, and so on. So this makes a consistent kind of picture.

Ehret: This is reminiscent of the life history of many annual plants. That is to say, onset of maturation may be followed quite systematically by the death of the plant. But then we can influence photoperiodic mechanisms (5), thereby delaying or postponing indefinitely the onset of maturation, and prolonging considerably the vegetative life of the plant.

Jarvik: One of the differences to be stressed here is that while there seems to be little or no senescence in the examples cited by Dr. Tyler and Dr. Ehret, what we are trying to explain in man is precisely this period of senescence. Why is there such a long period of senescence preceding death and, also, why do people age in a rather similar fashion? If we consider for a moment the signs and symptoms of senescence, is it not remarkable how limited their range is? Although the causes of death can be assigned to more or less distinct categories, aging persons exhibit a certain uniformity in over-all appearance.

It is difficult to fit this general resemblance of aged individuals to one another into an explanatory scheme based on the assumption that aging is due to the effects of individual genes, either singly, or combined in limited numbers. An alternative explanation might be advanced on the basis of chromosomal changes rather than gene mutations, in which case senescence may be said to represent the consequences of a progressive loss in chromosomal material resulting from mitotic errors. The occurrence of the same mitotic errors in different individuals could account for some of the similarities seen among the aged.

Thoughts along these lines have been plaguing me lately and stem directly from observations made in our new cytogenetics laboratory. The attempt to formulate a system on the basis of such preliminary ideas reflects the temerity of a novice, a student of psychological genetics suddenly given the opportunity to examine human chromosomes. Psychologists are intimately acquainted with variability and accustomed to dealing with measurements that vary around a mean. It was in line with past experience, therefore, to note that chromosome counts, too, appeared to vary around a central point.

Although 46 is the modal number of chromosomes in normal persons, some of the counts are above and some below that value. The general shape of the curve seems to indicate a skewed distribution with more counts in the lower than the upper range. Examination of published tables confirms these impressions. Most of the investigators seem to dismiss the aberrant counts as artifacts since it is well known that in

long-term tissue cultures mitotic errors are fairly common
and that, barring polyploidy, chromosomal losses occur more
frequently than chromosomal gains. Of course, only intact
cells are counted since damaged cells may well have lost
chromosomes artificially.

If we postulate, however, that such mitotic errors occur
in the intact organism as well as in tissue culture, then we
can say that, in a way, aging in the normal individual could
represent the accumulation of mitotic errors in those cells
that do divide repeatedly. If we classify cells as long-lived
or short-lived, repeatedly dividing ones would fall into the
short-lived category. I think that to date the cells that have
been studied most intensively with reference to aging are the
long-lived cells, like nerve cells, which are presumed to en-
dure more or less throughout the adult life span of an individual. These are the cells which show all the characteristic
histological changes of what we call aging, whereas the other
cells—such as lymphocytes and fibroblasts, hematopoietic
tissue and epithelial cells—are not considered suitable for
the study of age effects because they are new cells, young and
not old; they are consistently being replaced. If we look instead at how many generations a cell is removed from the
original zygote, then the situation is reversed: the nerve cell
becomes very young and the epithelial cell quite old. In such
an old epithelial cell, there have been many opportunities for
mitotic errors to occur and to be repeated. Since we only have
46 chromosomes instead of twenty thousand genes to deal
with, the statistical probability of duplication for any given
error is much higher than it would be on a purely genic hypothesis. Accumulation of similar mitotic errors in different
individuals would be expected to lead to similarity in aging.

Tyler: I didn't want to say "no senescence" in this particular case because I don't think we really know. I prefer
Dr. Fremont-Smith's term "very accelerated senescence."
We don't know, basically, that this is different from a very
gradual senescence. There may be similar changes at a very
accelerated rate.

Ehret: The difficulty is with "senescence." This unqualified term has been discussed repeatedly at earlier conferences but without lasting impact. The concepts of aging and
senescence are perhaps too closely related: aging places emphasis on all transitions in time; senescence emphasizes the
quality of the transitions and the accumulation of deleterious
ones. The deleterious effects occur as discrete events at different levels of organization within the individual. They may
occur at the macroscopic level as, for example, in the case of

organ failure. This is like a sudden catastrophe or accident, a splinter in the eye, being hit by an automobile, or something else obviously tragic. Or they may occur at a much lower level, as in accidents between photons and molecules, which are of quite a different sort. Then the sequelae may appear to develop slowly, even though the discrete event initiating the ultimate change was equally "instantaneous"; and, indeed, a consequence of such a "slow development" at one level may result later in the "sudden" cessation of operation of an organ or system at another level. The unqualified term "senescence" fails to attempt a distinction between the causes underlying very rapid deleterious changes and very slow deleterious changes.

Tyler: Should we distinguish between fast accidents and slow accidents?

Ehret: Not only that; the physical sites are different. They are alike only in their property of discreteness. The site may be a small particle—an organelle, a nucleotide—that interacts with other systems within the organism, each of which is "biological"; or a large particle—an organ or organ system—with other interacting potentials. Don't we want, in fact, to make such distinctions at this conference? Concretely, where are these physical interactions happening and, abstractly, at what levels of organization, when we talk about cell-aging, tissue-aging, organism-aging?

Tyler: As I say, I am not quite sure in my own mind. Is there a fundamental, basic distinction that we are making?

Ehret: It may be unfortunate that we have become this deeply involved in analogies with automobile accidents. However, since we have come this far, perhaps obsolescence theory in industrial technology can tell us about the aging or the life-expectancy of automobiles as a function of the durability of their fabrics. Suppose some fabrics have deteriorated even before the automobile is assembled—for example, a slow succession of discrete molecular accidents to the rubber of one tire. You drive out of the factory lot, and bang—the tire is flat, the car is out of action for good unless a spare tire is transplanted into place. On the other hand, after years of service the whole vehicle may fall apart like the wonderful one-horse shay. Or gross macroscopic destruction may occur at any time by the conventional catastrophic accident. Destructions of this sort are not without analogy in the organism, but, as we implied earlier, an analogy may provoke thought about mechanisms without serving to specify them.

Birren: In a sense, Dr. Jarvik led me down the garden path. She said aging was predictable and I was expecting a statement about the kind of predictable change. But she then said there were errors involved. I suppose either the chromosomal errors or defects are predictable and result in a pattern of changes, or else two systems of aging are being postulated: One, a senescence pattern resulting from the slow-turnover cells, and another one resulting from the faster-turnover cells. In any case, I felt a jump from an emphasis on a regular pattern of senescence, which I would certainly regard as likely, to a mechanism involving error. Perhaps I have difficulty with linking concepts of orderly senescence and error.

Jarvik: The errors occurring during mitosis could be due to any of the known mechanisms resulting in mitotic errors: non-disjunction, translocation, inversion, deletion, repetition, and the like. Although increase in chromosomal content can take place as well as decrease, a loss is more likely than a gain and, in general, a net loss is to be expected on theoretical grounds. Primarily, the fast-turnover cells would be affected and we would predict the loss of chromosomal material in those cells which multiply at a rapid rate.

As far as the slow-turnover cells are concerned, we can fall back on point mutation, induced by cosmic radiations and other mutagens. Those cells are available as targets for very long periods of time, because they don't duplicate, or not very much. The individual cells would be directly affected by "hits." Indirectly, the non-dividing or slowly dividing cells could also be affected by the changes taking place in the rest of the organism, secondary to the metabolic disturbances resulting from the greater variety in the karyotypes of the fast-turnover cells. After all, cells do not live as independent individuals but are influenced by all the other cells in the organism. Thus, changes in one system would be expected to produce changes in another. There might be an analogy here, when considering why unicellular organisms don't age. There aging is replaced by natural selection. If unicellular organisms are not fit for survival, they are eliminated from the population.

We can look at the multicellular organism as one kind of civilized society where less efficient and even defective cells are protected and aided by the other members of the community to the best of their ability, until a stage is reached eventually where interference with homeostatic mechanisms prevents the organism from coping with its responsibilities. When the defective elements interfere with a given level of functioning, the result is the death of the organism.

[After the conference, the paper by Jacobs, Court-Brown, and Doll (16) was brought to my attention as providing support for these speculations. The authors found that the proportion of aneuploid, specifically hypomodal, cells in cultures of human leukocytes increased with the age of the subjects.—L. J.]

Lansing: Do I understand that there are different mechanisms producing aging in rapidly multiplying cells—the intermitotic as against the postmitotic—and that these have separate mechanisms?

Jarvik: Yes, except the division into intermitotic and postmitotic is not strictly analogous. Some of the postmitotics are rapidly dividing cells; I think this group includes the lymphocytes.

Lansing: Let's leave the postmitotic and refer to the non-dividing nerve cells, which have a separate mechanism from the rapidly multiplying tissue.

Jarvik: I would think so. We don't know.

Lansing: These, indeed, may be immune to aging, and aging only occurs in epidermis and in liver, and in tissues in which there is relatively rapid multiplication. On that basis, a very nice experiment can be made. Experimental hepatectomy, if repeated regularly, could give very rapid senescence, at least of the liver.

Jarvik: The human liver cells are polyploid, which makes it difficult to compare the chromosomal content. They already have an abnormality.

Fremont-Smith: Have you by chance compared rapidly growing cells in tissue culture, taken from a very young individual, with the same type of cell taken from an elderly individual, and cultured it in terms of the chromosome?

Jarvik: Dr. Court-Brown told me he has some evidence on this point and it would contradict certain aspects of this theory, I think. But as would be expected, if the basic postulate of increased variability and net loss with age is accepted, he did find a loss with advancing age. Unfortunately, we can't make the other test, that of comparing the chromosome content of slow-growing cells with that of fast-growing cells, because we can't grow the former in tissue culture.

Fremont-Smith: Is there a greater or faster loss in the same type of fast-growing cell, taken from an elderly individual, than in that taken from an embryo or from a very young individual?

Court-Brown: The system we have been working with and, I think, that Dr. Jarvik may be working with, is an artificial system which causes lymphocytes to divide in culture. By and large, they only go through one division in the culture. There is quite clear evidence that the proportion of aneuploid cells in the culture increases with the age of the individual. It is debatable whether this is a cultural effect in terms of aging or whether, in fact, one is harvesting and sampling an increasing number of aneuploid cells.

Fremont-Smith: How about chromosome counts taken from the elderly, rapidly growing cells, and those taken from the very young individual, for instance, epithelial cells taken from an elderly person? Do they show a loss of chromosomes?

Court-Brown: No. The only work that has been done is on blood lymphocytes, simply because this is the only system that can be set up in a completely standardized way.

Fremont-Smith: Is it possible, with current techniques, to make chromosome counts, comparing an elderly individual and a very young individual, for the same type of rapidly growing tissue?

Court-Brown: It is possible only in terms of tissue fibroblasts, apart from the lymphocyte situation, which is quite artificial. The fibroblast situation ought to be an easy one to work with because there is considerable variability between samples; it should be easy to set up a culture in terms of the time required to produce an adequate number of cells in mitosis.

Brues: One of the difficulties in the mass culture of cells, of course, is that a great many of what we would consider errors probably have some adaptive value to this rather unusual environment in which the cells are growing. These can be cloned out and will perpetuate themselves. On the other hand, the cells in the mass culture are in continuous competition. Practically all of these anomalies grow more slowly than the wild-type cells. So they are continually eliminated. The situation is very complicated, and it has proved difficult to analyze.

Court-Brown: This objection doesn't operate in terms of blood cultures. We only got, on the average, one division.

Lansing: I keep coming back to Sonneborn's thesis (34) of some thirty years ago concerning the flatworm. The work involved successive selection of anterior products from the division of anterior products, and posterior products from the division of posterior products, with one basic difference in the two: there was virtually no cell division, no multiplication, in the anterior products that contained the brain and the pharynx, whereas the tail component had to regenerate most of the body, and so had a great abundance of mitotic activity.

The senescence occurred not in the posterior product with much division but in the anterior product with very little division. The anterior line had a short life span, whereas the posterior product, with great abundance of division, went on indefinitely. I think this is almost diametrically opposed to your notion, Dr. Jarvik.

Storer: I wonder if you are suggesting that the only possible way a cell can make an error is by division. Cells that don't divide can certainly accumulate errors in their information. Dividing cells in some situations may be given an opportunity to eliminate errors, whereas in the anterior portion of the flatworm, with practically no cell turnover, there is presumably little opportunity to eliminate the accumulated errors.

Fry: What are the criteria of aging in proliferative cells?

Jarvik: Maybe we have to have different criteria for different types of cells. With certain cells, we use the histological criteria that have so far been used. For other cells, such as the rapidly dividing ones, one could, for instance, use karyotype analysis, if we get to the point where we can identify each chromosome, or perhaps even have maps of chromosomal regions. Eventually, we may expect biochemical analysis of the DNA. I tried to look this up, but it seems that measurements are not yet accurate enough to detect the absence of a single chromosome, much less a portion of a chromosome, or the presence of an unusual combination with a total number of 45 or 46. Eventually, when more refined techniques become available, we may be able to tell aging by such biochemical and cytological means.

The other point to mention is that the rapidly dividing cells are the ones that are involved in neoplastic disease. It is extremely rare for nerve cells to undergo neoplasia. Yet, we all know that neoplastic disease increases with age. So possibly there might be some relationship.

Fry: There is no clear correlation between the incidence of neoplasms and the rate of cell renewal in a tissue. In the small intestine, cell renewal is very rapid but neoplasms are uncommon. In the large intestine, cell renewal is rapid and neoplasms are common. The cells of the corneal epithelium are renewed throughout life, but more slowly than those of the intestinal epithelium, and neoplasms are extremely rare and probably only occur secondary to ulceration. There might be, however, a correlation between the ability of tissues to eliminate abnormal cells and the incidence of neoplasms. Lipkin and Quastler (23) gave a single injection of tritiated thymidine to rats and mice and found, after 1 week, that the number of heavily labeled cells was greater in the colon and the stomach than in the small intestine. They noted that the rank order found for the retention of heavily labeled epithelial cells in these areas was the same as the rank order of the frequencies of malignant changes in the corresponding areas of the gastrointestinal tract of man.

To return to the question of aging, we have found that the rate of cell renewal in the small intestine decreases with age. It is, however, difficult to determine whether these changes are intra- or extracellular in origin.

Court-Brown: One has to be terribly careful about saying this is part of the aging process simply because one finds changes, such as changes in proportion of aneuploid cells with age. What we so badly need is some sort of objective way of saying: "Here is a person who looks much older than he ought to for his years," and then study him in terms of the degree of aneuploidy and see whether one can correlate the two.

Ehret: I am reminded of Graeme Welch's experiments with yeast cells in the chemostat (36), in which a certain flux of radiation delivered continuously to the cell population caused cessation of growth and "death" of the chemostat. But at lower dose rates or higher division rates the induced errors did not accumulate sufficiently for the chemostat to be stopped. The cell population was able to stand a dose of radiation each generation equal to about one-fourth the LD_{50}, and apparently throw out the errors that might have threatened the "survival of the chemostat" as a whole. If we can consider the chemostat as quasi-organism, then why not the organism as quasi-chemostat—in which it is not too surprising to find survival of the whole in the presence of widespread error in the parts? On the other hand, the analog in the organism for evolution in the chemostat (29) may be neoplasia—quite suitable for tissue culture but not for the whole organism.

Court-Brown: As far as the human lymphocyte is concerned, it is now beginning to look very strongly as if the whole thing can be explained. This whole increase in proportion of aneuploid cells with age is explained on the basis of errors in division, involving the sex chromosomes. The aneuploid cells in the male are clearly cells of which a great proportion are results of error involving the Y chromosome;

and, presumably, in females they are the errors involving the X. These may be mediated by some other homeostatic mechanisms in the body, secondary to changes taking place in the endocrines. I don't think one could say they are. One would be surprised if they have anything to do with the actual basis of the process of aging.

Quastler: I remember a case where there seems to be association between permanence of cells and pathology—the lens of the eye. Radiation causes chromosomal anomalies and, in most species, cataract; damaged cells remain in the lens. In the chicken and in the ground squirrel, chromosomal damage occurs as usual, but the damaged cells are removed, and no cataract develops (30).

Cottier: Does anybody know what happens if a rapidly proliferating tissue from a senescent animal, showing cellular abnormalities, is transplanted to a young animal of the same strain? Are the cellular irregularities of the transplant maintained or do they diminish? Perhaps such an experiment would shed some light on the problem of whether these abnormalities are signs of senescence inherent in the cells, or whether they are due to other factors, such as decreased vascularization, or both.

Ehret: We may consider transplantation in the higher plants. If the plant is young, a photoperiod sufficient to induce maturation in an older plant may not induce maturation in it; but if an old plant is grafted onto the young plant, then photoperiodic induction will cause the young plant to flower (38).

Sacher: I would like to return to Dr. Jarvik's hypothesis. If I understand her, the element of cellular structure which accounts for the observed phenomenon of aging uniformity is the chromosome rather than the gene.

Curiously, what she has done is to invert an argument which was used by Dr. Szilard (35). He said that in order to account for the shape of the life table on the basis of a genetic mechanism of killing, one must postulate the loss of whole chromosomes, because the accumulation of aging damage by recessive lethal gene mutations would lead to a spread of ages at death much narrower than is observed.

According to Szilard, the frequency distribution of the number of faults inherited accounts for most of the variance of ages at death. This again comes back to Dr. Kallmann in that Szilard placed great weight on Kallmann's data on mean difference in age of fraternal and identical twins, in which it appeared that the mean difference is considerably smaller for identical twins than for fraternals.

What is the evidence about the inheritance of longevity in fraternals and identicals, and what is the evidence for a theory of the inheritance of non-functional chromosomes?

Brues: Personally, I would be much interested to hear a little more about this, for it appears to indicate a heritable basis for longevity. I wonder if Dr. Kallmann would discuss that.

Kallmann: If the process of growing old is viewed in a biological perspective, aging represents "an essential function of a genetically regulated growth phenomenon which is linked with the reproductive requirements of the species" (22). According to Needham (28), the individual must age because there is a need for the reproductive replacement of a certain number of individuals. More specifically, it has been hypothesized that in the interest of balancing the survival capacity of the species, a certain death rate serves a positive selective purpose. The assumption is that without replacing the individuals lost by infertility, illness, and death, the species would not be able to survive (7).

Once again, I have some difficulty in applying these concepts and terms to human populations. If it can be said that a given death rate serves a positive selective purpose, a similar stipulation can be made regarding war or a certain crime rate. Perhaps I don't understand the evolutionary principles involved.

In man, the reproductive period is rarely utilized in full. Hence, even a doubled average life span would not lead to a material increase in the reproductive rate and could easily be absorbed without posing a threat to the survival of the species. In other words, I find it difficult to think of a relatively early death as something that is on the positive side rather than deleterious.

Dobzhansky: Deleterious to whom? To the fellow who dies or to somebody else?

Kallmann: Deleterious to the individual, as well as to society.

Fremont-Smith: If there were not enough food to sustain a population where all the people lived to the age of 150, but enough if they all died at 50, then it would be an advantage to society for them to die at 50, perhaps.

Kallmann: The same argument would lead to the conclusion that a positive selective purpose is served by war or criminality.

Fremont-Smith: Or flu epidemic. From the point of view of defining what kind of an advantage, as long as the nature of the advantage is specified, I think this could even be possible. If a flu epidemic had swept through and killed off all the Nazis, that would have been a great advantage, but it would be a very highly specific advantage.

Lansing: I think we have to distinguish between advantages to a population and advantages, or lack thereof, to the individual.

Fremont-Smith: Or group of individuals.

Lansing: I would be specific with the individual. When we talk of senescence, at least as biologists, we are thinking principally, but not exclusively, of the interest of the individual. As a side issue, there is an area where we do concern ourselves with advantages, or lack thereof, to society, or the population as a whole—whether it can entertain an increase in population or not. That is another issue. Senescence is an individual problem.

Tyler: We have gone from one level to another. These are big jumps for me—participating for the first time in a conference on aging—to go from aging at the molecular level to aging at other levels, such as the ribosome, the nucleus, the cell, the tissue, the organ, individuals, and the species. Is it assumed that similar concepts may apply at all levels?

Lansing: This is what we have been doing this morning. We have jumped from population senescence, and the interest of the population, down to molecular problems, and, in between, we stopped off with chromosomal aberrations, and so on. I think this is hard on anyone, no matter how many conferences he has attended.

Tyler: What general criterion of senescence does one use? Is it functional efficiency? Is it the ability of the molecular system, or of the nucleus, to do their job at their respective levels?

Lansing: We slipped over that area quickly. I think Dr. Fry asked what the criteria are in rapidly dividing cells? We really don't know what the criteria are. I wish I did know. Or we can refer to histological criteria, but as a professional histologist, I have trouble here, too. I don't know an old cell from a young one, or old tissue from young.

Tyler: What happens, for example, to conduction of a nerve impulse?

Lansing: I don't know of any data except that, in a few specific instances, lymphocytes behave differently. We don't know whether this is an expression of aging, as you point out, or whether it is a secondary factor associated with aging.

Although I seem to be taking a negative approach here, I think it is most important that we do establish or direct our attention to this basic question: What are the criteria of aging at any level, whether it be the organism or the organ or the cell, or component of the cell? I don't know what they are.

Brues: I am quite sure we will get back to Dr. Fry's question in a large way soon. At the moment I supposed we were discussing the role of senescence. As a horseman of the Apocalypse, I think Dr. Kallmann was leading into a discussion on the genetic matter.

Kallmann: In man, the clearest evidence for genetically potentialized longevity variations is derived from comparing mean intrapair life-span differences related to zygosity in same-sex pairs of twins. In our study of senescent twins and their sibs (22), such analyses were made biennially, from 1948 to 1959, on a slowly increasing number of pairs with two deceased partners. Our final data in 1959 were obtained from 192 pairs.

Expressed in months of total lifetime, intrapair differences in length of life were found in this study to be consistently greater in two-egg than in one-egg pairs, particularly in the female series, but with a diminishing trend in both sexes as the observational period progressed. Initially, members of one-egg pairs differed in their mean life span by about 3 years, while the corresponding difference in two-egg pairs was almost 6 years (Table 1). At the time of the last analysis, these differences had dwindled to 2.5 months in the male series and 25.5 months in the female series.

Along with the expected decline in intrapair life-span differences with increasing age, Table 2 (p. 41) shows that the expression of differences related to zygosity instead of being wiped out persisted beyond the age of 80 in both sexes. With all complete pairs arranged according to the age at death of the first-deceased twin, the variation between one-egg and two-egg pairs in the upper age group was 7 months in the male series, and 12 months in the female series. Corresponding differences varied from 17 to 113 months in the age group 60-64, and from 12 to 29 months in the age group 70-74. A unidirectional trend of this kind in a series of 10 comparisons would be a matter of chance less than once in a thousand times.

Retrospectively, it may be said that one of the unavoid-

TABLE 1

Mean Intrapair Differences in Life Spans of Same-Sex Senescent Twin Pairs over Age Sixty

(In months)

Year of analysis	Male		Female	
	One-egg	Two-egg	One-egg	Two-egg
1948	47.6	89.1	29.4	61.3
1950	48.0	73.8	18.2	41.3
1952	40.7[†]	79.1[†]	30.7[†]	69.5[†]
1954	50.6	68.9	22.9[†]	65.6[†]
1956/7	60.0	64.5	36.9[*]	68.2[*]
1958/9	62.5	65.0	55.4	80.9

[*] Equals difference between one-egg and two-egg pairs significant at 5% level.
[†] Equals difference between one-egg and two-egg pairs significant at 1% level.

Reprinted, by permission, from Kallmann, F. J. 1961. Genetic factors in aging: Comparative and longitudinal observations on a senescent twin population. In P. H. Hoch and J. Zubin (eds.), Psychopathology of aging. Grune and Stratton, New York.

able imperfections of our longitudinal twin study was a lack of information about cytogenetic and comparative-radiation data. Especially in one-egg pairs with considerable intrapair life-span differences, it would be of interest to know whether one of the twins received more extensive X-ray treatment during his lifetime than the other. Such data would now be obtainable and this should be ascertained.

For the purpose of this discussion, I have asked Dr. Jarvik to focus her report on our relatively small series of one-egg pairs who showed a marked life-span difference, with or without major differences in the environmental aspects of their life histories. This report will illustrate the difficulties encountered in a comparative study of this kind.

Jarvik: In the course of our longitudinal twin study we have been looking for identical twin pairs who had been exposed to large differences in environment, in order to see if such differences would be reflected in the physical and mental signs of aging. Such pairs were hard to find since most of the twin partners were exposed to very similar environments. Among the hundreds of pairs in our series, only a handful had experienced notable differences in life histories.

Some of you may already be familiar with the history of the one pair in our series which had the most outstanding differences in living conditions. We followed them for over 15

years and now they have both completed their life histories
(17).

These twins were separated at about the age of 18 years.
One of them married a local farmer, and the other one became a missionary. The married twin raised a large family,
six children, and in her entire life was never farther away
from her birthplace than ten miles.

The co-twin, soon after she finished a course in Bible
school, was sent as a missionary to the Orient and spent much
of her adult life in China and India. Consequently, there were
marked differences not only in climate and in diet, but also in
the socio-cultural milieu, as large a difference as anyone
would be likely to find in present-day society. Yet, when they
were reunited after the retirement of the missionary, at the
age of 65, they were so similar that people had difficulty in
distinguishing them by their appearance alone. This despite a
weight difference of 28 pounds in favor of the widow. If the
twins went out of the room and only one came back, we were
never sure which one it was. They had a series of psychological tests, and here again the resemblances were far more
impressive than the differences (Fig. 1).

The twins died at the ages of 92 and 94, respectively. The
exact difference was 28 months.

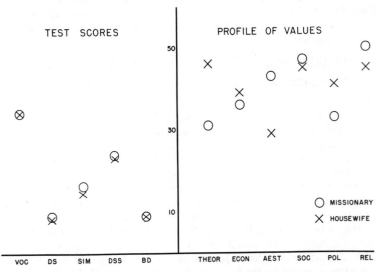

Fig. 1.—One-egg female twins separated for 27 years. Reprinted, by
permission, from Jarvik, L. F. 1962. Genetic variations in disease resistance and survival potential. In: F. J. Kallmann (ed.), Expanding goals
of genetics in psychiatry, pp. 10-24. Grune and Stratton, New York.

Fremont-Smith: Which one lived longest?

Jarvik: The widow. The missionary died first but she had broken her hip. So we are not really sure that hers was a natural death.

Brues: The heavier one lived longer?

Jarvik: That is correct. (Laughter) We have a pair of twin brothers who could be interpreted as saying "Hurrah" for the other side. Here, the divorced, remarried, and widowed twin continued an arduous schedule as a general practitioner for almost two decades after the death of his monozygotic twin brother. Differences in marital adjustment, professional demands, dietary habits, and medical care could all be adduced to account for the difference in their life spans of almost 20 years (235 months). The physician attributed his twin's premature death—at the age of nearly 70—to inadequate medical care, including the lack of dietary restriction which apparently allowed ad libitum consumption of milk and butter. While both succumbed to coronary thrombosis, the physician, who avoided lipids and cholesterol, showed the first signs of coronary heart disease at the age of 85, 15 years after the death of his brother whom he then survived for another 5 years.

Kallmann: What you did not mention was the physician's belief that the early death of his twin brother had something to do with the fact that he had a son who was an outstanding gerontologist.

Fremont-Smith: That is a dangerous thing to have!

Kallmann: In the opinion of the physician, it was. (Laughter)

Jarvik: Another pair of twins, concordant for death due to coronary thrombosis, showed numerous similarities in their life histories, including specialization in the same branch of medicine, a common office, and delayed marriage shortly before reaching the half-century mark. They resembled each other so closely that they had no difficulty in substituting for one another at any time they so desired, which was often. Nevertheless, there was a discrepancy of over 10 years in the time of their deaths. No history of differences in dietary habits was given in their case but, of course, at the time of gathering the information (over 15 years ago) no attempt was made to itemize intake of proteins, lipids, and carbohydrates.

The 10-year discrepancy in life span may not be as striking as it appears at first glance, inasmuch as the longer-lived twin had a cerebrovascular accident 4 years after his brother's death. Far from attributing his survival to expert medical care, this physician's wife ascribed it to <u>lack</u> of therapy since she believed that "physicians usually kill their patients with doctoring." He himself tended to emphasize the detrimental influence of his brother's change in residence, and those of us who are commuters can readily understand this point of view. Unfortunately, we do not have sufficient data to confirm or deny the postulated life-shortening effects of commuting.

Far from being facetious, this example merely illustrates the difficulties encountered in large-scale population studies. Regardless of the amount of time and effort spent to acquire as complete a dossier as possible on each case, the data accrued are limited by the extent of existing knowledge.

<u>Brues</u>: If you study a series of monozygotic and dizygotic twins, what sort of differences in life span do you see?

<u>Jarvik</u>: In the age group 60-64, the average difference was almost twice as large for dizygotics as for monozygotics: nearly 16 years versus 9 years (20). There is the difficulty that you have to compensate for the actual age at which the first twin dies because, as Dr. Kallmann pointed out, the greater the age, the less the difference we can expect. Yet, even at the age of 80, there is still a difference of about 1 year between the two zygosity groups. I think it is 3 years for one-egg and 4 years for two-egg pairs in the female series. In other words, if twin sisters both reach the age of 80 or over, and then one of them dies, the one-egg co-twin may expect to survive an additional 3 years and the two-egg co-twin a year more than that, or 4 years.

<u>Keys</u>: Was the environmental factor actually balanced out there? Are the environmental situations, the extent to which they may differ, the same for dizygotic and monozygotic?

<u>Jarvik</u>: We failed altogether to find large differences in the environment.

<u>Keys</u>: Such factors as separation, in terms of space, from the place of birth, and things like that? As far as I have seen in the Swedish study,* which was a very large series, as you know, the dizygotics move around and separate from each other much more than monozygotic twins. Therefore, this factor is not balanced out.

---

*Studies on twins in progress at the Swedish National Institute of Hygiene, Stockholm.

Jarvik: We tried to rate environmental differences in relation to separation but it became very difficult to evaluate. Let's say one of the twins moved away and lived in a different city. Would they be classified as different because they were separated by several hundred miles, or would they be called similar because they both lived in comparable urban areas? How about the pair where one stayed on the farm and the other moved to a city just a few miles away, or the pair where both partners lived on large farms, one on the West Coast and one on the East Coast? Which pair would be considered to have similar and which one dissimilar environments? I am sure such differences play an important role but we haven't been able to tease them out of our material so far.

Barrows: Do you find that the cause of death is the same, more frequently, in one-egg versus two-egg twins? In the three cases you cited it actually was the same. I am not quite sure what the two females died of; the two sets of males both died of coronary. Is it more likely that they will die of the same cause?

Jarvik: It is somewhat more likely that one-egg partners will have the same cause of death. We have not done a complete cause-of-death analysis as yet. A special analysis has been carried out for cancer deaths, and there we tried to be extremely careful in demanding verification of the presence or absence of neoplastic disease. Thus, of 161 twins reported to have had cancer, only 69 were acceptable for intrapair comparisons. We found just six pairs who were concordant for cancer, I believe. Usually, if one twin died of cancer, the other one did not. This may be because he died of something else first, before he could develop cancer. In three of our six concordant pairs it actually took from 12 to 15 years before they became concordant. Among them was a monozygotic pair where one twin showed the first symptoms of lymphosarcoma at the age of 58 years. His brother remained in good health for 13 years, and was 71 years old when symptomatic reticulum cell sarcoma was discovered (18).

Storer: After correcting for differences in survival time, based on whether the twins are old or young, is there a tendency for the twins who die at younger ages to show great differences in survival?

Jarvik: Yes, there is, but our youngest age group begins at 60 years.

Storer: Is this an arbitrary cut-off age?

Jarvik: Yes, this age was arbitrarily selected in the hope

that we would be able to follow the twins to the end of their lives.

Storer: Let's consider twins dying under age 75. Do they tend to show a greater difference then those who live beyond 75?

Jarvik: In general, yes.

Kallmann: With progression toward a lower and lower residual lifetime ceiling, the cogency of the difference between genetically similar and dissimilar zygosity groups seems to undergo little change with increasing age (Table 2). Apparently, the observed life-span differences between one-egg and two-egg series of twins remain essentially of the same order of magnitude at successive age levels in both sexes, below and over the age of 70.

TABLE 2

Mean Intrapair Differences in Life Span, Both Twin Partners Dying over Age 60 of Natural Causes (192 Pairs)

(In months)

Age group first deceased (In years)	Male		Female		Opposite sex
	One-egg	Two-egg	One-egg	Two-egg	
60-64	113	130	102	215	138
65-69	39	82	71	122	183
70-74	66	78	68	97	80
75-79	38	42	49	70	68
80 and over	35	42	36	48	68

Reprinted, by permission, from Kallmann, F. J. 1961. Genetic factors in aging: Comparative and longitudinal observations on a senescent twin population. In P. H. Hoch and J. Zubin (eds.), Psychopathology of aging. Grune and Stratton, New York.

We have found no evidence in support of the notion that the environmental circumstances differed far more in two-egg than in one-egg pairs of twins. Actually, one of the most pronounced differences observed in our study occurred in a one-egg pair, the farmer's wife and the missionary described previously. Even in this pair, various teams of our investigators failed to obtain significant psychological test differences. The neighbors were unable to tell the twins apart, and the grandchildren called both of them "Grandma."

Hence, I would say that there were just as many environmental differences in one-egg as in two-egg twins.

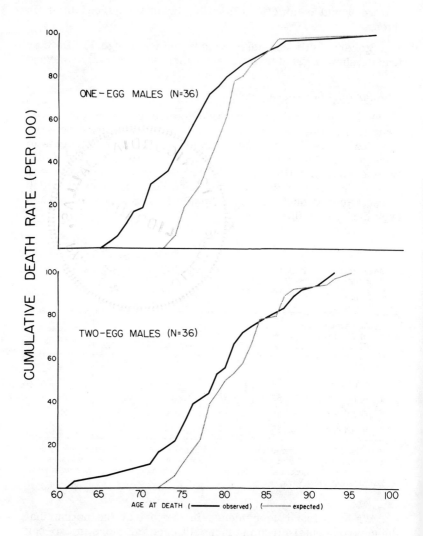

Fig. 2.—Cumulative death rate (per 100) of surviving same-sex co-twins compared with expected general population rate. Reprinted, by permission, from Kallmann, F. J. 1961. Genetic factors in aging: Compara-

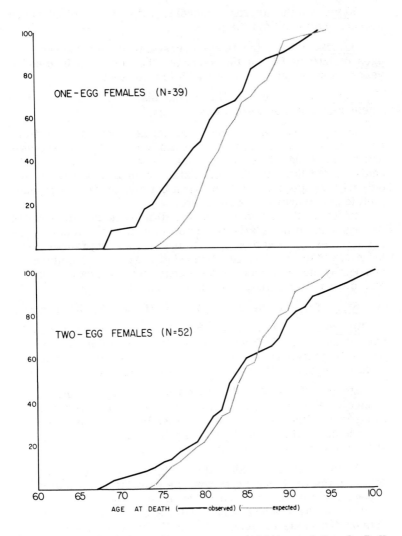

ONE-EGG FEMALES (N=39)

TWO-EGG FEMALES (N=52)

AGE AT DEATH (━━━observed) (···········expected)

tive and longitudinal observations on a senescent twin population. In: P. H.
Hoch and J. Zubin (eds.), Psychopathology of aging, pp. 239 ff. Grune and
Stratton, New York.

Keys: On the average, there is a difference of 10 years between individuals in the pairs.

Jarvik: Where the first-deceased twin died between the ages of 60 and 64, on the average, the second twin died 10 years later, which goes along with the life span.

Keys: With such a life span, that would be expected whether or not they were twins.

Jarvik: That is correct. You can see the larger differences in the two-egg pairs, particularly in the female series—and we have encountered this sex difference in many of the analyses we have done. The males seem to age earlier not only with respect to total life span but also so far as psychometric performance is concerned.

In Table 2, for instance, the difference in life span of two-egg males is relatively small, in contrast to that of two-egg females. It is comparable to that of two-egg females at a later age, as can be seen from the next-to-last column. In one-egg twins, too, we observe a consistent decrease in intrapair differences in length of life with advancing age.

Storer: After correction, do you still see the differences?

Jarvik: This is uncorrected. The age groups refer to the ages at death of the first-deceased twins, and the mean intrapair differences in length of life were entered in the appropriate categories. How do you want to correct it?

Storer: If one of the pair dies between age 60 and 64, the chance of the other one living for some time afterwards is fairly good. But if one of the pair dies between age 75 and 78, the chance of the other living very much longer is small. It should be possible to correct for these differences.

Jarvik: We have done this (Fig. 2). Taking the age at death of the first-deceased twin, we calculated the statistical expectancy for the survivor. We asked, "How long would a person, having reached a particular age, be expected to survive on the basis of actuarial data?" Of course, the expectancy is the same for the one-egg and the two-egg twin partners. It is not possible to correct for the fact that in one case it was the identical co-twin who survived and in the other case it was not—their expectancies are the same. Taking the actuarial predictions, we found that when a one-egg twin partner died before the age of 80, his co-twin's actual survival time was considerably less than the expected survival time.

Brues: Since we have been invited to bring various data to this conference, I have copied some very well-known data on the blackboard, derived from the Old Testament (Table 3) (6). I have put down on the left the reputed ages of the biblical patriarchs at death, beginning with Adam and running down through Jacob.

The figures on the right are their ages at birth of the heir or first-born son. Data on later children are not available. The biblical historians were mainly interested in the heirs.

Simms: Do you personally guarantee the authenticity of the data?

Brues: It is in one book many people believe is the most authentic. (Laughter)

One notices the quantum jumps from around 930 to 430 to 230 to around 100-plus. This has been a subject of interest among Old Testament historians, but not very much lately, as nearly as I can make out.

In the first column, with the exception of Enoch, who was translated rather than died, the variance is extremely small. I think Mr. Sacher pointed that out to me.

Dobzhansky: Should we conclude that mankind has degenerated because of accumulation of deleterious suspensions of natural selection, and so on?

TABLE 3

Genealogy of the Patriarchs from Adam to Jacob

Patriarch	Age at death	Age at birth of the heir
Adam	930	130
Seth	912	105
Enos	905	90
Cainan	910	70
Mahalaleel	895	65
Jared	962	162
Enoch	(365)	65
Methuselah	969	187
Lamech	777	182
Noah	950	502
Shem	600	100
Arphaxad	438	35
Salah	433	30
Eber	464	34
Peleg	239	30
Reu	239	32
Serug	230	30
Nahor	148	29
Terah	205	130
Abram	175	100
Isaac	180	60
Jacob	147	

Reprinted from Clarke, A. 1874. The Holy Bible: The text with a commentary and critical notes, vol. 1, p. 87. Nelson and Phillips, New York.

Brues: The biblical source attributed the deterioration to environmental factors—that mankind misbehaved.

Simms: Maybe we are more truthful now. Are you sure those aren't months, rather than years?

Brues: If that were the case, and it could be, it is a little difficult to fill in the intermediate ones which run around 400. That was directly after the Deluge. Shem was born before the Flood, and he went with his father on the ark. Everybody below Shem was born after the Flood.

Sacher: Evidence for the deleterious effect of inbreeding.
It may be appropriate to remark here that paleolithic man, and specifically Peking and Neanderthal man, could reach an age of 50 years, and neolithic man could exceed 70 years. This is based on osteological indications in the skulls.

Fenn: What about the population growth as a whole, with a very long life span of that sort? Would it be greater or would it be less? I believe it took many, many centuries to double the population of the earth in those early days. Now it doubles in about 35 years. Is this correlated with the reproductive age of the men, or what?

Brues: Which was sometimes rather delayed, as in the case of Noah whose first was born after he was 500. There are no good data on the rate of population increase, except that having gone on through those generations before Noah, there were people enough to fill several large and rather wicked cities in the world at that time, all of whom were presumably descended from Adam.

Fenn: It is rather remarkable that the population grew so slowly, with lots of room and no crowding.

Fremont-Smith: What was the background radiation at that time?

Brues: Insofar as the chronology is correct, it was very little different from what it is at present.

REFERENCES

1. Austin, M. L., D. Widmayer, and L. M. Walker. 1956. Antigenic transformation as adaptive response of Paramecium aurelia to patulin; relation to cell division. Physiol. Zool. 29: 261-87.

2. Beale, G. H. 1954. The genetics of Paramecium aurelia. Cambridge: Cambridge Univ. Press.

3. Blest, A. D. 1960. The evolution, ontogeny and quantitative control of the settling movements of some New World Saturniid moths, with some comments on distance communication by honey-bees. Behaviour 16: 188-253.

4. Blest, A. D. 1963. Longevity, palatability, and natural selection in five species of New World Saturniid moth. Nature 197: 1183-86.

5. Borthwick, H. A., and S. B. Hendricks. 1960. Photoperiodism in plants. Science 132: 1223-28.

6. Clarke, A. 1873. The Holy Bible: The text with a commentary and critical notes. vol. 1, p. 87. New York: Nelson and Phillips.

7. Comfort, A. 1956. The biology of senescence. New York: Rinehart.

8. Dobzhansky, Th. 1955. Evolution, genetics, and man. New York: John Wiley and Sons.

9. Dobzhansky, Th. 1956. What is an adaptive trait? Am. Nat. 90: 337-47.

10. Dobzhansky, Th. 1963. Mankind evolving; the evolution of the human species. New Haven: Yale Univ. Press.

11. Dunn, L. C. 1957. Evidence of evolutionary forces leading to the spread of lethal genes in wild populations of house mouse. Proc. Nat. Acad. Sci. 43: 158-63.

12. Ehret, C. F. 1960. Organelle systems and biological organization. Science 132: 115-23.

13. Haldane, J. B. S. 1932. The causes of evolution. London: Longmans; New York: Harper.

14. Hutchinson, G. E. 1959. A speculative consideration of certain possible forms of sexual selection in man. Am. Nat. 93: 81-91.

15. Jacob, F., and J. Monod. 1961. On the regulation of gene activity. Cold Spring Harbor Symposium on Quantitative Biology 26: 193-211.

16. Jacobs, P. A., W. M. Court-Brown, and R. Doll. 1961. Distribution of human chromosome counts in relation to age. Nature 191: 1178-80.

17. Jarvik, L. F. 1962. Genetic variations in disease resistance and survival potential. In F. J. Kallmann (ed.), Expanding goals of genetics in psychiatry, pp. 10-24. New York: Grune and Stratton.

18. Jarvik, L. F., and A. Falek. 1962. Comparative data on cancer in aging twins. Cancer 15: 1009-18.

19. Jarvik, L. F., and A. Falek. 1963. Intellectual stability and survival in the aged. J. Gerontol. 18: 173-76.

20. Jarvik, L. F., A. Falek, F. J. Kallmann, and I. Lorge. 1960. Survival trends in a senescent twin population. Am. J. Human Genet. 12: 170-79.

21. Jarvik, L. F., F. J. Kallmann, A. Falek, and M. M. Klaber. 1957. Changing intellectual functions in senescent twins. Acta Genet. 7: 421-30.

22. Kallmann, F. J. 1961. Genetic factors in aging. In Paul H. Hoch and J. Zubin (eds.), Psychopathology of aging, pp. 227-47. New York: Grune and Stratton.

23. Lipkin, M., and H. Quastler. 1962. Cell retention and incidence of carcinoma in several portions of the gastrointestinal tract. Nature 194: 1198-99.

24. Mather, K. 1943. Polygenic inheritance and natural selection. Biol. Rev. 18: 32-64.

25. Medawar, P. B. 1957. The uniqueness of the individual. London: Methuen.

26. Montaigne, M. 1580. Essais, II, 37: De la resemblance des enfans auz peres.

27. Morgan, T. H. 1919. The physical bases of heredity. Philadelphia: W. B. Saunders.

28. Needham, A. E. 1959. The origination of life. Quart. Rev. Biol. 34: 189-209.

29. Novick, A., and L. Szilard. 1950. Experiments with the chemostat on spontaneous mutations of bacteria. Proc. Nat. Acad. Sci. 36: 708-19.

30. Pirie, A. 1961. Difference in reaction to X-irradiation between chicken and rabbit lens. Radiation Res. 15: 211-19.

31. Robertson, O. H., M. A. Krupp, S. F. Thomas, C. B. Favour, S. Hane, and B. C. Wexler. 1961. Hyperadrenocorticism in spawning migratory and non-migratory rainbow trout (Salmo gairdnerii); comparison with Pacific salmon (genus Oncorhynchus). Gen. Comp. Endocr. 1: 473-84.

32. Robertson, O. H., and B. C. Wexler. 1962. Histological changes in the pituitary gland of the Pacific salmon (genus Oncorhynchus) accompanying sexual maturation and spawning. J. Morphol. 110: 171-85.

33. Roderick, T. H., and J. B. Storer. 1961. Correlation between mean litter size and mean life span among twelve inbred strains of mice. Science 134: 48-49.

34. Sonneborn, T. M. 1930. Genetic studies on Sterostonium incaudatum. I. The nature and origin of differences among individuals formed during vegetative reproduction. J. Exper. Zool. 57: 57-108.

35. Szilard, L. 1959. On the nature of the aging process. Proc. Nat. Acad. Sci. 45: 30-45.

36. Welch, G. P. 1957. Effects of chronic exposure to X-rays on a steady-state population of Saccharomyces cerevesiae. Univ. Calif. Rad. Lab. Report No. 3763. Berkeley: Univ. of Calif. Press.

37. Williams, G. C. 1957. Pleiotropy, natural selection, and the evolution of senescence. Evolution 11: 398-411.

38. Zeevaart, J. A. D., and A. Lang. 1963. Suppression of floral induction in Bryophyllum daigremontianum by a growth retardant. Planta 59: 509-17.

Genetics and Environment

PART II

Brues: We have asked Dr. Tyler to lead the next part of our discussion.

Tyler:[*] I shall discuss two general topics. The first is perhaps not likely to raise any special controversy, but the second may very well do so, especially as it deals with cancer. The first topic overlaps with material scheduled to be presented tomorrow. It concerns the life span of cells, particularly those cells to which the species owes such immortality as it has, namely, the eggs and sperm. I shall discuss some experiments dealing with the life span of the gametes themselves, as cells, under ordinary sorts of conditions that they would encounter. These include experiments in which I was engaged a number of years ago (21, 28, 36, 37, 39, 41, 42, 43, 44, 45). They deal mainly with sea urchins and other marine animals, since such animals provide isolated sperm and egg cells that are relatively easy to handle experimentally.

When sea-urchin eggs are shed into the surrounding sea water and are not fertilized, they have a relatively short half-life under ordinary conditions. This is of the order of a day or so at temperatures of around 20° C. It varies somewhat with the species. If the eggs are fertilized, however, they can live for a week or more without receiving any nutriment from the surroundings.

It was of interest, then, for us to attempt to learn what might be responsible for their death under ordinary circumstances. Our experiments indicated that under ordinary con-

[*] The preparation of this material, and original work of the author cited therein, was aided by a research grant (GM-06965) from the National Institute of General Medical Sciences of the National Institutes of Health, United States Public Health Service.

ditions they seem to die from bacterial attack. In one of these experiments, unfertilized sea-urchin eggs were collected with aseptic precautions and kept in sterile sea water. They survived and remained fertilizable for some 21 days instead of a day and one-quarter, which was the maximum survival of the controls in this experiment.

On the other hand, if one tries to shorten the life span by adding bacteria, using cultures of the organisms that one ordinarily finds around the eggs when they die, this doesn't have very much of an effect. It appears that the eggs are resistant to bacterial attack for a certain period of time. After this they become susceptible to attack by particular microorganisms that are likely to be present ordinarily in their surroundings. We did not determine which microorganisms, among those that are ordinarily present, attack the eggs of the species of sea urchins used in these experiments.

Fremont-Smith: What do you use as end point, inability to fertilize?

Tyler: Yes, and we also use the visible changes.

For the experiments on adding bacteria, the latter were obtained from a culture of dying sea-urchin eggs and grown on a medium recommended to us by Dr. Selman A. Waksman, of the Department of Microbiology, Rutgers University, as suitable for growing many kinds of marine bacteria. We used that medium enriched with a brei of sea-urchin eggs.

It was thought at one time that the death of the unfertilized egg might be occasioned by metabolic changes that spontaneously go out of control at a set time after the cells are shed from the ovary. In particular, a great increase in rate of oxygen uptake has been observed at the time of death. However, the experiments have shown that this great increase in oxidations is primarily due to bacteria. When the eggs are kept under sterile conditions, the rate of oxygen uptake remains at a low steady level, as shown in Figure 3. When, as in this experiment, after a period of prolonged survival of the eggs under sterile conditions, bacterial contamination later occurs, the oxygen consumption of the suspension rises correspondingly.

So it appears that under ordinary conditions the unfertilized egg cell doesn't suddenly run wild at a set time and start burning itself up at an accelerating rate; it simply becomes susceptible to bacterial attack when it has been on its own for a certain period of time—without nutriment and other factors that it had received in the ovary. Under sterile conditions no spontaneous increase in oxidation rate is observed during the prolonged survival of the unfertilized egg.

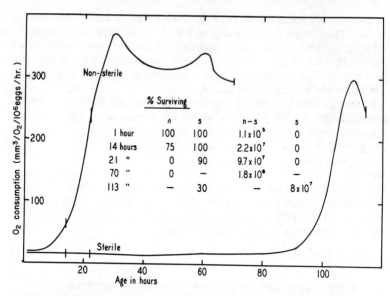

Fig. 3.—Rate of oxygen consumption and length of survival of unfertilized *Arbacia* eggs under sterile (s) and non-sterile (n-s) conditions. After Tyler, A., N. Ricci, and N. H. Horowitz. 1938. The respiration and fertilizable life of *Arbacia* eggs under sterile and non-sterile conditions. J. Exp. Zool. 79: 129-42.

The sperm have a somewhat different way of dying. They die apparently by intoxicating themselves with heavy metals that are present in trace amounts in their surroundings. They have evolved an efficient mechanism for complexing heavy metals. Apparently this has become so efficient that they will bind enough to inactivate constituents that are essential for their survival.

Fremont-Smith: Is this also the case for sperm of other species?

Tyler: The experiments have been done with sperm of sea urchins, roosters, and bulls. First, I should mention a basic phenomenon, known as the dilution effect, that has mystified investigators for some time. If a sample of sea-urchin semen is kept undiluted at room temperature, the sperm will live ordinarily for about a day. If the semen is diluted 10 times with sea water, the sperm may live for a couple of hours. If diluted another 10 times, survival is generally a few minutes, and after still another 10 times, it is only a few seconds. In early experiments on this problem it was thought that, since sperm are motile cells, they would need a lot of energy to keep them going. Dilution might then mean a relative loss of components of the energy-supplying system. So sugars, ATP, amino acids, etc., were tested and it turned out that amino acids were highly potent in overcoming the dilution effect and prolonging the life of the sperm. However, the experiments showed that the added amino acids were not metabolized by the sperm. This leads us to consider other possible ways in which they might act, and it seemed that a possible way could be by chelation of heavy metals, since amino acids (as well as proteins, which also prolong the life of sea-urchin sperm) are known to possess this property in marked degree. A number of other metal-chelating agents, including the special amino acid, ethylene diamine tetraacetic acid (Versene®), which is commonly used for metal chelation, were then tested; these prolonged the life span of sperm of various marine and land animals even more effectively than did the various ordinary amino acids (Table 4).

The analysis thus led us to conclude that the heavy-metals present in trace amounts in the natural media in which the sperm is shed, or in ordinary salt solutions with which semen may be diluted for experimental purposes, are primarily responsible for the rapid aging.

Incidentally, before the loss of fertilizing capacity and motility, there is another sign of deterioration of the sperm. This is revealed by the behavior of eggs which have been fertilized by aged sperm. The initial response of the egg, as indicated by elevation of the vitelline (fertilization) membrane, is poorer with the aged sperm. The prolongation of life span with metal-chelating agents also delays that phase of the aging process.

Finally, I should remark that, while the experiments show that effects of trace metals may be very important in the rapid aging of sperm that occurs upon dilution, there are probably several other factors also involved. These may well be diffusion of nutrients or other essential constituents out of the sperm, along with depletion of their reserves of metabolizable substrates accelerated by increased activity upon dilution.

Ehret: Are the chelators effective on eggs also?

Tyler: The experiments show an effect on eggs, but not to the same extent as on sperm.

Keys: What about a synthetic medium without the metals?

Tyler: Artificial sea water, low in trace metals, is better for sperm and eggs than natural sea water. It can also be better for the whole animals and for their development. We have raised embryos and kept various species of marine animals

TABLE 4

Action of Various Metal-chelating Agents on Life Span of Sea-Urchin Spermatozoa at 19°-22° C

Substance	Species	Semen concentration, %	Number of experiments	Half-motile life* and half-fertilizable life† in hours, in solutions at the following concentrations in sea water						
				0	10^{-2} M	10^{-3} M	10^{-4} M	10^{-5} M	10^{-6} M	10^{-7} M
Versene[1]	Strongylocentrotus purpuratus	1	8*	2.9	0.3	21	22	13	7	7
	Strongylocentrotus purpuratus	1	3†	1	<1	20+	20+	10-15		
	Strongylocentrotus purpuratus	0.1	4*	0.2	<0.1	3	10	1.5	0.3	0.2
	Lytechinus pictus	1	4*	3.2		21	27	29		
	Lytechinus pictus	1	2†	0.8		24+	24+	24+		
	Lytechinus pictus	0.1	1*	0.2		18	22	13		
DEDTC[2]	Strongylocentrotus purpuratus	1	3*	5.6	2.5	17	5.5			
	Lytechinus pictus	1	8*	5.8	2.7	22	32			
	Lytechinus pictus	1	2†	1			30+			
	Lytechinus pictus	0.1	1*	<0.5	1	4	2.5			
Oxine[3]	Strongylocentrotus purpuratus	1	3*	2		16	14	2		
	Strongylocentrotus purpuratus	0.1	1*	0.1		2	2	0.1		
	Lytechinus pictus	1	2*	0.4		4.5		1.5	0.8	0.5
Cupron[4]	Strongylocentrotus purpuratus	1	2*	1			6	8.5	5	
	Strongylocentrotus purpuratus	0.1	2*	0.3		2	2	2	0.3	

[1] Ethylenediaminetetraacetic acid   [2] Diethyldithiocarbamate   [3] 8-Hydroxyquinoline   [4] α-Benzoinoxime

Source: A. Tyler 1953, Biol, Bull. 104: 224.

for long periods of time in an artificial sea water which, in addition to being low in trace metals, contains only the major chemical constituents of sea water; namely, Na^+, K^+, Ca^{++}, Mg^{++}, Cl^-, $SO_4^=$, and HCO_3^- (Table 5). They do very well in this. Of course, one can't add the animal without adding a reasonable amount of some trace elements that it ordinarily needs. But evidently they don't need the amounts that would be supplied by natural sea water in order to survive for prolonged periods of time. Fertilization and development, and also the production of eggs and sperm, can occur in such a simple artificial sea water as that shown in Table 5.

TABLE 5

Composition of an Artificial Sea Water Suitable for Prolonged Survival of Spermatozoa, Eggs, Embryos, and Whole Organisms (37)

Substance	Volumes
0.55 M NaCl	1000
0.55 M KCl	22
0.37 M MgCl$_2$	195
0.37 M Na$_2$SO$_4$	103
0.37 M CaCl$_2$	35
bring to pH 8.2 with:	
0.55 M NaHCO$_3$	ca. 6

In conclusion, I believe that when one now discusses the "fitness of the environment" as an expression of the effectiveness of natural selection, it should be noted that there are experiments that show, at least for marine animals, that one can replace the natural environment with a simple artificial environment to which the animals are better fitted as far as life span and reproductive activities are concerned.

I shall turn now to another aspect of aging that relates to the second part of the title of this conference, namely, biological organization. For this I would like to talk about neoplastic disease, which pertains to this particular conference as one of the manifestations of aging, and as a manifestation of some sort of biological disorganization. First, to connect it with the work I have just discussed, it may be noted that there is evidence for some role of the so-called trace elements in the neoplastic process. At least there have been many papers written on the subject. I am not going to dwell on this, but it is clear that accumulation of certain of the heavy metals, in trace amounts, can alter the physiology of the cell, or induce changes of specific types, one of which could be in the direction of neoplasia. But the analysis of neoplasia that I wish to discuss comes from a different direction.

In connection with studies on the problem of differentiation in normal development, I have often been puzzled, as have many others, about the development of tumors. The neoplastic tissue is often cited as an example of growth without differentiation or with eventual loss of whatever differentiation may have been present initially. In a sense this could serve as a control for many experiments on differentiation. Conversely, studies of normal development may be expected to contribute to our understanding of the neoplastic process.

There have been many theories about neoplasia, about cancer, based on developmental phenomena. None, so far, seems to offer much possibility for experimental testing. Recently I have published (38, 40) a developmental, immunogenetic concept that does indicate directions in which tests of validity may be made and that provides an outline of a unified theory of cancer. Perhaps it won't satisfy you, but it may induce you to think about the problems from a somewhat different point of view than you had done previously.

At present, most oncologists apparently think there are just two main theories about cancer: the virus theory and the theory of genetic mutation, as such. Since viruses and genes are now recognized to be very similar in essential properties, the two main theories are very similar. Proponents of both express their views in terms of a modification of the phenotype of the cell (determined intrinsically by infecting virus or by mutated gene) such that it proliferates continuously and fails to differentiate, or, if differentiated, eventually loses its specific differentiated characteristics. These views assume that the neoplastic cell has a peculiar property because of something it possesses intrinsically in the form of an unusual DNA or RNA. This could be the DNA or the RNA of a so-called tumor virus, or the DNA of a mutated gene. It could also be a mutation of a host-cell gene induced by virus. These views assume that the neoplastic cell would retain its neoplastic properties, if transplanted to other hosts, so long as it was not rejected and could keep such properties outside the animal as well as inside. The idea, common to both virological theories and mutational genetic theories, is that the cells intrinsically possess determinants in the form of the DNA or RNA of the virus, or in the form of a mutated gene, so that this abnormal property will be manifested in the same way as cells manifest the action of "normal" genes. Thus the neoplastic cells would be expected to behave differently from normal cells in tissue cultures. This has been reported by many investigators, as is now well known. Most authorities do not claim that the cells grow more rapidly than normal in culture, but they are reported to grow differently (more three-dimensionally) and to grow for a longer period of time. One can induce this type of growth in cultures of cells by polyoma virus and by Rous sarcoma virus. One can also do it with other viruses which are not considered ordinarily to be tumor viruses. There are a number of other objections to a simple view of neoplasia considered as a phenotypic expression of a virus. These objections relate to the fact that the tumor-inducing virus may disappear or at least become unidentifiable in the cells of the tumor that it has induced.

There is another school of thought—and perhaps I am the only one who represents this at present: this is the notion that a neoplastic cell is not intrinsically a bad cell, but is one that has become altered in such a way that its neighbors exert a bad influence on it. It then responds to this influence by continuous proliferation and by aggressive action against the host. In culture, the cell wouldn't be particularly different from the corresponding normal cells. The alteration in question is considered to be gene loss or gene inactivation. The particular genes involved are considered to be those that determine the histocompatibility antigens of the organism.

Simms: May I point out one exception to that? Rous sarcoma cells, when planted in tissue culture, start to grow instantaneously, without any lag period, whereas the normal fibroblast from the same animal has a lag period of about 3 days before growth begins.

Tyler: I believe one can account for that difference by noting that, while growing as a tumor in the organism, the cells have already received a stimulus to growth from their host. I will discuss later the nature of the stimulus. At present I would say that the cells coast along on this stimulus temporarily. After some time in culture, this difference is lost. So this is an initial difference. Of course, there are also other initial differences. For example, there are differences in metabolic properties, such as glycolytic capacity in some tumors. As Paul (26) has shown, these also vanish after a while. The high glycolytic activity is evidently dependent on the tumor having grown as a large, poorly vascularized mass of tissue for some time. One can reproduce the metabolic properties with ordinary tissue cells by simulating such conditions.

After reviewing much of the evidence from various sources, I have come to the conclusion that there are no intrinsic differences between normal cells and so-called malignant cells of corresponding type, with respect to metabolic and proliferative properties, but that the neoplastic property is simply a response to the action of materials from other cells of the organism by cells modified in a particular way, namely, by loss of a histocompatibility gene. These materials encourage the cell to proliferate; that is, they add a proliferative stimulus of some sort, and the now neoplastic cells also manufacture noxious materials in turn.

The first question to be raised is why does the host tolerate this? Ordinarily, the body has mechanisms for disposing of all kinds of foreign materials, including foreign cells. Why doesn't it dispose of the neoplastic cells? This question is answered very simply by the theory.

It rests simply on the results of experiments dealing with transplantation between inbred strains of animals and their F_1 hybrids. As is well known, tissues can be transplanted successfully between members of the same inbred strains but not between the strains, nor from the F_1 to either of the parents. They can also be transplanted successfully from either of the parents to the F_1 hybrid. In the latter case, the A-strain parent does not possess an antigen foreign to the F_1 host, and neither does the B-strain parent. So tissue from A, or from B, will be tolerated by the F_1 hybrid. In the same way, if cells of an organism have lost a histocompatibility gene, or if the gene has been inactivated, the cells will still be tolerated.

In the transplantation experiments, when cells of an inbred parental strain are transplanted to the F_1, the grafted cells, while tolerated by the host, may themselves react against the foreign antigens of the host. So these cells will try to reject the host; that is, they will react immunologically against the host if they are immunologically competent cells. If the transplanted tissue contains only a small proportion of immunologically competent cells, it would presumably be only the latter that would respond to the foreign antigens of the host.

This is the graft-versus-host reaction that was discovered by Simonsen (31, 32) and by Brent and Billingham (3, 4) and termed "runt" disease by the latter investigators. Since it is not restricted to transplantation to immature, or fetal, hosts that tolerate foreign cells, but can occur also in adult F_1 hosts receiving cells from inbred parental strains or in irradiated or cortisonized hosts, the term "transplantation disease" has been proposed for all these cases (38). Our theory proposes, then, that cancer is analogous to transplantation disease. In other words, the neoplastic tissue behaves as though it were a transplant from an inbred parental strain to the F_1 hybrid, and as though it contained immunologically competent cells. In connection with immunological competence, I would consider that any tissue that can be allergically sensitized contains immunologically competent cells. Either a certain proportion of the cells is immunologically competent, or perhaps all of them are capable of assuming, at some time and under appropriate conditions, a state of immunological competence. The basic theory assumes only that the histocompatibility-gene loss or the gene inactivation occurs in a cell that is immunologically competent or that can become competent.

The characteristic reaction of the immunologically competent cell to a foreign antigen is to proliferate. Since host antigens are foreign to the cells that have lost a histocompatibility gene, and thus the corresponding antigen, this antigen in the host serves as a proliferative stimulus. The altered cells now receive an added stimulus to proliferation; that is, it is added to stimuli ordinarily received, and is given to the cells in chronically continuous fashion from the surrounding tissues.

Normally, there are probably a number of factors which control the rate of proliferation of the cells of a particular tissue. In this situation something more is added to these factors; namely, that the altered cell and its progeny will be exposed to materials from the host that they now regard as a foreign antigen. The exposure is likely to be irregular in time and dosage, presumably depending upon many factors that may control the extent to which host-cell antigens may be liberated, or produced, so as to reach the altered cell, and possibly on the physical state of the material. But there is no escape for the altered cells. As long as they remain in the organism, some of the "foreign" antigenic material will reach them from time to time in one form or another. The cells thus receive this added stimulus to proliferation in continuing, though perhaps irregular, fashion. The response, namely proliferation, is one that is known to be characteristic ordinarily of immunologically competent cells upon exposure to a foreign antigen. However, in the case of the cell that has undergone the loss or inactivation of a histocompatibility gene, the "foreign" antigen is continuously at hand in the surrounding tissues.

Dobzhansky: Why then do hybrid cells not act as tumor cells in the parental strain?

Tyler: They are rejected. The host cells will react immunologically against the hybrid cells, and the result will be a homograft rejection reaction, as it is in transplants between the two strains.

Dobzhansky: If you postulate that the neoplastic cell contains more antigens and, consequently, is stimulated to grow, isn't a neoplastic cell in the original organ then the same as A cells in A-B host?

Tyler: So far, I believe, I haven't really called the cell that has undergone the gene loss or inactivation a "neoplastic cell," have I? I regard it as an initially normal cell characteristic of the tissue in which it is located.

We can, however, call the "gene-loss" cell and its progeny neoplastic cells, but they are neoplastic only if they are located in a host that possesses a histocompatibility gene that they lack, and does not lack any histocompatibility gene that these cells possess. So the assignment of the designation neoplastic to them depends upon their location; if these cells were transplanted to a suitable host, they would presumably behave normally.

Fremont-Smith: Are any cells at the top level potentially neoplastic?

Tyler: Any tissue of the body that is capable of reacting immunologically presumably contains immunologically competent cells.

Fremont-Smith: They would be neopotential.

Tyler: That means most tissues of the body, because I guess there is hardly a tissue that can't be sensitized in some way.

Storer: Are you saying, in other words, that the cells that become neoplastic simply don't have the complete complement of antigens that the host has?

Tyler: That is right. They haven't gained anything, just lost something; namely, one of the particular surface proteins which we designate as histocompatibility antigens. These are presumably mediators of interactions between cells.

In mice, there are some 14 genetic loci known where there are detectable histocompatibility genes. Presumably there are as many, or more, in human beings. Let us consider an individual heterozygous at one of the histocompatibility loci, and represent the genes at that locus as A and B. Assume that gene B has somehow or other been inactivated or lost in one of the cells. The corresponding antigen will then not be formed. Previously, this cell has been forming the B antigen. So it has B antigen on its surface. However, in the course of the normal turnover of cellular materials it will, after a period of time, lose the B antigen. This loss will occur early if the gene loss occurs in a dividing cell. In a non-dividing cell it might take years. Once lost, the B antigen will not be replaced because the cell doesn't have the genetic information to make the appropriate messenger RNA serve as a template for its synthesis.

Brues: May I go back before this step and try to restate it so I can be sure to understand the argument? The reactions you are talking about are of two kinds. In both cases they are a reaction of the cells that do not contain some factor against cells which contain a factor to which they are sensitized. Where the lacking one is the whole organism, it rejects the graft; where the lacking one is the graft, it responds in a peculiar manner. Is that your hypothesis?

Tyler: Right.

Quastler: The cells are supposed to lose the tolerance they previously had?

Tyler: According to certain theories about tolerance, the altered cells might be expected to be tolerant of the other tissues of the host, having arisen in the presence of the "foreign" antigen. I don't think a discussion of this subject would be very fruitful at present, but I should remark that many investigators consider tolerance to be a quantitative matter, not an absolute thing. With living cells, it can be manipulated to be essentially a permanent condition. But, ordinarily, the immunological suppression is found to be temporary.

On the basis of a clonal-selection theory of antibody formation, tolerance can be attributed to a destructive effect of excess antigen on those lines of immunologically competent cells that normally manufacture a protein (antibody) that is complementary to the foreign antigen. If this view is accepted we would interpret the failure of the altered, immunologically competent cell to become tolerant as meaning that there is not at any one time a sufficient amount of the foreign antigen present, in appropriate form for action, around the altered cell so as to exert a destructive effect. The smaller amounts serve simply as the proliferative stimulus that is the common effect of ordinary amounts of foreign antigen on immunologically competent cells.

Incidentally, one of the proposed therapeutic measures, on the basis of our theory, is the administration of an excess of the antigen that the tumor cells lack, so as to induce such allergic destruction of the cells. Evidence for the occurrence of allergic death of antibody-forming cells in a graft-versus-host situation has been presented by Gorer and Boyse (8).

Simms: I said a few minutes ago that the Rous sarcoma cells placed in a tissue culture start to grow immediately, whereas the normal cells have a lag period. We found the reason for that to be due to the fact that normal cells produce an inhibitor which apparently coats the cells and prevents further growth, whereas the tumor cells either don't produce the inhibitor or else are not affected by it. How would that fit in with your discussion?

Tyler: I wouldn't have a very special interpretation of that, other than to assume, as probably you and others have done, that the inhibitor represents one of the factors ordinarily responsible for growth regulation in the organisms, and that it can continue to express itself in culture, at least for a while.

Simms: The inhibitor in dormant tissue keeps the tissue in normal state.

Tyler: That is right. I know there are these properties, and contact properties, too, which are supposed to be altered in tumor cells. As I mentioned earlier, the tumor cells initially, upon explanation, may be coasting along on the stimuli they have received in the organism. Also, the loss of surface antigen may well affect contact properties. Further, we should note that unless one is dealing with clones derived from a single tumor cell, the cells in cultures derived from a tumor may be mixtures of neoplastic and normal cells.

The neoplastic cells might thus continue to receive, in culture, the added proliferative stimulus in the form of "foreign" antigen from the normal cells. The same considerations probably apply to experiments in which a tumor-inducing virus causes cells, in a normal tissue culture, to transform into cells that may have neoplastic characteristics. Again, this may be a matter of interaction between infected and uninfected cells, with the virus being responsible only for causing a gene loss or inactivation of appropriate type in the cell it invades.

When comparing cultures of tumors and of normal tissues, it is also important to be sure that one is comparing corresponding types of cells. This, I understand, is not easy to ascertain, especially as plating efficiencies in primary cultures are generally quite low.

Quimby: Dr. Tyler, it had always appeared to me that a cell in tissue culture keeps growing, regardless of whether it is neoplastic or normal, and does not differentiate.

Tyler: Yes, ordinarily that is true.

Simms: With normal tissue in culture, the colony will develop up to a certain point and then stop; the tumor cells keep on growing.

Tyler: Holtzer et al. (11) have reported some interesting experiments on growing cartilage cells in culture. Upon restricting the medium, the cells will redifferentiate and form cartilage. When well fed, they resume growth and division. Apparently this can be done only a few times. After several subculturings, whatever the cell contained that determined it to form cartilage is lost. I think this bears on the question of anaplasia. This is the question of why, after prolonged growth or repeated transplantation, a tumor loses most or all of the specific differentiated characteristics it may originally have had.

I think there are two factors involved which embryologically are termed intrinsic determinative factors and specific inductive factors. The former represent whatever particular agents appear in a cell when, embryologically, it has been determined to develop into a particular tissue. We think of this in terms of something that decides that only a certain part of the genome will be operative in cells of any particular tissue. The inductive factors are those influences from the surrounding tissues that induce a cell to differentiate in a particular direction. in a growing tumor, the multiplication of the cells and the increase in mass of tissue, in effect, progressively lessen the influence of these factors. Thus it can be assumed that the intrinsic determinative factors are diluted out as the cells continue proliferating. Also, as the mass of the tissue becomes progressively greater, the inner cells are less accessible to inductive agents supplied by the surrounding tissues.

The general proposition is that, at the start, a tumor is likely to continue to produce the particular materials characteristic of the tissue or cell of origin; but, as the tumor grows, the cells become less and less differentiated, and the tumor progresses toward anaplasia.

A unified theory is supposed to explain everything about cancer. It should explain the cause and the pathology and should offer some sort of cure as proof that the theory is essentially correct.

As for the cause, we consider this to be the loss or inactivation of a specific gene; namely, one of the histocompatibility genes. The loss or inactivation can come about in any one of a number of ways: radiation, chemical carcinogens, viruses, inactivation-by-position effect, or any one of a number of mechanisms that Dr. Dobzhansky has detailed for us more adeequately than I can.

The assumption of a loss or inactivation accords with a number of findings. For example, it is well known that there are chromosomal aberrations in most tumors, even leaving out of consideration, for the moment, the Philadelphia chromosome. Diverse kinds of chromosomal aberrations are present, in many instances, in the same kind of tumor. This would be difficult to interpret if one were to assume a specific mutation or the addition of specific chromosomes, or parts there-of, as the causative factor. On the other hand, if one assumes the loss of a gene, and also that this can be at any one of a dozen or more loci in the chromosomes, then it is readily un-derstandable that diverse kinds of chromosomal aberrations can include a loss at one or another of these loci. Further, there need not be a microscopically visible deletion, and, for that matter, these same effects (failure to produce a particu-lar histocompatibility antigen) can be obtained by some gene-inactivation process involving no loss of chromosomal mate-rial at all.

Generally, the chromosomal aberrations encountered in tumors represent gains of chromosomes, or parts thereof, rather than losses. One may, then, raise the question whether or not this can be reconciled with the idea of a loss. The answer is that by virtue of increasing the number of repre-sentatives of a particular chromosome, or a part thereof, the cell is more likely to be able to tolerate losses in this part of the genome.

The argument would be as follows. Presumably, for ade-quate functioning, a cell must have most genes doubly repre-sented. Until recently it has been generally held that the pri-mary reason haploid cells or haploid embryos die is because of a balanced lethal situation in the original diploid organism. Thus a lethal gene, which would ordinarily be covered up by the normal allele in a heterozygous diploid, could express it-self in the haploid condition. Recent investigations have shown that haploid frog eggs that have, in early cleavage, undergone a regular doubling up of their chromosomes, thus becoming homozygous diploids, will develop perfectly normally, whereas those that remain as haploids die at time of gastrulation. This work has been done by S. Subtelny (34) and P. Grant and P. M. Stott (9).

The diploid set of genes—or perhaps the diploid set of most genes, since we know that the X chromosome can be hap-loid—seems to be essential for appropriate functioning of the cell.

If, then, one wants to induce a loss of a particular gene by the deletion of all or part of the chromosome carrying the particular gene, it would certainly help to have another repre-sentative of this chromosome present. For example, let us assume we have an individual heterozygous at some histo-compatibility locus, say the H-2 locus in mice. We can desig-nate this individual H-2^a, H-2^b. If one of these chromosomes, say the one carrying H-2^a, doubles up, then the cell could more readily sustain the loss of all or part of the chromo-some carrying H-2^b. Thus the latter gene would be lost to the cell, but all the other genes that might have been lost with it would still be represented in diploid or triploid condition, depending on whether the whole chromosome or only a part thereof is lost.

In this connection it should be noted that mongolism (Down's disease) predisposes toward leukemia. Since individuals afflicted with Down's disease are known to be trisomic for one of their chromosomes, the increased incidence of leukemia would be consistent with the expectation on the basis of the type of mechanism mentioned.

Another area of investigation providing information that has seemed consistent with our views is that of ionizing radiation. We know that such radiation causes malignancy of various sorts. In studies of the manner in which the frequency increases with dose, there are differences of opinion as to precisely what the relation is. I believe it was Drs. Court-Brown and Doll (6, 7) who first proposed that there was a linear relationship between incidence of leukemia and the dose of radiation to which various populations of individuals subjected to irradiation were exposed.

Court-Brown: I should intervene. We found the linear relationship to satisfy our working model. We are now dissatisfied with our working model. (Laughter)

Tyler: I didn't think you were going to let that go by. At about the same time Drs. Court-Brown and Doll reported their analysis, one of our colleagues, Dr. Edward Lewis (19), examined similar data and he also observed a linear relationship for the data obtained on human beings. Dr. Brues (5) has analyzed these and other data, including much from experiments in his laboratories, and has indicated that the relationship between dose and incidence in most cases is non-linear and thus not likely to provide evidence for a one-hit, no-threshold situation. The gene-loss hypothesis offers a resolution of the divergent findings and interpretations.

The resolution would simply be this: both linear and non-linear relations can be obtained. It depends on the genetic makeup of the material being irradiated. If we are dealing with an organism that is heterozygous for histocompatibility alleles at one or a number of loci (it may also be homozygous at some loci), then a single hit would be sufficient to create a gene loss for one of these alleles and thus to induce a neoplasm. So such heterozygous animals should exhibit a linear dose-incidence relationship if there are not too many homozygous loci. Human beings, notably non-inbred animals, and presumably also Sprague-Dawley rats fall in this category, but not the highly inbred strains of mice. It is of interest that the data obtained with human beings and with rats largely show a linear relationship. With the inbred lines of mice, the data seem to be interpretable mostly on a two-hit or multi-hit basis. The supposition on our hypothesis is that, since the inbred animal is homozygous at all histocompatibility loci, two hits are needed at any one locus to knock out both alleles, which would be necessary so that the cell would then regard the remainder of the body as foreign.

Obviously, these views suggest further experimentation and analysis. Dr. Brues has informed me that in the course of related work he plans sometime to initiate some experiments along this line; namely, to determine whether or not the frequency of induction of tumors in response to a given dose of radiation is greater in the F_1 hybrid than in either of the two parental strains of inbred animals. This could be done either with widely different strains or with co-isogenic strains.

Similarly, the frequency of spontaneous tumors would be expected to be greater in the F_1 than it is in the two inbred strains. This assumes that we are dealing with inbred strains that have not been genetically selected for factors which can induce high percentages of tumors. As is well known, there are many inbred lines of mice that regularly develop certain types of tumors in high frequency. This may be attributed to specific genes which will induce chromosomal alterations (involving histocompatibility-gene loss or inactivation) in cells of certain tissues. By selection, of course, one can obtain that. For the proposed type of experiment, it would be preferable to take precautions to avoid use of such strains of animals.

Ehret: As I understand it, you expect somatic mosaics. What sort of end points can you use?

Tyler: Dr. Atwood has demonstrated the occurrence in human red blood cells of losses of blood-group antigens. One might expect that the progenitor cell, or cells, would be neoplastic.

Atwood: How do you get around it?

Tyler: In this case we don't know just what happened to the cell in which the loss occurred. If it simply lost its nucleus and became a mature erythrocyte it would not be expected to behave neoplastically.

I don't know of any accounts in mammals of loci of the kind Barbara McClintock has described (22, 23) in corn, which have such drastic effects on the behavior of the chromosomes. Probably those causing very extensive chromosomal aberrations are more readily eliminated by selection in mammals, but those inducing minor changes may well persist.

For our purposes, such effects would be expected on occasion to involve the loss of one or another of the histocompatibility genes and should thus result in neoplasia in such cells where there are not other concomitant chromosomal losses or other changes that are lethal to the cell. In most mammals, there are a good many histocompatibility genes. In mice, it is now known that the Y chromosome has such a locus. The same analysis leads us to suppose that the frequency of cancer in males of an inbred line should be greater than in the females. I don't think this has been properly investigated yet.

Atwood: How do you explain a graft from parent to F_1 that is not neoplastic?

Tyler: I consider runt disease to be a form of cancer.

Atwood: You won't find any tumors if you open up the animal.

Tyler: Generally not, but some tumors have been reported in experiments along this line in several laboratories. In some of these, the host was irradiated and this complicates the situation. However, tumors did arise from non-irradiated parental cells. We have done similar experiments with irradiated cortisonized and untreated F_1 hosts given parental cells and have obtained a few tumors.

Atwood: Runt disease doesn't always occur.

Tyler: That's true; with some combinations of strains the usual parent-to-F_1 transplantation rarely gives runt disease even when the host is a very young animal.

Atwood: Enough has to be put in, and it has to be done at the right time, and so on.

Brues: A very attractive feature of a hypothesis of this sort is that it has built in it the indication that one doesn't just push a button and get a tumor, that a setup has to be created in which there is an interaction between the host and the abnormal cell. This is really essential for any sort of mutational theory. If we look at the probability, as you have, Dr. Tyler, of developing red cell precursors with certain deletions, we should be having tumors all over us all the time, if there were not many other factors involved. The introduction of the host as a reacting factor in this picture, I think, serves to bring into consideration a good many of the physiological factors we know about development. Isn't it true, for instance, that in the somewhat analogous case of Rh incompatibility it takes a while before the fetuses reject it, and the length of this interval may vary from one individual to another, owing to something we call competence?

Tyler: The work to which I referred, in which some tumors arose following transplantation of normal tissue to a tolerant host, was done by Kaplan, Hirsch, and Brown (14), Law (18), Barnes et al. (1), and Vos et al. (46). These investigators all used X-irradiated hosts, except that Vos also used non-irradiated F_1 hosts.

Atwood: What kinds of tumors were they?

Tyler: Generally lymphomas. Transplantation tests that were done in some of these experiments indicated that many of the tumors could be grafted successfully to the donor-strain animals, indicating that the tumor was of donor-cell origin.

According to our theory, the tumors should take in the donor strain and grow for a while by coasting along on the stimulus they had previously received, but they should not be malignant growths in the donor strain. The exception to this would be the situation in which the original cells, upon growing as a tumor in the tolerant host, suffered loss of histocompatibility genes. However, if the original donor were highly inbred and homozygous for such genes, this event would be expected to be relatively rare since both alleles would have to be lost in the same cell.

The cited experiments do not provide critical information concerning this point. Experiments by the Kleins (15, 16, 17) contribute further information which is largely consistent with our views but, again, not entirely critical. They produced tumors in F_1 hybrid mice and tested the transplantability of the induced tumors. For the most part, they grew in other F_1 animals, but some of them were found to "take" also in animals of one or the other of the parental strains. Some of these are called false positives because they don't continue to grow as malignant tumors. One can interpret these cases as due to the loss of a histocompatibility gene at a heterozygous locus in the F_1 hybrid. This would cause the cell to grow as a neoplastic cell in the F_1 hybrid and to take as a false positive in one of the parents.

Atwood: They should no longer be tumors when transplanted to the parent. But when this is done, they do turn out to be tumors.

For example, the Kleins' ascites tumors are purposely originated in the F_1 heterozygote from parents that differ only in the histocompatibility alleles at a single locus. Such cells, when the allele from one parent is lost, grow as tumors in the other parent.

Tyler: Some do grow progressively as tumors but some don't, even though they take.

Atwood: Supposedly, whenever one of the alleles is lost, the tumor will grow in one parent.

Tyler: In some cases there may be several losses. Those that grow progressively in one of the parents may have suffered additional histocompatibility-gene losses.

Atwood: The rates, of the order of 10^{-5}, do not suggest that more than one event is necessary.

Tyler: There may be some secondary losses that occur in the tumor itself. Under the conditions in which cells grow in a tumor it is quite conceivable that additional chromosomal aberrations may occur.

Atwood: You can't have it both ways. The Kleins created a tumor that will grow both in the F_1 and in one parent, and this is against your theory.

Tyler: No. For simplicity, I illustrated the situation initially as involving only one locus.

Atwood: You require additional unobserved histocompatibility differences to be present.

Tyler: In the Kleins' experiments, the strains that were used were thought to be highly inbred and co-isogenic. Unfortunately, this was evidently not quite the case, according to more recent papers published by Linder and Klein (20) and by Snell (33). The strains involved had been retrieved from other laboratories by the Jackson Memorial Laboratory after the fire at Bar Harbor. Evidently the inbreeding had not been maintained too effectively, as judged by skin-transplantation tests. In any case, the principal points of the experiments, for the purpose of the present discussion, are still valid; namely, tumors induced in F_1 hybrids may often lack parental strain antigens, whereas such variants are rarely obtained with tumors induced in the (partially inbred) parental lines.

At this point, I should present the results of the first preliminary experiments we have conducted to test the possibility of obtaining tumors by transplanting normal tissue from parental strain animals to the F_1 hybrid.

We obtained three tumors out of 48 F_1 animals in the experiment. The experiment involved about 500 animals, half of them as donors of the cells. These were dissociated cells, comprising, after straining off the undissociated tissue, the equivalent of perhaps half the cells of a single spleen. They were injected subcutaneously.

Atwood: How did this compare with the spontaneous?

Tyler: The controls consisted of all the isologous and homologous transplants with these two strains (C57BL and A/J) and the F_1, as well as transplants from a third strain into each of these. There were no other tumors except the three in the F_1 animals. These all involved strain-A donor cells. The results are just sufficiently encouraging to warrant our undertaking more experiments. As a matter of fact, I suspected in advance that it would be very naive for one to expect to get anywhere near 100% of tumors in F_1 animals receiving parental cells. In fact, in one series we tried to stack the cards. As I mentioned, Kaplan and others (14) who had earlier obtained tumors had pre-irradiated the F_1 host. So I supposed that X rays in the host make some tissue space available for the transplanted cells by destroying host cells. We used cortisone for this purpose in one series of animals. However, only one of the tumors arose in a cortisonized animal.

Court-Brown: One very important thing you have to explain in your hypothesis is the change in probability of development of the tumor following a given carcinogenic insult from year to year.

Tyler: That is, successive ones.

Court-Brown: No, given a single dose of radiation. Let's go back to the unfortunate human being. The probability of the emerging of leukemia rises to a peak in 5 or 6 years and dies away again after about 10 or 12 years. How do you explain that?

Tyler: I would relate the latent period to the properties of the particular type of cell involved, with respect to changes also in the physiology of the host. For example, we may consider the case of the differentiated nerve cell. Antigenic loss might be very slow, following gene loss. Protein turnover is likely to be slow, and the cell may ordinarily never divide in the lifetime of the organism. So even with an appropriate gene loss a tumor is not likely to develop.

In other kinds of tissue there may well be a higher probability that the affected cell will, sometime or other during the life of the organism, turn over its protein sufficiently to lose the surface antigen in question. Then it will have the abnormal relation with its neighbors whereby the antigen possessed by the neighboring cells is now foreign to the altered cell and serves as an additional, and continuing, proliferative stimulus to it.

If we are dealing with a tissue that is under some hormonal control, then hormones that are supplied naturally or artificially at some time after the gene loss would accelerate protein turnover and the antigenic loss.

Again, I should remark that the "foreign" antigen provides an additional proliferative stimulus. This, of course, isn't the only proliferative stimulus that a cell may receive. However, in the postulated situation it is a continuing one. That is what puts the neoplastic cells out of harmony with the rest of the body.

Quimby: Will you explain the experiment whereby you obtained three neoplasms out of 48? It seems to me there should have been 48 out of 48. (Laughter)

Tyler: On the basis of the simplest form of the theory, that would be the expectation. But, just as one often fails to get runt disease in the appropriate situation, we should not ordinarily expect 100% of tumors in the present experiments.

Returning to the question of why we do not get tumors in 100% of the F_1 animals that receive parental cells, some experiments by Gorer and Boyse (8) may have a bearing on this. Mice of strains A and C57BL were pre-immunized against sheep cells, so that their antibody-forming cells were labeled by virtue of making anti-sheep-cell antibody. When transplanted into the F_1, the A strain cells increase considerably in number but the C57BL cells show no proliferation. In fact, there is a loss or complete disappearance of the C57BL cells. Gorer and Boyse suggest that they have suffered an "allergic death." This is a phenomenon that can be demonstrated in cultures of cells of a tuberculin-sensitive organism when exposed to the antigen. Perhaps C57BL cells are particularly sensitive. In any case, it serves as an example of suppression of transplanted cells that should be tolerated genetically.

This phenomenon of allergic death provides a basis for one of the methods that I have proposed for destroying or suppressing a tumor; namely, the administration of large amounts of the antigen that they lack and to which they have become sensitive. This should damage or kill the cells by allergic shock.

Another proposed therapeutic measure consists in repair of the antigenic loss by administration of the appropriate messenger RNA or, by genetic transformation, by administration of the appropriate DNA.

Brues: That, by the way, has been put on a more or less quantitative basis by using mixtures of the two types of cell, say, a mixture of 20 parts of C57BL cells and one part of the A strain cells.

Atwood: I don't see how you put over the idea that any cell is immunologically competent.

Tyler: It is not necessary to assume that any cell is immunologically competent or can become so. The primary assumption would be that any tissue of the body in which a neoplasm can arise contains some immunologically competent cells. With respect to the possibility of transformation of cells from one type to another, this is part of the general question of whether or not differentiation is irreversible. I think that most biologists assume that it is. However, there are a number of experiments that demonstrate changes from one cell type to another. Also, nuclear transplantation experiments would indicate that, as far as the nucleus is concerned, one from a presumably differentiated cell can give rise to all, or almost all, other types of cells of the organism.

Storer: It isn't clear to me why the direct approach to this problem won't work. The deletion of an antigen is required. One could start with two strains of known genotype with respect to the histocompatibility loci. If the hybrid was then produced and tumors were induced in these hybrids, one could test for which antigens were present by cytotoxic techniques or by agglutination techniques.

Tyler: This would be essentially an extension of the experiments that were done by the Kleins, using other methods in addition to transplantation for identifying the antigenic loss. I agree that this would be worth doing.

Storer: One would expect, I think, to find isoantibodies in these tumor-bearing animals. What is the situation there?

Tyler: Several investigators have demonstrated the presence of Coombs' positive red cells.

Storer: Not in the graft-versus-host, but in the spontaneous tumor situation.

Tyler: There have been several investigations in which this has been demonstrated (2, 10, 40). The fact that such tumors are frequently found can be considered to be of more significance than the failure to demonstrate the presence of the antibodies in many cases. This is because one is dealing with a situation in which there is present a great excess of antigen (from the rest of the body), which would certainly militate against ready demonstration of the antibody.

Brues: To bring cancer and aging closer together, I am going to show a simple curve (Fig. 4). No doubt we are all familiar with this, but it is worth thinking about. When either

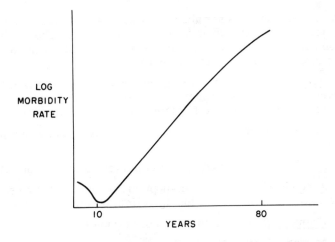

Fig. 4.—Diagrammatic graph of human cancer evidence against logarithm of age. Adapted from Simms, H. S. 1946. Logarithmic increase in mortality as a manifestation of aging. J. Gerontol. 1: 13-26. (Note: As indicated in the text, tumors of different sites may show differences in the relative proportions of the descending [juvenile] and ascending [adult] portions of the curve. Also, tumors under endocrine control may show inflections of the latter portion of the curve.)

cancer incidence or total mortality rates are plotted against age, the result is a curve such as that in Figure 4, which passes through a minimum in youth and suggests that there may be two things going on, one of which one is "born with" and the other of which develops progressively with time and with what we used to call "wear and tear." On the theory we are now discussing, this involves primarily the development of immunological trouble as one gets older.

Lansing: What tumor are you plotting the age incidence for?

Brues: Certain tumors occur in youngsters, and others occur later as an increasing function of age. They fall into two fairly discrete groups: Wilms' tumor of the kidney, for example, is completely characteristic of youngsters. In addition, there are some, such as osteogenic sarcoma, where we see a fair incidence at both ends of life, while the curve is depressed in between.

Lansing: Some fall off with advancing age, too, I believe.

Brues: Yes, it may be. The increase may not go on forever. This is a point that perhaps someone else could speak about more competently than I. I could believe it worked either way. The evidence is not absolutely solid as to whether the incidence keeps going up with age or tapers off. The problem arises of diagnostic skill not being exercised as much on very old people as it is on younger people.

Fremont-Smith: If this figure were drawn as a family of curves, one for each specific cancer, wouldn't some of the cancers of infancy drop off completely, or nearly completely?

Brues: Dr. Simms, as a matter of fact, did that in a publication some time ago (30).

Lansing: I think Saxton (29) collected some data on this.

Atwood: Changes in cell-population size of the tissue of origin may explain part of the age effect on incidence.

Fremont-Smith: Is that true of uterine cancer?

Atwood: I think it is.

Brues: There are situations with both uterine and breast cancer where, ordinarily, there would be a fairly simple exponential function or logarithmic function, whichever it is. These two undergo a break at middle life, which is undoubtedly due to endocrine influence on the process.

Tyler: I hesitate to stick my neck out farther and include aging with cancer except to say, as you indicate, that there is a correlation.

Brues: We are going to make up mathematical models later, but I believe we ought to have this in mind and be thinking about it.

Tyler: If we want to consider them in the same context, then we might interpret both as being due to an immune response primarily, involving production of circulating antibodies and of immunologically aggressive cells.

Atwood: Your theory predicts that there will be no neoplasms in animals that are completely immunologically incompetent. I read somewhere that myxinoids are this way; they accept grafts from one another and have no demonstrable antibodies.

Tyler: Several of the lower vertebrates have been explored.

Steinbach: Isn't it the hamster?

Atwood: Hamsters are immunologically competent.

Tyler: There are special conditions in the cheek pouch.

Fish are known to develop tumors. Also, fish are known to be immunologically competent.

Fremont-Smith: Are elasmobranchs immunologically competent?

Tyler: I don't know of any skin graft experiments.

I think I have spoken about most of the items that I had intended to discuss here, including suggestions as to measures that might be explored for the treatment of cancer. The theory indicates a few possible procedures. One would involve restoration of the lost histocompatibility antigen by administration of the corresponding DNA or messenger RNA. Another is to destroy or damage the tumor cells by administering shocking doses of the antigen. We can also conceive of ways of employing radiation more effectively. But, by and large, this would involve substituting one type of cancer for another, and one could not keep this up very long. One can also think of using appropriate immunologically aggressive foreign cells that react aggressively against the tumor cells but are themselves later destroyed by the host. These and other suggestions are more fully discussed in my previous papers (38, 40) on this subject.

Brues: There is one thing that might come up in connection with discussions of physiology and pathology. Since you led into it, Dr. Tyler, what should we think of the notion that some of the changes in aging might be explained by the gradually developing mutual hostility of cells, in general, owing to one-by-one deletion of these immunologically determining factors in somatic cells?

Tyler: This does provide a mechanism for obtaining deleterious effects. If there is a simple mutation, involving a change to another histocompatibility gene, the organism has a way of taking care of the situation; namely, it disposes of the cell. The altered cells could perhaps do some damage for a while as they respond immunologically to any host antigens that they may have lost, but at the same time the host responds to them. Of course, the host, being bigger, wins out.

Atwood: How do you save your hypothesis against the early thymectomy business? Here it is possible to get an animal that will accept the various grafts.

Tyler: This is actually supporting evidence since thymectomized animals, generally speaking, show greatly decreased ability to develop tumors in response to radiation.

Atwood: How generally speaking?

Tyler: Dr. Brues can undoubtedly tell us more about Kaplan's original experiments (12, 13) on thymectomy. How well protected are the animals from induction of tumors by radiation?

Brues: They are well protected from one particular set-up which has been tested.

Atwood: Naturally, the one that comes from that cell of origin, but what about all the rest?

Cottier: I don't think we have much information on this. Many mice that are thymectomized shortly after birth start to waste within 2 to 5 months.

Tyler: One could probably keep them alive longer by avoiding natural infection.

Quastler: Two weeks would be enough to induce tumor with MCA or DNBA.

Atwood: I want to make a prediction: the tumors will be inducible.

Tyler: Thymectomy does not destroy all immunological reactivity on the part of the host.

Atwood: It is possible to do both the bursa and the thymus on the chicken; that is its advantage. Again, tumors will be induced by the standard agents, I would predict.

Tyler: I believe there would be a very great lowering of the incidence.

Atwood: If your theory is right, wouldn't there be an abrupt change in tumor incidence when inbred lines are crossed? The kinetics of induction have to be different. You pointed out that mutations have to be multiple or double for the inbred ones, but not for the crossbred. This would make a very large difference to the incidence, other things being equal. Do you have evidence that such things happen?

Tyler: I referred earlier to some, and I reviewed some of the evidence in my previous papers (38, 40). I think it needs further testing, precisely from the present point of view. One must also avoid certain pitfalls, such as the use of high-tumor lines that may produce up to 100% of spontaneous tumors.

Atwood: Isn't it a bit of a contradiction to get a high-tumor line by means of inbreeding, according to your hypothesis? What does one have to do?

Tyler: One need only assume the operation of one or another of the known genetic mechanisms by which chromosomal aberrations may be induced. Barbara McClintock and other cytogeneticists (22, 23, 35) have provided many examples of genes which will cause a variety of chromosomal aberrations.

Keys: In your experiment, you were disappointed because you only got three out of 48 in the expected high-risk group, contrasting with the fact that in the two homozygous parental strains you didn't get anything. Isn't that right?

Tyler: Yes; the other controls were also negative.

Keys: Statistically, this isn't of any significance at all, is it?

Tyler: I would say it has a low level of significance if related to the expectation of 48 out of 48. However, it may well be highly significant for appropriate modifications of the basic hypothesis.

Keys: You obtained three events distributed in three classes, each of 48, or a total of 144, actually. It doesn't seem to mean anything.

Sacher: There must still be some threshold that this sort of immunological aggression would have to surpass before a tumor could be established. Do you have any estimate of the magnitude of the resistance of the body to invasion?

Tyler: Those are some of the factors that one would want to avoid introducing at the start. However, it does appear that we will now have to introduce them. I mentioned one possibility; namely, allergic death of the cell as indicated in the experiments of Gorer and Boyse (8). Parental cells in the F_1 may thus be overwhelmed by a foreign antigen. This could be an important factor in explaining why we did not get 100% tumors in our experiment, and got none at all in some combinations.

Sacher: In regard to tumors in man, how do you interpret the fact that the immune capacity of the body, at least as measured by the isoagglutinin titer for the ABO blood groups, seems to have as a function of age almost an inverse relationship to tumor susceptibility?

The titer rises to a maximum at about 10 years of age and then decreases. Log titer decreases linearly with age from about 20 to 100 years.

Brues: In the case of retinoblastoma, which Neel (25) and others have studied, this is definitely, and rather simply, heritable. I think the picture is one in which a certain population is destined to get retinoblastoma, and that population will be wiped out in the course of the first few years. This may be true of some of the others, but retinoblastoma has been shown to be heritable. Neel has, indeed, calculated a mutation rate for it, from the incidence of retinoblastomas in those without indication of it in their forebears.

Tyler: This is a case of specific genes affecting a particular tissue.

Brues: That is the simplest case, and I am suggesting it as one where there is a simple genetic situation, without additional complications.

Dobzhansky: In case of retinoblastoma, it can probably be accounted for by supposing this particular gene increases the probability of loss of antigens in certain tissue.

Tyler: Yes, that would be the assumption. One can cite an example of this kind of phenomenon; namely, chromosome diminution. As is well known, this occurs regularly in many species of animals. In most species it is the somatic cells that undergo this process, and it occurs at particular stages of development.

Brues: Another instance where there is apparently some sort of clear-cut relationship between the genic material and neoplasia is the situation you mentioned, Dr. Tyler, the chromosome change, or the trisomy, that is peculiarly conducive to chronic leukemia. Also, I believe there is a relation between mongolism with trisomy and aging, or aging of parents. I know that Dr. Court-Brown has some material on this.

Court-Brown: The situation at present—and I won't pretend to quote it accurately—is that, with the exception of the XO type of female, there appears to be a parental age relationship, as with all other types of constitutional chromosomal aberrations. The most accurately worked out, of course, is for what is known as regular mongolism. The risk for this has been well worked out by Penrose (27), in which the probability of conceiving a mongol by women of age 20 is, roughly, about one in two-thousand-odd conceptions. This rises very slowly, and then starts to rise fairly fast after the age of 35. Ultimately, for women 35 years and over, its probability is something like one in 40 conceptions.

It is also becoming evident, from not quite so extensive data, that paternal and maternal age at conception is important in relation to the risk of conceiving XXX females or XXY males, and quite markedly so for trisomy involving 17-18, and trisomy involving one or other of the pairs of 13, 14, and 15.

There is another situation which may or may not be relevant to this. A great deal of work is going on in various places in which an attempt is being made to work out the sequence in which the various autosomes complete their DNA replication.

It appears that all the chromosomes which get involved in trisomic states are, in fact, late DNA replicators. The latest of the lot, of course, is the X chromosome, which by the Lyon hypothesis is an inactive one. I wonder if anyone has any views on the possibility that age itself may in some way influence the speed at which DNA replication occurs—whether it is not possible that the older one gets, some of these autosomes every now and again may fail to complete replication before division takes place and thus lead to subsequent errors in chromosome numbers.

I think, also, from the data we have on aging, it is interesting that in males it seems to be mainly the Y which is lost with age; presumably deletions of the X increase in females. Also the Y is a late replicator, not quite as late as the X. I am wondering if anyone has any views on this particular situation.

Brues: This is a rather remarkable rate of increase of a phenomenon associated with aging. The probability of a mongoloid child seems to go up with doubling time of, perhaps, 3 years, and most of the phenomena of aging, based on death rates, double every 10 years or so. Of course, we can't extrapolate this much beyond 45.

Tyler: Is there no such effect in the male?

Court-Brown: There is so far as 21-21 fusion is concerned. This is related to paternal age.

Tyler: This is clear now?

Court-Brown: This seems clear.

Atwood: How do you know the Y is lost more frequently as the male ages?

Court-Brown: From cytogenetic analysis of cells with 45 chromosomes to determine which chromosome is missing.

Fry: There is evidence that the duration of DNA synthesis is longer in some of the cells of old animals. Would the prolongation of DNA synthesis without some other alteration explain the failure of a chromosome to replicate before the onset of division? Have you any information on the sequence in which the autosomes replicate?

Court-Brown: I don't know what the time sequence is.

Quastler: The total time spent in DNA replication varies more in old animals than in young ones, which indicates some loosening of controls; this may help to explain a rare loss of a chromosome.

Birren: I wonder, in relation to the disappearance of the Y chromosome, whether this is possibly related to the general superiority of the female, in terms of resistance to almost all diseases? It may be a little irrelevant, but I am curious about a possible genetic basis for the somewhat better mortality picture for women than for men, and indeed for females of most species. Could this possibly be related to the chromosome phenomenon you mentioned?

Court-Brown: I don't know what the explanation is. Can I describe our observations on the increase of aneuploidy with age?

We used the blood culture technique after Morehead et al. (24), and counted, unfortunately, only 30 cells per culture. We did not have a very satisfactory population of males, about 125 varying in age from less than 10 to over 65 years.

The males yield quite satisfactory data, however: a fairly linear increase of aneuploidy. The female situation is more difficult. The female points follow the males up to about the age of 45, and then they start to shoot up rapidly. This population is a very unsatisfactory one, in that it cannot be said to be a random human population, based on volunteers, hospital inpatients, and parents of mongols, and such as that. We are now in the process of getting a random sample of the human population.

When one analyzes hypodiploid cells, the cells of 45 chromosomes, one finds the entire change in the male is explained by the loss of Y chromosomes. One gets very significant slopes. As far as the females are concerned, the entire increase of hypodiploidy is explained by loss of a medium-sized chromosome, which we are presuming at the moment is the X.

This is the type of finding. Whether it has anything to do with the greater ability of women to withstand pressures, I don't know, but one's first hunch is that this is related in some way to changes in sex-hormone status.

Atwood: One possible reason that these changes involve only X or Y is that in both cases the hypodiploid is in an XO cell. This is the only kind of hypodiploid cell known to be permanently viable. Maybe the others are just selected out.

Court-Brown: We would think the others have been selected out.

Dobzhansky: To make it quite clear, does that mean that these aneuploid cells are in the circulation or does it mean that aneuploids arise in tissue culture sooner in aged persons than in young ones?

Court-Brown: We don't know whether, in fact, this is mediated by age differences in behavior of cells in tissue culture (remembering that the cultured cells only divide once), or whether the older individual has more aneuploid cells in a sample from the circulation.

Dobzhansky: That, needless to say, would be extremely interesting to find out.

Atwood: Did you find that the frequency of other types of aneuploids has no relation to age?

Court-Brown: Yes. When you plot frequency of cells lacking the other chromosomes—other than the medium or small acrocentric, that is—against age, you get completely random relations.

Atwood: This is interesting to me because the loss of group antigen on red cells seems to be independent of age. I had thought at first it would be age-dependent because deficient stem lines would accumulate with time. But apparently if whole chromosome losses are the basis for loss of group antigen, they are selected against so completely that we see only the rate of origin, and not any accumulated lines. The rate of origin is, on this basis, around one in a thousand cell divisions.

Tyler: I am not clear about this. Don't you expect an increase even if they are selected against?

Atwood: No, if hypodiploids (other than XO) will not continue as stem-line cells, then the constancy with age is well explained as a constant rate of non-disjunction in the last divisions before maturation of red cells.

Tyler: I thought one would still expect more stem lines with lack of Y.

Atwood: But none of the markers are on the X or Y. If I could use one that was on the X, its losses would probably turn out to accumulate with age.

Tyler: Do you have some of the antiserum for the X chromosome antigen, the XGA?

Atwood: No. I doubt that enough is available to do one-tenth of one experiment.

Brues: That probably doesn't fully cover the point Dr. Birren raised, that is, the question of the greater viability, or greater longevity, of females as opposed to males. This might be related to the difference between the X and the Y, or the existence of the unpaired chromosome in the male. Was that something you were thinking about? I learned quite recently that in birds, where the female has the unpaired chromosome, the female nevertheless has greater longevity.

Sacher: A lot of this is due to nurture. In the human race, it is only in the past few centuries that the life expectation for women has exceeded that for men. In mice, greater longevity is shown for virgin females only.

Tyler: Dr. Court-Brown, don't you feel compelled to offer an explanation for the effects of the Philadelphia chromosome?

Court-Brown: I haven't got one. (Laughter)
I was very concerned to know whether, in fact, for instance, you regard the establishment of the Philadelphia chromosome as the initiating cause of chronic myeloid leukemia. At a meeting at the New York Academy of Sciences last week, I heard Dr. Peter C. Nowell state quite dogmatically that this is the case. We remain skeptical about this; we have had the unfortunate and absolutely fascinating case of chronic myeloid leukemia in a patient who actually had four well-established cell lines in his blood. He had an XY Ph-positive line and an XY normal line, an XXY Ph-positive line and an XXY normal line. With pencil and paper, one can, by postulating quite a number of successive errors in division, get to this state. One can also get to the state by postulating that the Philadelphia chromosome has arisen at least twice, once in either cell line.

Atwood: Did it look as though it were the same length?

Court-Brown: It was exactly the same size.

Atwood: Whereas among different leukemias it can be different lengths.

Court-Brown: It varies between individuals but tends to be the same in any one individual.

Atwood: Most likely, then, it had a single origin, followed by a non-disjunction of X in the same line.

Brues: Are these leukemia cells?

Court-Brown: The ones with the Philadelphia chromosomes are the leukemia cells. We have two cell populations in the sample of peripheral blood in this case. There are the immature granulocytes which are dividing, and the normal lymphocyte population which is quite definitely negative. But the erythrocyte precursors and granulocytes are all positive. I am not prepared to offer an explanation of what Ph. 1 chromosome was doing.

Tyler: I think that the occurrence of this deficient chromosome in the leukemic cells of individuals with chronic myeloid leukemia is consistent with the gene-loss theory of neoplasia that I have tried to develop. The fact that it seems to be associated with this type of leukemia is, as you say, difficult to explain. The direction of differentiation of a particular cell may be determined by other factors than its own chromosomal constitution. For example, it is quite possible for XX germ cells to produce spermatozoa, either upon transplantation to an XY host or after appropriate hormonal treatment of the fetal or neonatal animal. Possibly, in the case of the Philadelphia chromosome, the deleted material contains genes concerned with the differentiation of cells in a non-myeloid direction. Its loss would then permit more myeloid cells to form, assuming that the deletion also entailed loss of a histocompatibility gene that would make the cell susceptible to the proliferative stimulus proposed in our theory.

REFERENCES

1. Barnes, D. W. H., C. E. Ford, P. L. T. Ilbery, K. W. Jones, and J. F. Loutit. 1959. Murine leukemia. Acta Unio Intern. Contra Cancrum 15: 544-48.

2. Betts, A., P. G. Rigby, and G. H. Friedell. 1962. Serological abnormalities in transplanted and spontaneous cancer. In M. J. Brennan and W. L. Simpson (eds.), Biological interactions in normal and neoplastic growth, pp. 619-23. Boston: Little, Brown.

3. Billingham, R. E., and L. Brent. 1956. Acquired tolerance of foreign cells in newborn animals. Proc. Roy. Soc. (London) Ser. B 146: 78-90.

4. Billingham, R. E., and L. Brent. 1957. A simple method for inducing tolerance of skin homografts in mice. Transplant. Bull. 4: 67-71.

5. Brues, A. M. 1958. Critique of the linear theory of carcinogenesis. Science 128: 693-99.

6. Court-Brown, W. M., and R. Doll. 1956. Incidence of leukemia among the survivors of the atomic bomb explosions at Hiroshima and Nagasaki (Appendix A). In The hazards to man of nuclear and allied radiations, pp. 84-86. Cmd. 9780. London: HMSO.

7. Court-Brown, W. M., and R. Doll. 1957. Leukemia and aplastic anaemia in patients irradiated for ankylosing spondylitis. Med. Res. Council Special Report Series No. 295, p. 50. London: HMSO.

8. Gorer, P. A., and E. A. Boyse. 1959. Pathological changes in F_1 hybrid mice following transplantation of spleen cells from donors of the parental strains. Immunology 2: 182-93.

9. Grant, P., and P. M. Stott. 1962. Effect of nitrogen mustard on nucleocytoplasmic interactions. In M. J. Brennan and W. L. Simpson (eds.), Biological interactions in normal and neoplastic growth, pp. 47-73. Boston: Little, Brown.

10. Green, H. N. 1959. Immunological aspects of cancer. In G. E. W. Wolstenholme and M. O'Connor (eds.), Carcinogenesis: mechanisms of action, pp. 131-64. Ciba Foundation Symposium. London: J. A. Churchill.

11. Holtzer, H., J. Abbott, J. Lash, and S. Holtzer. 1960. The loss of phenotypic traits by differentiated cells in vitro. I. Dedifferentiation of cartilage cells. Proc. Nat. Acad. Sci. 46: 1533-42.

12. Kaplan, H. S. 1950. Influence of thymectomy, splenectomy, and gonadectomy on incidence of radiation-induced lymphoid tumors in strain C57 black mice. J. Nat. Cancer Inst. 11: 83-90.

13. Kaplan, H. S. 1959. Some implications of indirect induction mechanisms in carcinogenesis: a review. Cancer Res. 19: 791-803.

14. Kaplan, H. S., B. B. Hirsch, and M. B. Brown. 1956. Indirect induction of lymphomas in irradiated mice. IV. Genetic evidence of the origin of the tumor cells from the thymic grants. Cancer Res. 16: 434-36.

15. Klein, G., and E. Klein. 1959. Cytogenetics of experimental tumors. In Genetics and cancer, pp. 241-70. 13th Annual Symposium on Fundamental Cancer Research. (M. D. Anderson Hospital and Tumor Inst., Houston.) Austin, Tex.: Univ. of Texas Press.

16. Klein, G., and E. Klein. 1959. Nuclear and cytoplasmic changes in tumors. In D. Rudnick (ed.), Developmental cytology, pp. 63-82. New York: Ronald Press.

17. Klein, E., G. Klein, and K. E. Hellström. 1960. Further studies on isoantigenic variation in mouse carcinomas and sarcomas. J. Nat. Cancer Inst. 25: 271-94.

18. Law, L. W. 1961. Immunological aspects of carcinogenesis. Acta Unio Intern. Contra Cancrum 17: 210-14.

19. Lewis, E. B. 1957. Leukemia and ionizing radiation. Science 125: 965-72.

20. Linder, O., and E. Klein. 1960. Skin and tumor grafting in coisogenic resistant lines of mice and their hybrids. J. Nat. Cancer Inst. 24: 707-20.

21. Lorenz, F. W., and A. Tyler. 1951. Extension of motile life span of spermatozoa of the domestic fowl by amino acids and proteins. Proc. Soc. Exper. Biol. Med. 78: 57-62.

22. McClintock, B. 1951. Chromosome organization and genic expression. Cold Spring Harbor Symp. Quant. Biol. 16: 13-47.

23. McClintock, B. 1953. Induction of instability at selected loci in maize. Genetics 38: 579-99.

24. Moorhead, P. S., P. C. Nowell, W. J. Mellman, D. M. Batipps, and D. A. Hungerford. 1960. Chromosome preparations of leucocytes cultured from human peripheral blood. Exp. Cell Res. 20: 613-16.

25. Neel, J. V., and H. F. Falls. 1951. The rate of mutation of the gene responsible for retinoblastomas in man. Science 114: 419-23.

26. Paul, J. 1959. Environmental influences on the metabolisms and composition of cultured cells. J. Exper. Zool. 142: 475-505.

27. Penrose, L. S. 1961. Mongolism. Brit. Med. Bull. 17: 184-89.

28. Rothschild, Lord, and A. Tyler. 1954. The physiology of sea urchin spermatozoa. Action of Versene. J. Exper. Biol. 31: 252-59.

29. Saxton, J. A. 1952. Cancer and ageing. In A. I. Lansing (ed.), Cowdry's problems of ageing, pp. 950-61. Baltimore: Williams and Wilkins.

30. Simms, H. S. 1946. Logarithmic increase in mortality as a manifestation of aging. J. Gerontol. 1: 13-26.

31. Simonsen, M. 1953. Biological incompatability in kidney transplantation in dogs. II. Serological investigations. Acta Pathol. Microbiol. Scand. 32: 36-84.

32. Simonsen, M. 1957. The impact on the developing embryo and newborn animal of adult homologous cells. Acta Pathol. Microbiol. Scand. 40: 480-500.

33. Snell, G. D. 1960. Note on results of Linder and Klein with coisogenic resistant lines of mice. J. Nat. Cancer Inst. 25: 1191-93.

34. Subtelny, S. 1958. The development of haploid and homozygous diploid frog embryos obtained from transplantations of haploid nuclei. J. Exp. Zool. 139: 263-305.

35. Swanson, C. P. 1957. Cytology and cytogenetics. Englewood Cliffs, N.J.: Prentice-Hall.

36. Tyler, A. 1942. Developmental processes and energetics. Quart. Rev. Biol. 17: 197-212 and 339-53.

37. Tyler, A. 1953. Prolongation of life-span of sea urchin spermatozoa, and improvement of the fertilization-reaction, by treatment of spermatozoa and eggs with metal-chelating agents (amino acids, Versene, DEDTC, oxine, cupron). Biol. Bull. 104: 224-39.

38. Tyler, A. 1960. Clues to the etiology, pathology, and therapy of cancer provided by analogies with transplantation disease. J. Nat. Cancer Inst. 25: 1197-1229.

39. Tyler, A. 1961. The fertilization process. In E. T. Tyler (ed.), Sterility, pp. 26-56. New York: McGraw-Hill.

40. Tyler, A. 1962. A developmental immunogenetic analysis of cancer. In M. J. Brennan and W. L. Simpson (eds.), Biological interactions in normal and neoplastic growth, pp. 533-72. Boston: Little, Brown.

41. Tyler, A., and E. Atkinson. 1950. Prolongation of the fertilizing capacity of sea-urchin spermatozoa by amino acids. Science 112: 783-85.

42. Tyler, A., and F. W. Dessel. 1939. Increasing the life span of unfertilized Urechis eggs by acid. J. Exper. Zool. 81: 459-72.

43. Tyler, A., N. Ricci, and N. H. Horowitz. 1938. The respiration and fertilizable life of Arbacia eggs under sterile and non-sterile conditions. J. Exper. Zool. 79: 129-43.

44. Tyler, A., and Lord Rothschild. 1951. Metabolism of sea urchin spermatozoa and induced anaerobic motility in solutions of amino acids. Proc. Soc. Exper. Biol. Med. 76: 52-58.

45. Tyler, A., and T. Y. Tanabe. 1952. Motile life of bovine spermatozoa in glycine and yolk-citrate diluents at high and low temperatures. Proc. Soc. Exper. Biol. Med. 81: 367-71.

46. Vos, O., M. J. de Vries, J. C. Collenteur, and D. W. Van Bekkum. 1959. Transplantation of homologous and heterologous lymphoid cells in X-irradiated and nonirradiated mice. J. Nat. Cancer Inst. 23: 53-73.

Changes in Structure and Performance of Cells and Tissues with Age

PART I

Simms: We have been making studies on the mechanism of longevity for a number of years. I would like to discuss our findings and the methods that we used to obtain them. First of all, I should like to describe the conditions that were necessary to obtain satisfactory results.*

To achieve uniform conditions, we need uniform temperature, uniform humidity, and uniform light throughout the life span of the animals. We call our rat quarters the "rat palace" because of the unusually fine conditions. We feel that these are essential for long-term studies.

One of the things that requires the most planning is to get uniform light. The rooms in which the animals are housed are so arranged that there are two rows of cages down the center of each (Fig. 5), each row of cages facing a wall. In that way, they don't get any direct light. The windows are closed off so that no light enters from outside. If we had open windows, the rats would have a short day in the wintertime and a long day in the summertime, and that would have a physiological effect on the animals. The lights are overhead, projected onto the wall by means of parabolic reflectors. The rats get indirect light and, as closely as possible, the same amount of light in every cage. In our quarters, the fluorescent lights are on 12 hours during the day and off 12 hours at night throughout the year.

*The research described here has received financial support from the Josiah Macy, Jr. Foundation, the Albert and Mary Lasker Foundation, and National Institutes of Health grant H-945.

87

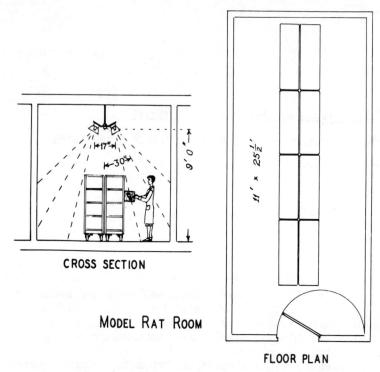

CROSS SECTION

Model Rat Room

FLOOR PLAN

Fig. 5.—Ideal rat room with cages facing walls and receiving only the light reflected from the walls. Reprinted from Laboratory Animal Care, 1963.

In the first part of our studies, we had a large number of rats under uniform conditions throughout their life span, until the time they became moribund. When they were thought to be moribund we killed them, did a complete autopsy, and made sections of the various tissues. In that way we obtained an understanding of the lesions present in each animal, and these we studied in relation to age.

Figure 6 shows a logarithmic mortality curve. This is not for rats, but for humans. I think you are all familiar with Gompertz' equation and with the fact that the logarithm of the probability of death, or death rate, in humans is known to go up almost in a straight line after the age of 30. This has been known for nearly 140 years.

Figure 7 is a summary of our findings on the lesions in rats. It represents the per-cent incidence of the lesions of the five major diseases found in male rats, as a function of age.

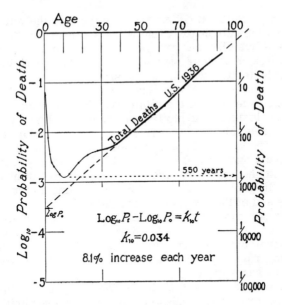

Fig. 6.—Logarithmic mortality curve—human data. Reprinted from J. Gerontol. 1: 13-26, 1946.

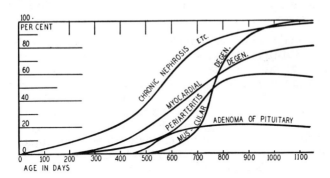

Fig. 7.—Per cent incidence of five major lesions of male rats—total of all degrees of severity in each age group. Figures 7, 8, 10, 11, and 12 are reprinted from J. Gerontol. 12: 244-52, 1957.

Lansing: What do you mean by "muscular degeneration"?

Simms: That is degeneration of the muscle, particularly in the hind legs. It has been described by Dr. Berg, our pathologist (5).

Quimby: Gross atrophy or pathological finding?

Simms: Both. It is a gross effect as the animal gets older, and the pathological finding on sectioning of the muscle.

These five diseases are: chronic nephrosis and glomerulonephritis, muscular degeneration, myocardial degeneration, periarteritis which, while similar to the periarteritis found in humans, is a more serious disease in the rat, and one tumor, adenoma of the pituitary. The incidence curves of these five lesions are plotted in Figure 7. Each curve has three characteristics, the first of which is the maximum height of the curve. Figure 7 shows that the total incidence at maximum age, in two cases, is 100%. With myocardial degeneration, however, we know that regardless of how old the rats get it would not reach 100%. The same is true of periarteritis and of the adenoma of the pituitary.

Thus we can get curves which approach either 100% or a lesser level, depending on the disease. Those that approach a lesser level indicate that our animal colony is not uniform, that some rats are resistant to the particular disease, and others are susceptible.

The second characteristic is the sharpness of the curve. The curve for chronic nephrosis and glomerulonephritis starts practically at birth and does not reach its maximum until beyond 1,100 days. On the other hand, that for muscular degeneration is not observed until after 500 days and then it goes up sharply.

Lansing: I am very much impressed by the fact that two disease entities, if you wish to call them diseases, reach the 100% level later in the life of the rat. This may have some real meaning with respect to what happens when an organism grows old. But it also makes it imperative, I think, that we define these disease entities. I still don't understand what you mean by "muscular degeneration." How objectively can one measure this? What are the criteria? If we lack objectivity it is very easy to arrive at a 100% level. Also, what do you mean by "chronic nephrosis"?

Simms: A more accurate term for this disease is glomerulonephritis. I accept Dr. Berg's findings. He does the autopsies and examines the slides.

Lansing: And the muscular degeneration?

Simms: The criterion for the muscular degeneration is the observation under the microscope, rather than the gross finding.

Lansing: What does one see under the microscope?

Simms: I will have to refer you to Dr. Berg's description of that (5).

Fremont-Smith: Could we ask, in the same context, how much of any one of these conditions has to be present in order to count it? If you could find any muscular degeneration at all, would this be on the curve, or must there be a certain numerical amount of quantity of muscular degeneration to count it?

Simms: It is any degree of degeneration.

Fremont-Smith: Even one cell?

Simms: Yes, the smallest amount observable. We did, at the same time, make studies of the lesions of different degrees, and we got curves like those in Figure 8. This shows the incidence at different ages of marked lesions, medium lesions, and the first observable lesions.

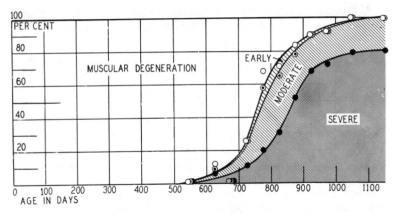

Fig. 8.—Example of lesion incidence curves of a major disease in rats. The top curve is identical with the muscular degeneration curve in Figure 7. In this disease the lesions are late in appearing, but there is a rapid rise in incidence, reaching 100% at 1,100 days.

Fremont-Smith: Could you tell us, roughly, what kind of curve marked lesions for muscular degeneration would give? Does it approach 100%?

Simms: Yes, all the curves for this disease approach 100%. The bottom curve in Figure 8 represents the marked lesions.

Fremont-Smith: At different points?

Simms: We have to keep the animal until it's a lot older in order to get marked lesions up to the 100% level.

Keys: Can we take it that none of these conditions is a lethal disorder in the rat?

Simms: They all contribute to death. We have given up trying to decide what causes death because that seems to be an impossible thing to do and is not important for the interpretation of the data.

Keys: Some of the rats die, don't they, before you decide they are moribund and knock them over the head, or whatever you do?

Simms: A few, and they are autopsied, if they are in sufficiently good condition to permit it. But with the majority, we can tell in advance when they are about to die and we kill them off in order to get the tissue in good condition.

Cottier: Do your rats develop hypertension?

Simms: Yes, some of them do, but we can't observe that on autopsy; so I am not presenting hypertension among the lesions (7).

Cottier: Does the presence of hypertension correlate with the development of necrotizing periarteritis?

Simms: No.

Jarvik: Are these rats from inbred strains?

Simms: They are what we call random inbred, in that we started four lines from a group of Sprague-Dawley rats in 1945. Two lines were random inbred and two were closely inbred. But we gave up the closely inbred lines because they did not survive well. These figures represent the random inbred rats from an original group of about fifty.

Among these rats, to begin with, we had one anomaly that we had to breed out. That was an eye anomaly that we didn't want.

Then, as in all rat colonies, we had a high incidence in the beginning of pulmonary infection. Dr. Berg was not with me then, but, when he did join me a couple of years later, he succeeded in getting rid of the pulmonary infection by simply weeding out every rat that showed symptoms, or any suggestion of such symptoms.

To return to the three characteristics about each curve: as for the steepness, it is a measure of the homogeneity of the colony.

If we had 1,000 rats that were exactly identical, the curve would be like that in Figure 9. The fact that the curves in Figure 7 are not like that in Figure 9 indicates that the individu-

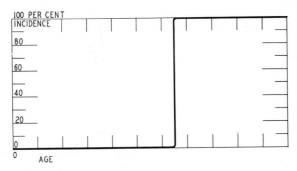

Fig. 9.—Hypothetical curve representing a population in which all individuals are identical with respect to the onset of a given disease.

als are not identical in respect to those diseases. Therefore, Figure 7 shows that there is much greater uniformity in the colony with respect to muscular degeneration than there is in regard to kidney disease.

All of these are endogenous diseases; they do not represent infectious diseases. We succeeded in getting rid of all the infectious diseases at the time these data were obtained. Now infection has returned again.

Fremont-Smith: About how many rats were involved in the curves in Figure 7?

Simms: About 1,400 male rats.

Quimby: With the exception of muscular cellulitis, it looks as though there were survivors after 1,100 days. That is a pretty long life expectancy for a rat.

Simms: Yes, we did get some surviving beyond that point. I don't recall the age of the oldest rat, but I know we had them for over 1,200 days. I recall one rat that was very old, with practically no lesions whatever: but that is a very rare thing.

Fremont-Smith: It is, I believe, a very unusual rat colony in which all infectious diseases have been eliminated.

Simms: Figure 10 shows the slopes of the curves in Figure 7—in other words, the incidence of new lesions, the probability of acquiring a new lesion within the next 100-day period. It can be seen that the muscular degeneration, with its compressed curve in Figure 7, has a very sharp curve in Figure 10. These represent the distribution of the onset of lesions, of the different diseases. All the peaks come within a range of between 550 days and 750 days.

I picture the onset of lesions in the rat as somewhat

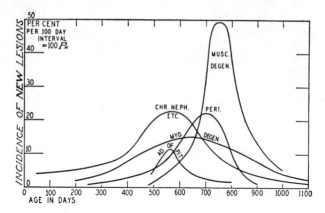

Fig. 10.—Probability of onset of new lesions among the total number of rats alive in each age group. The values represent the slopes of the curves in Figure 7.

analogous to a situation where we have 1,000 alarm clocks that do not keep very good time. If they were all set to ring at 6:00 A.M. and if there were considerable variation between the clocks, they would go off in a manner something like the curves in Figure 10. By analogy, I look upon the rat as having a predisposition to the onset of these lesions at some time in its life, but the individuals vary as to the exact age. As I said earlier, if they were all identical, they would all appear at the same moment.

Now, getting back to the question of the Gompertz equation (Fig. 6), we know the probability of death rises logarithmically with age. In Figure 11 we see that the logarithm of the probability of onset of lesions also rises with age in the same manner as the death rate. The bottom curve is the curve for mortality of the rat, and is approximately a straight line.

Fremont-Smith: They are all quite parallel, aren't they?

Simms: They are not exactly parallel, and they are not exactly straight, but they approximate a straight line. We could get straighter and more parallel lines if we made correction for the fact that they don't all approach 100%.

Lansing: I am a little disturbed; I am still concerned with the disease entities that we started with. We are expressing quantitatively data that are subjectively collected. Unless we have an objective measure of the disease entity we are referring to, I think we get into difficulty when we take these data and convert them into quantitative expressions.

Unless I can understand and have an expression of the

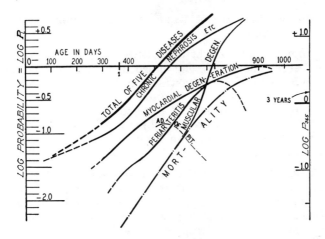

Fig. 11.—Logarithm of the probability of onset of new lesions among rats having no lesions (of the disease in question). Certain curves would be straighter if correction were made for the fact that the incidence of some lesions did not approach 100% (see Fig. 7). Also, the top curve represents the sum of the probabilities of five diseases. The bottom curve is the mortality curve of male rats.

quantitative measure of change in myocardium, I find it difficult to translate this observation into a Gompertz equation, or any other equation. I don't know what is meant by "muscular degeneration." Again, this has to be defined for me, objectively and quantitatively, if the data are to be used quantitatively.

Similarly, I am not a pathologist, I do not know what "nephrosis" is. I would like to know, with respect to the distal convoluted tubule or the proximal convoluted tubule, what happens specifically, with some quantitative measure of change in the kidney that then can be applied to quantitative expression.

Simms: It is qualitative; it is not a measure of the amount of change. It is the first observable change under the microscope, in each disease. The data become quantitative when we plot the number of individuals that have observable lesions.

Lansing: But I have to know what we are observing if I am to plot these analytically.

Simms: I will have to refer you to Dr. Berg's descriptions (47).

Keys: If you had better microscopes, or looked at more

sections, would you not expect to change these incidences, these dates of onset?

Simms: There might be a little difference if there were two different observers, but these are all observed by one pathologist, Dr. Berg. Of course, the age at which he first observes a change does not mean the change started then. It is merely the age at which it has become big enough to be observable. Probably, if we had some way of detecting the preceding changes, the curve in Figure 7 would be over to the left a little further.

Keys: I am not surprised that radiologists disagree with one another, but what was interesting to me was that when they were resubmitted the same films, the reproducibility by the individual radiologist of his own previous finding was about 60 per cent on such a simple matter as left ventricular hypertrophy.

Fremont-Smith: This is well known. We had studies on cirrhosis of the liver by a group of experts, with the same outcome. It seems to me we have to accept this, that there is no absolute end point, that it is very hard to say how much of a beginning is a beginning. It is what Dr. Berg saw, and it is in his paper (47). Don't you think we should leave it at that, recognizing this as an inevitable weakness when one is dealing with detection of pathological processes?

Simms: Figure 8 is an example of the curves we get in plotting the different degrees of severity. The lowest curve represents the severe lesions, the middle area shows the moderate lesions, and, above that, a few of the slight or "early" lesions.

Fremont-Smith: They are very parallel.

Simms: Yes. As I said, plotting these this way gives us curves that are parallel with the mortality curve. We also showed that the period from the onset to the severe lesions is about the same, regardless of age of the animal (47).

Figure 12 gives further evidence of the relationship between the probability of onset of lesions and probability of death. Both are plotted on a logarithmic scale. The solid line represents the actual data. The dotted line is what we would get if there were perfect correlation. It isn't perfect, but it is pretty close.

Keys: These represent all of these diseases put together?

Simms: Yes, it is the onset of all lesions of five major

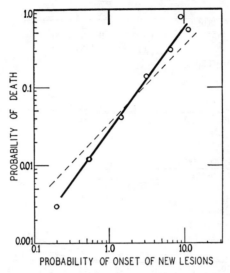

Fig. 12.—Log-log plot of probability of death versus onset of new lesions (see top and bottom curves in Fig. 11). The dotted line corresponds to perfect correlation.

diseases added together. The probability of onset is parallel with the probability of death, or very close to it.

Figure 13 gives us a comparison between the rat and man (49). We have plotted on one age scale, rather than two, the data on the incidence of lesions in rat, and the incidence of such major lesions in man. The lower chart shows the probability of onset in the rat and in man.

Keys: The upper diagram really shows prevalence, doesn't it, rather than incidence? Surely, those curves don't go up to 100%.

Simms: It is per-cent incidence. Unfortunately, the word "incidence" has more than one meaning. We use the word here to mean the percentage of animals having observable lesions at different ages. The word "prevalence" can be used instead if it is defined this way.

You will note in Figure 13 that rat and man behave alike as far as the onset of lesions is concerned, except that in the rat all the lesions occur in the first 4 years, and in man there is a long lag period before the onset of major lesions. It is observable in both charts. So there is a species difference in the susceptibility or resistance to the onset of major lesions. Of course, the diseases in man are not identical with those in the rat, but they represent the same organs and there is no

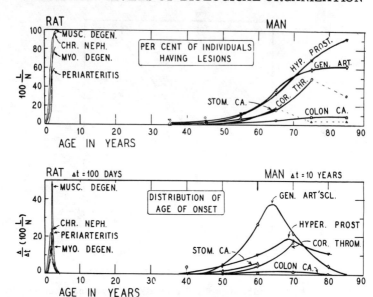

Fig. 13.—Lesion data of rat and man plotted on the same age scale. The left end of the top chart has the same curves as Figure 7, but laterally compressed. The lower chart has the same curves as in Figure 10, also compressed. Reprinted from Ciba Foundation. 1959. Symposium on the life span of animals, pp. 72-79. London.

reason to think that they differ entirely in character.

Quimby: I don't understand your procedure. Did you sacrifice a given number of animals every so often?

Simms: We had to in the lower age brackets.

Quimby: How do you discover a lesion?

Simms: By autopsy and examination of tissue section. Beyond 500 days the data represent rats that were all moribund or died spontaneously. In order to get data below 500 days, we had to kill off a couple of groups to get the curves down in the lower chart. The criticism might be raised that there is a certain amount of selection here, that the rats studied in the upper age brackets were selected automatically as those that were not killed off at an early age. That may affect the shape of the curve a little.

Quimby: That was my point. The first part of the curve is developed by animals deliberately sacrificed, and the last part develops from animals which are obviously moribund for one reason or another.

Simms: Yes, that is true. However, the two curves run into each other without any observable break.

So much for healthy animals under normal and favorable conditions.

We next tried one variation of the condition: that is, reduced food intake. We reduced the food intake of some rats by about 33% and of others by about 46% of what they would eat if they were allowed to. Although fewer rats were used in this experiment than in our control studies, and we couldn't get complete curves, we did get some points which indicate the trend.

Figure 14 shows the effect of food restriction on the lesion of glomerulonephritis (this is the same lesion as "chronic nephrosis," etc., in Fig. 7). One group of rats was restricted by 33%, in other words, they were given 67% of the food they

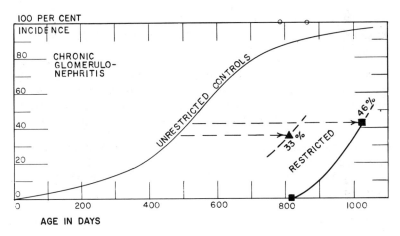

Fig. 14.—Lesion incidence of chronic glomerulonephritis in male rats on restricted food intake as compared with ad libitum-fed controls. The solid curve for the controls was previously obtained from 1,400 rats, and the circles represent concurrent data on a few control rats. Figures 14 through 21 reprinted from Geriatrics 17:.235-42, 1962.

wanted, weighed out and given each day in the form of pellets. Then another group was restricted by 46%; they got 54% of the food they wanted. The lesion onset of the group of 33%-restricted rats at this one age is quite far over from the original curve (obtained from the 1,400 male rats studied earlier), and you will notice a further delay in the onset of lesions in the 46%-restricted rats.

Figure 15 shows the same sort of thing for myocardial degeneration—in both the 33% and 46% groups. We have every

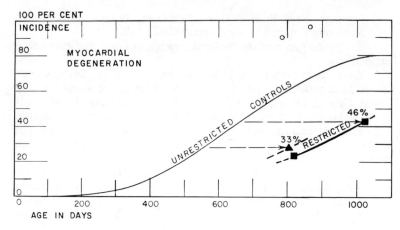

Fig. 15.—Similar data on myocardial degeneration

reason to think that if we had complete curves they would run parallel with the controls.

Figure 16 represents periarteritis in 33%- and 46%-restricted rats as compared with the unrestricted controls. The circles represent some controls run at the same time, and do not coincide with the curves because there were just a few animals, and that difference is not statistically significant.

Figure 17 indicates the effect on muscular degeneration for the 46% group only. No observations were made on the muscles of the 33% group. The curves for tumors are not shown, but most of the various tumors were delayed in the same way.

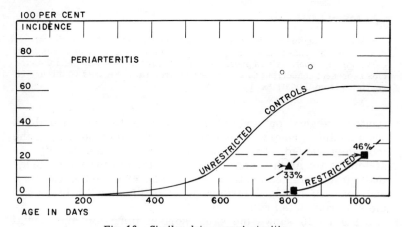

Fig. 16.—Similar data on periarteritis

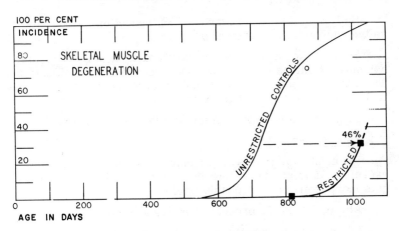

Fig. 17.—Similar data on skeletal muscle degeneration. There were no data on this disease in the 33%-restricted animals.

The observations mean that, as a result of one change in the conditions, namely reduced food intake, we have affected the age of onset of all major diseases of these rats.

Atwood: Did you start restricted intake at an early age, as McCay did (36), or late?

Simms: I think McCay started some of his rats early and some late (36). We started food restriction at the time of weaning—at 28 days of age.

Fremont-Smith: Was the food restriction sufficient to cause a delay in the rats reaching their full weight?

Simms: The restricted rats reached a lower level of maximum weight than the control (ad libitum-fed) rats. The weights were studied as compared with the weights of normal animals, and there was a constant difference throughout. The restricted rats were not obese, whereas the control rat—and by "control" I mean those on ad libitum food intake—all had subcutaneous fat and could be called obese.

Kallmann: If the food intake remains unrestricted, do all animals tend to eat the same amount?

Simms: Pretty close to it, yes.

Kallmann: Do you call this overeating?

Simms: Yes, we do. Of course, that is a comparative term, but we considered it overeating—at least it is "over" in terms of what is best for the animal.

Kallmann: Do you regard a 33% reduction in food intake as the equivalent of a starvation diet?

Simms: No, it is not a starvation diet. It is a better diet, not only as far as survival is concerned: the rats look better. The fur is smooth, and they look a lot younger than the control, ad libitum–fed animals of the same age.

Fremont-Smith: Dr. Simms, did they have any exercise?

Simms: No.

Fremont-Smith: A rat, in nature, would get a lot more exercise. It might be eating the same amount, but because it gets more exercise it probably would be leaner.

Atwood: It would probably not live any longer.

Ehret: As an example of a method of restricted diet, Dr. R. W. Swick uses a special device to permit the administration of isotopically labeled nutrients around the clock (53). These rats get a small amount of isotope in the food every hour. Since they are not fed to satiation, they are always apprehensive, waiting for the next bit of food to appear. Is an underfed animal different in cycle of activity?

Simms: It is different in that as soon as it hears the girl coming with the food, it gets to the front of the cage and is extremely eager to get at the food.

Barrows: We have tried to measure the activity of the restricted animal versus the animal fed ad lib. The results are a little confusing. If the total random movements are measured in what we could call a jiggle or suspension cage it will be found by this measurement that the restricted rats are a lot less active, although they give the impression, as Dr. Simms says, of being active. There is an increase in activity preceding the feeding period. Nevertheless, there is a reduction in total activity, which makes sense. If the animal is getting less food, I don't see how it could be more active.

Fremont-Smith: Would this be true if it had a wheel?

Barrows: We also did this in the wheel, where one finds the opposite.

Fremont-Smith: I was going to predict that. Therefore, the first one didn't make sense.

Barrows: In the wheel the restricted animals run more.

Ehret: Do they run more, or are the integrated periods of running time longer?

Barrows: The number of revolutions is greater. In other words, in the situation where voluntary activity is measured, the restricted animals will run more. Interestingly, again the increase in activity precedes the time of feeding. At present, we cannot interpret these results.

Fremont-Smith: Couldn't a survival pressure be involved in this, if the rat were in nature and restricted in food? Because food wasn't available to it, for one reason or another, it would likely be more active in search of food. It would seem to me this tendency for a hungry rat to show increased running activity, when there was a chance to run, would fit in at least with the idea of survival pressure to seek out food in nature.

Barrows: Here, again, in the random-movement cage the total energy expenditure, if it could be calculated, would be a lot less. So I really don't know, from these data, what the impact of increased activity is on longevity. We had hoped that perhaps we could tie this together.

Atwood: Didn't Selye investigate that? I think he found that exercise is bad for one, actually.

Barrows: This was his conclusion, but there were very few animals in his study, as I recall. The more active animals died sooner, I believe. Is that not right?

Atwood: That seems intuitively right, too. (Laughter)

Quastler: How about the effort spent? The skinny rat spends less effort running once around the wheel than the fat one does.

Barrows: Here is another problem with which one is faced when there is the size differential. There is a lack of controls. In a similar fashion, what effect does a difference in the pace of the animal have on the measurement of activity? We don't know. However we did add ballast to the cages to compensate for differences in the weights of the animals. Nevertheless, such variables may introduce bias into activity measurements.

Birren: Dr. Anton Carlson[*] told me, in relation to the effects of physical activity on aging, that he had the idea that increased activity consequent to food restriction might lead to improved longevity in animals. Together with a reduced diet, he fed a group of rats shredded cellophane. The idea was that the distention of the stomach would reduce the rat's hunger

[*]Former Professor of Physiology, at the University of Chicago— a personal communication.

drive. Apparently, the rats' activity was reduced but they showed the same benefits of greater longevity. He told me informally that he concluded it was not primarily physical activity but diet restriction. I am not sure if this study was reported in the literature.

Fremont-Smith: McCay's rats were heavily infected with pulmonary disease, with otitis media, and with pyelonephritis. This was only discovered when a pathologist was introduced into the program by the Macy Foundation. That is why I happen to know about it. The interesting contrast here is that this is the only case I know of in which a somewhat parallel restriction study was done, with somewhat the same favorable results, in a colony in which these common infections were eliminated.

Barrows: Dr. Morris Ross (43) has done a similar study. The complete data have not yet been published.

Simms: With regard to longevity, Figure 18 shows our calculations of life expectancy. The left-hand line represents the logarithm of the mortality of the control (ad libitum–fed) male rats while the right-hand line is for the 46%-restricted male rats. These lines give the logarithm of the probability of death, the same sort of thing we plot with the Gompertz equation for the unrestricted and for the restricted rats. These follow the simple equation

$$k \triangle t = \triangle \log P_t,$$

and the slope $\underline{k}$ of each of the two curves is used in calculating the life expectancy, at birth, from this equation (46):

$$t = 1/k \; [(1.6k/P_0) + 1],$$

where $100 \log P_0$ is the intercept at age zero. Obviously, these two curves must meet at the age of birth because the rats were presumably identical at that time, but the curves spread apart afterwards.

The life-expectancy values of the males, computed by the equation above, were 802 and 1,005. That is about 200 days difference in the life expectancy. With the females, it was 950 compared with 1,244—in other words, about 300 days, increase in life expectancy as a result of the restriction of the diet down to the 54% level.

Barrows: You had two levels of restriction. Could you tease out the difference in longevity on the basis of how much

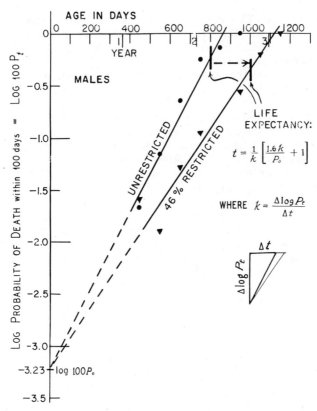

Fig. 18.—Logarithm of the mortality data of restricted and control rats. The slope of the lines gives the values of k used in computing life expectancy from the equation.

they were restricted? Your charts showed that the onset of these observed microscopical changes occurred later in the rats which were more restricted. Can you indeed demonstrate differences in longevity between the two groups of restricted animals?

Simms: I didn't do it, but I would expect that the life expectancy of the 33%-restricted rats would be in between.

Barrows: The reason I ask is that in McCay's early work (37) the length of time he restricted his rats did not actually have much effect on the over-all life span. Admittedly, the number of rats in McCay's studies was small.

Simms: Yes, and his rats were not free from lung infection.

Barrows: The restricted rats lived longer than the ad lib–fed animals. However, whether they were restricted for 100, 300, or 500 days, all the experimental animals died at essentially the same time.

McCay fed the same diet to all the animals, but fed the restricted rats smaller quantities of carbohydrate. In the work of Ross (43), with which I am sure you are familiar, the animals were fed diets of different compositions. Dietary restriction can be effected by feeding, for instance, on 8% protein diet ad lib. Ross showed that such animals will voluntarily eat less food but will live longer.

The other groups were fed smaller amounts of food than the control rats which were fed Purina Laboratory Chow ad lib. The growth curves of the various groups of restricted rats differed markedly from that of the control animals. One group grew at a rate of about 10%, two groups grew at 30%, and one group grew at 50% of that observed in the control rats. The differences in maximum body weight were essentially of these same orders of magnitude. Yet, in terms of mean life span, or 50% mortality, there were no marked differences among the restricted groups.

Fremont-Smith: They were all better than the unrestricted?

Barrows: Oh, yes. The unrestricted rat lived about 750 days. The increase in life span in Ross's restricted rats was about 250 days. In order to attempt to demonstrate differences among the restricted groups, Ross has calculated specific mortality rates. The difficulty here, of course, is that it is not possible to get any estimates of variability. The specific mortality rate can be obtained at any given time, but not a measure of variance. Although some of the rats seemed to have a greater life expectancy later in life, it really can't be proved statistically.

Simms: He didn't have infection-free rats, did he?

Barrows: No, but by the same token I don't see that the longevity of the 33%-restricted rats is any different from the 46%-restricted animals. You say you feel it is. I think this is important.

Simms: I can look up the data and calculate it.*

---

* Subsequent calculations on the data of the 33%-restricted rats showed that there were too few animals to tell us whether the life expectancy was significantly different from that of the 46%-restricted rats.

Barrows: My point is that it looks like an all-or-none phenomenon, which we detest in any biological system.

Atwood: McCay (36) always created the impression that the cessation of the restriction was the time from which the life span had to be measured. Is that wrong?

Barrows: Yes. If one takes McCay's own data and subtracts the times of cessation of restriction from the life spans, the values are not constant.

Atwood: Is there a trend in that direction?

Barrows: No. Actually, it goes down. The longer the animal is restricted, the shorter is the time between the time of cessation of restriction and death.

Fremont-Smith: The refeeding was a very short period, if they had been restricted for very long.

Barrows: I don't know how the concept has gotten about on the basis of McCay's data. Has anybody looked at the data? My impression is that there is not a fixed amount of living after cessation of restriction.

Simms: Unfortunately, we didn't have very many animals in the 33% group.

Barrows: That was when you ran into the difficulties of moving into a new building.

Ehret: Are there any data on the influence of temperature on longevity?

Simms: Johnston et al. (29) have shown that rats at 83° F live longer than those at 48° F—a rather extreme temperature range. We tried to get the temperature the rats liked best. In the beginning, we tried different temperatures. We found that if they were too hot they would come to the front of the cage and gasp to try to get air. If they were too cold, they would go to the back of the cage and huddle together. We selected a temperature in between.

We first chose a temperature of 76° F with a humidity of about 60% throughout the year. We have now raised that somewhat. We have a different type of cage, made of aluminum and stainless steel. Under these conditions, they seem to require a little higher temperature. We go up to 77° or 78° F, with a 60% humidity. But change in temperature is not one of our experimental variables.

Barrows: The only systematic study in this regard was done by Kibler (31) in the rat. If the temperature is reduced rather markedly the rats will die much sooner.

Quimby: They certainly will. I had this happen to 200 rats. (Laughter)

Simms: We had very elaborate temperature controls put in by a well-known manufacturer. They are supposed to keep the temperature within half a degree, plus or minus. It's fine as long as it works, but it doesn't work all the time. (Laughter) It is too sensitive and goes haywire. We have had the maintenance man up from the manufacturer many times to make adjustments and corrections. Our intentions are to keep the temperature very close to the one at which the thermostats are set.

Now may we go on to the next logical development from our studies? This is the theoretical consideration of various ways in which life span can be altered (48), either extended or shortened. There are three main ways in which we can affect life span.

One theoretical way to extend it is to reduce the incidence of disease, as shown in Figure 19; in other words, reduce the number of individuals that are susceptible. If this is done, we get a curve such as the one shown for the incidence of lesions and probability of onset. In humans, we do this when we vaccinate against smallpox or protect against some other infectious disease.

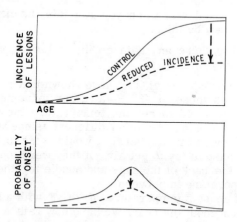

Fig. 19.—Theoretical mechanism for altering average life span—reduction of number of individuals susceptible to a disease.

Figure 20 shows the second way in which life span can be altered. The left-hand curves represent lesion incidence and onset under ordinary conditions; and the middle curves represent the resulting death. However, if we can delay the time of death after the onset occurs, we get the right-hand curves,

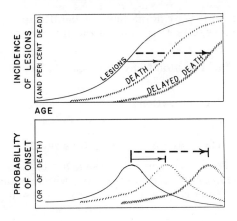

Fig. 20.—Alteration of average life span by delaying death after the on-set of a disease.

representing delayed death. That is what happens when we treat pernicious anemia, for example, with liver extract, or a diabetic with insulin. We don't affect the onset of the disease but we do delay death after the onset.

The third theoretical way to prolong life span is by de-laying the onset of lesions, as demonstrated in Figure 21. This is what we believe we have done in the case of dietary restriction. There are probably other ways in which this can be accomplished. We are attempting now to use other influ-ences, one being stress, which we expect will push the exper-imental curves to the left instead of to the right. We have also started treating another group of rats with thyroxin to deter-mine whether that will push the curves to the left or not.

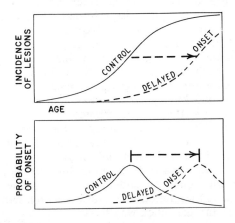

Fig. 21.—Alteration of average life span by delaying the onset of lesions

Lansing: Is it your point that probability of death in your rat population results from one of the five disease entities in Figure 7?

Simms: No, I wouldn't say necessarily from only one of them.

Lansing: A combination?

Simms: Yes.

Lansing: There are no other factors involved?

Simms: There are other diseases, but these are the most prominent ones. There are tumors, too, which in the female is the mammary tumor. But most of the tumors in the rat are benign.

Lansing: At least in this population the rats die of specific disease entities. The phenomenon that some people have euphonically called "endogenous aging" doesn't operate here?

Simms: I don't think the rats die from aging, if that is what you mean. Aging, as I see it, affects the onset of the lesions. They die from the lesions; they don't die directly from aging.

Barrows: Isn't this muscular dystrophy, as you call it, really a morphological change?

Simms: Yes.

Barrows: It is hard for me to see how a rat is going to die by virtue of lack of skeletal muscle.

The second thing is cardiac degeneration. As I recall from Dr. Berg's data, this is restricted almost entirely to the apex of the heart, and is quite minimal. Here, again, it is possible for an animal to die of cardiac failure; nevertheless, when one analyzes tissues for a variety of components, one never finds marked changes, at least so far.

Similarly, nephritis is diagnosed on the basis of histological changes rather than functional changes. We know that we can remove one kidney from a 22-month-old rat and the rat will regenerate the second kidney quite adequately and still survive with 50% less functioning kidney tissue. So it is difficult for me to conceive of these animals dying from the five diseases in Figure 7. Wouldn't it be just as correct to say that, as age increases, there is an increasing probability of seeing cellular changes under the microscope as to say that this was a frank, functional disease which caused death. Is this going too far the other way?

Fremont-Smith: The question we are asking Dr. Simms, as I understand, is this: Is it possible that the lesions that Dr. Berg measures, which are parallel with probability of death, are only coincidental and not causal?

Barrows: Indeed, these morphological changes may be an expression of biochemical changes at the cellular level.

Simms: Going back to question No. 1 (laughter), the muscular dystrophy contributes to death in an odd way, in that the rat can't get food because its muscles become so weakened that it can't get at the feeder. Less food, to a certain extent, is good for it. Beyond that, it tends to starve.

Fremont-Smith: Were they not eating their food?

Simms: Not when their muscular dystrophy became severe. As for the changes in the heart and kidney, as I am not a pathologist, I can merely reflect Dr. Berg's views. He feels that if the renal lesions get severe enough, they affect the animal to the point that they cause death. He does not believe there are any generalized cell changes that are a reflection of age, except the changes in the lesions I have mentioned.

A number of papers have been published with which Dr. Berg strongly disagrees—putting it mildly. In them, certain changes have been described in the muscle that have been ascribed to aging rather than to disease. His feeling is that those changes are all properly called disease.

Barrows: Yet, on the other hand, both Dr. Berg and Dr. Andrew (2), I think, agree on what they see in these sections. Berg decides that this is disease, whereas Andrew and our group take the position that this is a manifestation of aging. If they both agree that these are typical changes, perhaps the problem is merely a matter of semantics.

Birren: One might have also included coarsening of the fur, since older animals show a coarsening as well as a thinning of the fur. One might then have plotted a measure of fur, and likely it would have shown a similar plot; yet this does not fit our notion of a lesion. Furthermore, one might have taken the tendon from the rat tail, as Verzar (54) has done, showing a close relationship with age and the changes in the tendon. These observations add up to a collection of diffuse morphological changes. The notion of disease or lesions somehow does not help us very much.

Barrows: That is essentially what I am trying to say.

Simms: I have already expressed myself on this. Our

opinion is that all the changes that we observe in these organs are disease changes rather than age changes.

[Editor's Note: Dr. Simms wishes to add the following "afterthought" to his remarks at the conference:

[It so happens that the two lesions (in the kidney and the muscle) about which we have this controversy are the only two diseases which reach 100% incidence, as can be seen in Figure 7. If Dr. Barrows were to question some other lesion, such as periarteritis or myocardial degeneration, we would have a stronger case since these do not approach 100% incidence and, therefore, they must be diseases and cannot be age changes (since all animals age). It seems to me that one cannot properly pick out the two morphological changes that have 100% incidence and claim that these are not disease.

[Dr. Berg wishes to make the following comment: According to Andrew et al. (2) the skeletal muscle degeneration and accompanying loss of muscle fibers which develop in older rats represent an aging process of tissue composed of fixed post-mitotic cells. On this basis, Yiengst et al. (56) described marked changes in chemical composition of the gastrocnemius muscles, and Rockstein and Brandt (42) observed alterations in enzyme activity. However, it is difficult to accept the hypothesis that skeletal muscle degeneration is the result of an aging process for the following reasons: (a) lesions develop only in the hind-leg muscles, so that the process would have to be highly selective; (b) lesions consist of degeneration, necrosis, and fatty infiltration of muscle fibers and are typical of the disease described as muscular dystrophy in humans; (c) distribution of lesions is patchy, and degree as well as extent of involvement varies greatly in different fibers; and (d) onset of lesions is delayed by dietary restriction (10).]

Fremont-Smith: You also feel, as I understand it, that in addition to these being disease changes there are also mutually contributory causes to death?

Simms: Yes, several diseases. In general the animals showed more than one type of lesion on autopsy.

Fremont-Smith: There isn't some other underlying, not yet discovered cause or probability of death in these animals — so that these diseases are not crucial, so far as longevity is concerned?

Simms: Only that rats do have hypertension, which, of course, is not measured on autopsy. Dr. Berg at one time made a study of hypertension (7). With rats, as with humans, many individuals retain a normal pressure, while a certain percentage get an elevated pressure.

Fremont-Smith: What about heart weight? This would tend to go up, I would think, in hypertrophy of the heart, with sustained hypertension.

Simms: Yes, the heart weight does go up in some cases.

Cottier: This seems to be a rather unfavorable strain in which to study aging. Both chronic glomerulonephritis and periarteritis are definite diseases. I do not know if and to what extent the muscular and myocardial degeneration you mentioned depend on the vascular changes. It may be that because of the development of these diseases most of the rats do not reach a stage of senescence as we know it from many human cases and certain strains of mice.

Simms: All rodents and all strains of rats die within a 4-year period; whether they have the same proportional relationship between the lesions is another matter. But these seem to be the principal diseases that affect our rats. The ratio of incidence of the disease may be different in other strains, just as the incidence of tumors varies with the strain of mice.

Cottier: You corrected your data for leukemias, for instance. The question arises of whether one has to correct, also, for definite diseases such as glomerulonephritis or periarteritis nodosa? This is a very serious question because later I will show degenerative changes in mice which have 100% incidence. They probably are not lethal, but they are pretty typical for very old mice.

In a few animals that are left without specific disease, only these changes might be found and nothing else. Does one have to correct for these diseases in establishing a converse curve, or not?

Sacher: The mortality table is the outcome of a competition among several disease processes, and we must make some assumptions about the nature of the competition in order to calculate "corrected" incidences. If, for example, we assume that the various diseases are statistically independent, then the age-specific mortality rate is the appropriate basis for describing the age-dependence of a disease process.

Cottier: Would you, for instance, in a strain of mice that produces amyloidosis in middle age, correct for this?

Sacher: I have not done so, but I can see no objection. We have on occasion removed the lymphoma mortality so we could see how mortality from other causes is influenced by ionizing radiation exposure. Kimball (32) has given a statistical discussion of a procedure for computing lifetime incidences of specific diseases corrected for the mortality from other diseases.

Cottier: If the age-dependent mortality rate for amyloidosis is not corrected, one may get a broken curve. This represents a serious problem since amyloidosis in mice usually sets in prior to 20 months of age. Past the age of 2 years, the animals do not seem to be susceptible any more to de novo amyloid formation. It may well be that glomerulonephritis shows a similar age-dependency. Does this have any relation to real senescence? As I understand it, you don't regard the changes you mentioned as being typically senile.

Simms: That is right.

Cottier: You don't consider the list of diseases you gave to be characteristic of senescence?

Simms: No, we do not. Furthermore, we don't attempt to assign a single cause of death but feel that all the lesions present may contribute to the death of the animal.

In our early work, we tried to assign one disease as the cause of death, as is done with human data, but we gave that up. Now we merely list whatever lesions are shown; we do not attempt to say what killed the animal.

Keys: In general, these animals did not die spontaneously. You killed them, didn't you?

Simms: Practically, they died spontaneously. We waited until they were moribund. If we had waited 2 days longer, they probably would have died during the night and then been autopsied the next day.

Keys: When they were allowed to die naturally, what was the actual mechanism of death? Something happened. Did they die in uremia, in cardiac standstill? Did they have fibrillation, respiratory failure? What happened?

Simms: They die chiefly from uremia and/or complications caused by tumors, periarteritis, and muscular degeneration.

Storer: is it your thesis, then, that aging is not a lethal process? If we correct for all disease incidence, then presumably there would be no mortality rate.

Simms: Yes and no. I would say that aging brings on the disease, and the disease causes death.

Fremont-Smith: You are saying that aging causes death by virtue of the disease it brings on.

Simms: Yes.

Fremont-Smith: So you are saying that death is due to aging.

Simms: Indirectly.

Fremont-Smith: Therefore, we haven't seen aging free of disease.

Simms: No, although in very rare cases an autopsy on an old person has been reported to show no lesions.

Kallmann: How do you expect thyroid extract to accelerate the occurrence of fatal lesions?

Simms: It will speed up the metabolism, and it is important to know whether this will affect the age of onset of lesions.

Kallmann: How would a speed-up in the metabolism lead to such lesions as muscular degeneration?

Simms: I don't know. I don't know, either, why restricted food intake delays the onset of the lesions, but it does.

Fremont-Smith: Have you any indication that thyroid will accelerate it?

Simms: We don't know; we are going to try it out. Of the various possible experiments that we have considered, it is very difficult to pick anything that is simple because even the simplest experiment becomes complex before we get through with it. Even this would be complex. It will, of course, speed up the metabolism and presumably increase pulse rate; it may or may not affect the age of onset of the disease.

Stress is another thing we have been studying. Stress, which has been studied considerably by Selye (45), is not a simple matter. We have tried blinking lights and noise, which did not have any effect. We are now trying crowding within cages. But we don't know just how that is coming out.

Jarvik: Dr. Keys inquired about the mechanism of death in individual rats; even in humans, where we do have careful individual observation, I think we very rarely know the ultimate cause of death. Frequently we may wonder why they haven't died before. Another point that struck me was your mention of respiratory standstill. I have the impression that respiration is usually the last function to give out-patients continue to breathe who, to all intents and purposes, are already dead, unless there is pulmonary edema or something of the sort. If I recall correctly, it is rare for an older person to die of what would be a primary neurological deficiency. We tend to find circulatory and other failures instead. This was one of the reasons that made me wonder whether, for instance, aging in nerve cells leads to loss of function. Purely neurological causes of death are common in the upper age groups.

Simms: Dr. Abner Wolf (11) has been examining our rats and has found a myelin degeneration which does not parallel the incidence of muscle changes; we do not feel it is correlated or that it is a cause of death.

Atwood: Does it parallel the muscular degeneration?

Simms: No. We made a particular point of determining whether or not there was a correlation, but none was found.

Atwood: Does it precede it at all?

Simms: No, the rats that have one may or may not have the other.

Atwood: Are you looking at the appropriate nerve? For example, you could count the fibers in the appropriate nerve supply to see if they are fewer when the muscle is degenerated.

Simms: The myelin sheaths were involved but not the axons.

Atwood: As shown by actual counts, or by just looking?

Simms: No, there was no occasion to make counts. Dr. Wolf and Dr. Berg both examined the sections but found no correlation.

Lansing: Dr. Simms, according to Dr. Berg's paper (47) which some of us were looking at, the lesion in the kidney does not appear to be a glomerular lesion at all; the area of scarification that is illustrated is very gross. That suggests a disease other than one restricted to the glomeruli. This might be consistent with a massive damage to the kidney, because of some factor as yet undetermined, which could give rise to the hypertension you described as existing in the rat population. It is also consistent with the appearance of a periarteritis, and this in turn could well be responsible for the muscular changes by way of the changes in circulation, including the myocardial change.

So it seems as if you have here a package that is consistent with a single major disease entity in the population.

Cottier: I agree with Dr. Lansing.

Simms: Dr. Berg is in a better position than I am to comment on the nature of the lesions.

[Editor's Note: Dr. Berg would like to add the following supplement to Dr. Simms' remarks at the conference:

[Five major diseases, namely, chronic glomerulonephritis, periarteritis, degeneration of skeletal muscle, myocardium, and myelin sheaths develop with age in our Sprague-Dawley rat strain. Various types of spontaneous tumors also occur in this rat strain. The commonest neoplasms are adenoma of the thyroid, adenoma of the pituitary, fibroadenoma of the female breast, and pheochromocytoma of the adrenal. Detailed descriptions of lesions are given in papers from our laboratory (5, 10, 11, 12, 47). Muscular and neural lesions are unrelated. All of the diseases, including tumors, have their counterparts in humans. The principal cause of death is uremia. Other major causes of death are periarteritis and pituitary adenoma. The remaining conditions are contributory causes.]

I might point out, too, for anyone setting up an animal colony who is interested in our specifications, that we have a paper on this subject which will soon be published (50).

Dr. Berg and I feel very strongly that any experimental work which involves the study of life span, as a result of experimental treatment, should include complete autopsies for the determination of lesion incidence in relation to age, in order to determine whether the experimental treatment affects the onset of one or all of the lesions to which the animal is subject. This, of course, necessitates the co-operation of a pathologist, but we feel that it is essential in order to have a complete picture of what happens as a result of the experimental treatment.

One other point Dr. Berg wanted me to stress is that weight curves be kept of animals throughout their lives. As the animals grow older, there is usually a point where they begin to lose weight. That should not be considered as a result of aging but, rather, as an indication of disease. In every case involving many animals, when they were killed at the point when they began to lose weight, we found that disease had set in sufficiently to affect the animal's weight.

Keys: The same thing happens in man. Do you think that is disease, too?

Simms: I wouldn't want to say. Man is not under the uniform conditions that we have in our colony. It might well be an indication of disease.

Brues: What is basic in what happens in man? Is it disuse of muscles? Is it trouble with teeth, or trouble affecting food intake? Or is it not specific at all?

Keys: I think it happens very frequently in persons whom we would judge, from every criterion we have at the present time, to be in the best of health. Nevertheless, they grow thinner, and the fact that they lose weight probably is a good thing. In any event, are we to take it this is some sort of disease proposition? I don't see any reason at all to say that this is the case in man.

Atwood: There is less muscle, too.

Keys: No, the muscle loss begins long before.

Atwood: Muscle loss in man has a regular component that is clearly not disease. The Los Alamos group (1) has measured total body potassium, which is really a measure of muscle, and this declines throughout adult life at a constant rate.

Lindop: I don't agree with Dr. Berg. We have done body weights of all of our colony. What we call the senescent weight loss begins at about 72 weeks. Only about 10% of our control population has died. In other words, 90% of the population survives, and these probably continue up to about 173 weeks. They all show weight loss.

We have been doing serial killings, and I can't see that the groups showing this senescent weight loss have got frank disease processes.

Simms: It has been our experience that whenever there is a loss of weight in our colony, there is disease present which accounts for it. Dr. Berg believes that the weight loss is an indication of disease, rather than an indication of aging.

Lindop: If an individual animal suddenly shows a rapid decrease in body weight, this might be indicative of disease. If body weight changes are being taken as a measure of population aging, then I don't think the decrease in the mean body weight of the population is indicative of disease; I think it is a reasonable senescent change.

Simms: All I can say is that Dr. Berg doesn't agree with you.

Cottier: It seems reasonably well established that both humans and animals show a weight loss of a number of organs as they reach a very old age, even in the absence of detectable disease. In our strain of mice there is, for example, a rather steep drop in the liver-weight curve at an age beyond 900 days. In other strains, this organ seems to undergo a gradual weight loss even earlier, as Dr. Lindop indicated. In our mice we often could not find any disease that would explain the liver atrophy.

Simms: Are we talking about animals free from respiratory disease or other infections?

Cottier: In very old mice there was always a weight loss of the liver, even if they had no other detectable disease.

Lindop: Everitt (21) has made a careful study of the weight loss which occurs independently of diseases. He showed this was probably of adrenal cortical origin. That was his interpretation. He made a very clear difference in the weight changes which he got in animals in which he could see disease process and those which showed the weight loss without any disease process being present.

Simms: I am acquainted with Dr. Everitt's work. He worked a while with us. He does not claim to be working with animals free from respiratory disease. Respiratory disease may account for weight loss.

Lindop: If animals are serially killed as Everitt's were, they can be divided by straightforward pathological diagnoses into those which have apparent disease and those which haven't. In his group that did not show apparent disease, he still observed weight loss after a certain age. This, I would have thought, was reasonably good objective proof that there is a change in weight with age which isn't necessarily indicative of disease.

Simms: Dr. Berg very definitely does not agree. One of you is right and the other wrong.

Fremont-Smith: Perhaps Dr. Berg would make a comment on this question for the publication; that would be very useful to have.

[Editor's Note: Dr. Berg would like to make the following comment:

[Body-weight curves of male rats reach a peak at about 500 days of age. At this age, lesions begin to develop and a plateau appears in the curve. Incidence and severity of lesions increases and, at 800 days, the weight curve falls. A sharp drop in body weight may occur as a terminal event. As long as rats remain free from disease, there is no loss of body weight (6, 8, 9, 50).

[Everitt (22), on the other hand, attributed the senescent loss of body weight to an aging process. However, in his rats, unlike ours, there was a high incidence of lung abscesses. It is important to note that endemic lung infection may exist for a long time without causing clinical symptoms and that the infection may be overlooked unless the lungs are examined carefully at post mortem. Complete gross and microscopic findings at autopsy were not reported by Everitt except for a few grossly observed tumors. Lindop (35) also attributed weight loss of older mice to aging, although a high percentage of her animals had infected lungs as well as renal, hepatic, and intestinal lesions.]

Lansing: I wonder if someone could help me. I was thinking, as we talked about this apparent loss of muscle with the passage of time—later in life. Let's assume for a moment that this phenomenon does occur, and that it is not related to disease. Is there any information at all in the literature, does anybody know, whether old muscle can make more muscle? I am thinking now of the protein synthetic process in muscle. The young man, when he exercises, experiences hypertrophy of individual muscle fibers by way of accumulation of protein. Can the old man do this, or the old rat? Can old muscle make more muscle by way of hypertrophy? Certainly in man, I don't think this happens.

Atwood: Maybe they don't try hard enough.

Keys: There is a point of no return.

Atwood: It certainly happens in cardiac muscle.

Fremont-Smith: The former dean of Rochester Medical School, G. H. Whipple (55), did an interesting experiment with dogs. He found that muscle myoglobin could be increased only as the result of exercise. He tried a variety of diets, and so forth, but nothing other than exercise would increase muscle myoglobin. This bears on the subject indirectly, I think.

Lansing: Will exercise do it in the old dog?

Fremont-Smith: I don't know. I can't remember whether his report dealt with old dogs. Anyway, it would be important to remember this, if one is going to try it, because the animals will have to be exercised to make a fair experiment.

Lindop: I think one could get some preliminary data on this, for instance, from the physiotherapy of polio cases or patients who have had accidents and undergo muscle retraining. Muscle measurements are taken continuously.

Lansing: That injects another problem, the general phenomenon of atrophy of disuse, for example, as the result of a limb being in a cast for a long period of time. One finds, after removal of the cast and with exercise, at any age, there is recovery from the atrophy. But this may or may not be a different mechanism from the hypertrophy that I am referring to. I am curious, can old muscle make more muscle?

Fry: Dr. G. Goldspink (23) in the Department of Zoology, University of Dublin, is interested in this problem. He found that in biceps brachii of the mouse there were two populations of muscle fibers. In the adult mouse, the distribution of muscle fiber diameters had two distinct peaks at 20μ and 40μ. In the young mouse, only small fibers are present but, as the body weight increases, so does the number of large fibers. The level of nutrition, age, and exercise alter the ratio of large to small fibers. He hopes to determine whether or not exercise will also increase the number of large fibers in old mice.

Barrows: Will he attempt this with the aid of a treadmill?

Fry: He is using a system in which the mice have to pull a weighted cord to obtain food.

Barrows: Dr. Gordon Ring* and I have discussed this. I don't think there is any question that it is something worth doing. Dr. Ring felt it would be very difficult to get the animals to exercise enough to produce hypertrophy, that they just couldn't be made to work that hard. I don't know whether that is true or not.

Quastler: Is myoglobin synthesis in old muscles normal?

Barrows: We did not find any difference in the turnover rate of total proteins in the muscles of rats of different ages (4).

Cottier: It might be of interest to recall Dr. Spraragen's studies (52) on adult rabbits that had been fed a diet rich in cholesterol. The myocardium of the left ventricle was hypertrophic but it also contained a higher relative number of muscle cells that incorporated label after an injection of tritiated thymidine. This finding indicates that, besides the hypertrophy, there was also a slight increase in the number of muscle cells. Thus in young adult rabbits the heart muscle apparently can produce new elements upon some sort of stimulation.

Lansing: The labeling was in the nuclei?

*Gordon C. Ring, Department of Physiology, University of Miami School of Medicine, Coral Gables, Florida.

Cottier: Within the muscle-cell nuclei.

Lansing: And not in the interstitial cells?

Cottier: Not only. I remember his slides very well. There was definite labeling over muscle-cell nuclei.

Lansing: That is fascinating.

Cottier: As far as muscular hypertrophy in the old individual is concerned, there is hardly any doubt that this occurs. Paralysis of the legs at old age and consequent stress of the arm muscles result in a remarkable hypertrophy of the latter.

Sacher: We have been discussing a very interesting area of aging regarded as disease or susceptibility to disease and its morphological change. I wonder if we could ask our psychologist colleagues to talk about aging as loss of function. This is ultimately the problem that confronts us in aging, the gradual diminution of ability to perform.

Birren: I have been wondering how I would relate behavior of the nervous system to a kind of hierarchical concept of aging.

Obviously, we see aging in unicellular organisms as well as in multicellular organisms. One's criteria of aging may have to shift, in a sense, with the level of complexity of the organism with which one is dealing. By this I mean that the most complicated organism shares mechanisms of aging with the simplest unicellular organism, assuming for the moment that such mechanisms exist. However, the multicellular organisms have additional features of aging as well.

Thus one might expect to find extracellular aging, aging of the fibers in the extracellular space, which is not seen in the unicellular organism. Similarly, in mammals one sees phenomena of aging of the nervous system which may not have a counterpart in the lower metazoa. This means that the most complicated animal may show all the manifestations of aging of the simplest organisms, but show additional ones as well as a consequence of its evolved complexity.

Behavior, as well as anatomical or physiological properties, are very significant in determining which organisms survive. Therefore, it is successful behavior which survives in genetic lines. To look at it the other way round: the genetic lines become a function of successful behavior.

In small organisms, for example, successful behavior is related to speed in avoiding predators. In the wild state you rarely see the rat, because its predators will capture it very soon if escape behavior is less efficient. Any failure of the nervous system, in terms of speed of behavior, will result in the animal's death.

In the laboratory situation, we remove these predatory influences and we observe aging at a different level of complexity than in the naturally occurring states.

I have also been groping for another principle which expresses the view that, because of the hierarchical organization of the organism, the nervous system has a potential for intruding into any process at a lower level, including phenomena of aging. The issue is not, then, whether the nervous system can intrude its influence—it certainly can—but the frequency with which it does. The extent to which it does, in any particular instance, is the question. To cite one example, one might mention Curt Richter's (41) study of deaths in wild rats under unusual circumstances. He had rats swim in a small tank while being exposed to a stream of water. There were a substantial number of unexplained deaths. For some reason the animals just gave up; they didn't drown. The "spontaneous" deaths would seem to be some very unusual or uncommonly evoked function of the nervous system. I only want to emphasize again that the nervous system can intrude in any subordinate process in the body. The issue for research is this: how often and to what extent does it do so in aging in man? This means, I think, that we should see some duplication in man of phenomena of aging that we see in other mammals, but we should expect to find additional ones as well.

I would like to illustrate some of the work we have done. Figure 22 concerns age differences in the performance of the rat. This figure shows the swimming speed of the rat as a function of age. The ordinate is the time taken to swim a tank approximately 12 feet long. The distance the rat swam was 11 feet 6 inches. On the ordinate is plotted the swimming time in seconds, and on the abscissa the age of the rats in months (17).

Fremont-Smith: That is time taken to swim the length of the tank and get out?

Birren: From the start to the time it placed its front paws on the end ramp. Rats don't like water very much and they swim very fast—somewhat faster than 1 ft/sec. The lower curve represents the curve for female rats. Fastest swimming time of five successive trials shows a little increase at an age of 24 months. The ordinate is median swimming time of five successive trials.

Fremont-Smith: Old or adult?

Birren: In my colony, 24 months is old. Perhaps we don't

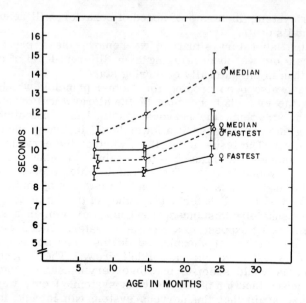

Fig. 22.—Swimming time of the albino rat as a function of age and sex. Time is reported in seconds to swim 11.5 ft. Measurements were based on 109 rats of different age and sex and were taken of the fastest time and the median time of 5 trials. Vertical lines are plotted as ± one standard deviation about the mean.

have as favorable environmental conditions as Dr. Simms has. We have about 50% survival to 22 months.

Fremont-Smith: Do the old rats swim slower because they take a longer time, or swim faster?

Birren: It takes the older males about 14 sec to swim the tank length, compared with 10.8 sec for young adult males. Interestingly, this is about a 20-30% slowing which is about the same order of magnitude for simple reaction time in humans over the adult age range.

Lindop: Isn't your sex difference surprising, that the female should be faster than the male?

Birren: Yes.

Keys: It should be slower. It takes longer to get there. Isn't that the way it went?

Birren: This is the length of time to swim approximately 12 feet. The female does it faster. The oldest female takes just about 11.4 sec; the oldest male takes about 14 sec.

Jarvik: Your age groups are the three points along the abscissa?

Birren: The age groups are 7-10 months, 12-17 months, and 22-27 months. One should remember that body size is so much different in the rat. The 1-year-old female weighs an average 300 g, and the male 480 g.

Keys: See how much more work he has to do.

Birren: We were interested also in the effects of fatigue in successive trials. I think this bears upon some of the points raised previously in relation to muscular performance.

Figure 23 shows the median swimming time in the first five trials for young females, young males, old females, and old males. These are just two age groups now. Notice that the young female has a very consistent performance here, showing little fatigue in 30 consecutive swimming trials. In resistance to fatigue the young males are almost as good. The older females and males differed more. The vertical lines represent the fact that some of the older males could not complete their performance and had to be taken out of the water when they were making no further forward progress before they drowned. Beginning at about 16 trials, some of the older ani-

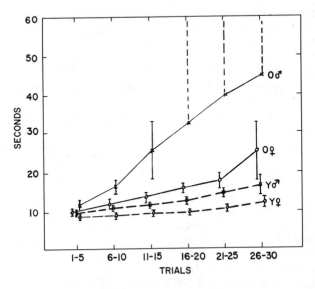

Fig. 23.—Fatigue effect on swimming times. Curves are drawn through median values for each block of 5 swimming trials. Swimming time is given in seconds to swim 11.5 ft. Forty rats were used—10 in each sex and age group.

mals were simply unable to go on, whereas in none of the younger animals did this happen; also it didn't occur in the old females.

Brues: I take it these rats are motivated, in that they have to sink or swim, is that it?

Birren: That's right. That's precisely why we wanted to study this kind of performance—where there seemed to be control over motivation.

Tyler: What drove them to the opposite side?

Fremont-Smith: Why didn't they go back to where they started, rather than to the other end?

Birren: This was part of the training. In the early trials we had a jet of air that they had to face if they turned around and swam to the starting point. Rats don't like air blasts, you know.

Cottier: How do you interpret the findings? It is somewhat embarrassing to see that the males lose the race. Is this because the females are more afraid of water? Is there any indication of why the females are faster? They are usually not as strong as males.

Birren: Perhaps it is strength in relation to body size, since the male rat is so much bigger. I don't know. Within the sex groups, we plotted swimming speed as a function of body weight, and we did not see any correlation. Some of the heaviest animals had the best performance within each sex group. I just can't make any statement about the basis for the rather large sex difference.

We were also interested in the extent to which the fatigue we produced was transient. To study this after the fatigue trials, we gave the rats 5 min rest, and then gave them five consecutive trials. Figure 24 shows some evidence for short-term recovery. Mind you, approximately 5 min earlier, these old males were unable to swim. They recovered, as you see, after 5 min rest and were able to swim at a median of about 22 sec, obviously slower than when they first started. There was a residual effect of fatigue and the curves show that they are again fatiguing, so there is a residual or cumulative effect. By the fifth trial, almost none of the old males were able to continue swimming. By contrast, the young females were almost all improving a little bit under these circumstances.

Lansing: In each case there was a 5 min rest period before the next trial?

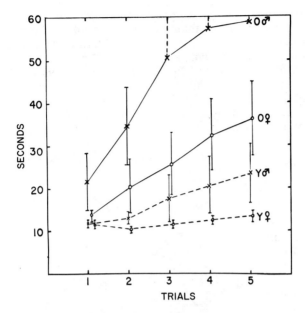

Fig. 24.—Recovery from fatigue of 5 trials following a 5-minute rest after 30 trials of continuous swimming, or failure.

Birren: There was a 5 min break between the 30 consecutive trials and the subsequent 5 consecutive trials. We wanted to see how rapidly this was reversed.

In another set of data, we gave these animals 12 consecutive days of training at 15 trials a day. Perhaps this introduces the issue of a possible hypertrophy of the muscle. After 12 days of practice, all the old animals were able to complete 30 consecutive trials successfully. So it looks as if the fatigue is to some extent a reversible disuse phenomenon (30).

I was interested in the fact that, while the fatigability was relatively reversible, the speed aspect was not. The age difference in speed of average or fastest performance did not change with practice, whereas the fatigue did. Perhaps we are faced with a muscular phenomenon and a neural phenomenon here, with speed being largely a function of the central nervous system.

Although we established the fact that the older animals were somewhat slower in performance, the next issue was how well they would learn a water maze. In this study they had a two-choice water maze to learn. In the first experiment there was an age difference (13). This difference seemed largely due to an interference with what might be regarded as a tropistic tendency on the part of the older animals. The older animals tended, more than the young, to follow the wall of the tank when swimming. This made it a different kind of choice situation for the age groups.

In the second study (Fig. 25) I used a two-choice T-maze. In this case the old and the young and middle-aged animals learned at approximately the same rate. Hence, one sees a difference in swimming speed with age, but not a difference in learning performance, at least of a two-choice task. Learning

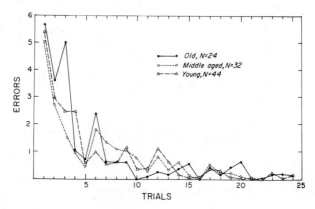

Fig. 25.—Mean errors per trial, by age groups, in learning the two-choice T water maze.

was expressed as errors as a function of trials. I am not saying that under some circumstances age differences in learning performance are not found, but I am suggesting that when you find differences in learning performance, it may be a function of some other aspect of the situation than acquisition or learning per se. I don't want to elaborate on that point since it has already been discussed by Jerome (28).

There is a long-standing issue in the literature, whether or not habit reversal is more difficult in the older animal. Figure 26 shows learning when the learned choices have been deliberately reversed. If the rat had learned a right-right choice maze to a criterion, then the maze would be reversed to a left-left maze. The three age groups were matched for initial learning. As you see, a true interference effect was obtained. However, the reversal effect was no greater in the older animals. When they were exposed to new conditions, all of them showed about the same increase in errors compared with their initial learning.

Under these circumstances, the analysis of the data shows

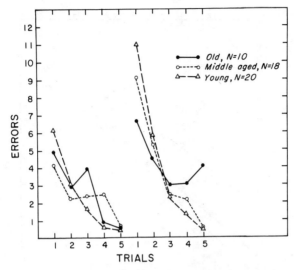

Fig. 26.—Mean errors per trial, by age groups, for learning of original and reversed maze. Age groups equated for original learning. Errors per trial for learning original maze shown on the left; errors per trial for learning reversed maze shown on the right.

there was no age difference in habit interference or learning reversal. From the data, one might expect that the results were going rather in the opposite direction, with old rats being somewhat better. However, from the gross statistical analysis, one merely concludes there is no age difference in reversal.

Now I would like to shift to some data on age differences in speed of human performance. In this work there were three age groups of human subjects: 80 to 89, 50 to 59, and 20 to 29. Along the abscissa are plotted the number of addition operations performed in problems of various length, that is, problems in two digits, three digits, up to twenty-five digits. The total time taken to do the problems is plotted as the log of the number of operations in the problem, with a two-digit problem considered as involving one operation (Fig. 27) (14).

The main point I wish to make is that at the intercept one sees a significant age difference. That is, for a problem of zero difficulty there is an age difference in speed of processing. Thus the data imply some fundamental timing difference in the older nervous system, in that it takes longer to process a problem of zero difficulty. It could well be that in difficult problems this timing acts disproportionately or as a power or exponential function, depending upon the number of elements of information one is handling.

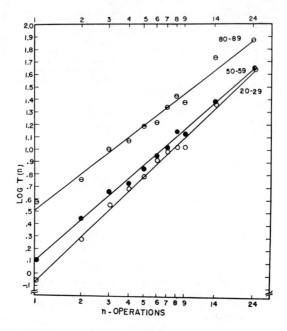

Fig. 27.—Time per problem, T (n), as a function of problem length, n. Mean values and lines of best fit are given for 3 age groups. Data are plotted in the form log T (n) = log K + m log n.

Fremont-Smith: There is very interesting work being done on the alerting reaction which can be measured by various vegetative responses and also by brain waves. It is conceivable that there has to be an alerting reaction to the central nervous system before it can enter into any new function. It is conceivable that one can distinguish whether the delay is in alerting reaction or in the actual performance, once it is started. This, I think, would be susceptible to current experimental studies.

There have been some very interesting Soviet studies (51) on the alerting reaction, which is quite sharp and discrete.

Birren: You must have been looking into my data because I have some information which seems to be related, although I wasn't planning to talk about it. The interesting thing we found was that the speed of reaction is tied in with the cardiac cycle. We get differences in highly alerted simple responses in humans, depending upon the phase of the cardiac cycle in which the stimulus is presented.

What we do is have the human subject react as quickly as possible by raising a finger as soon as he hears an auditory signal. We then analyze the data in terms of the phase of the cardiac cycle in which each of 100 successive stimuli are presented. Taking a simultaneous electrocardiogram along with the measurements of reaction time, we can plot the speed of response as a function of the phases of the cardiac cycle. Stimuli presented during the P phase, for example, are reacted to significantly faster than stimuli presented in the QRS phase (Table 6; Fig. 28) (16).

<u>Fremont-Smith:</u> What about age difference?

TABLE 6

Mean Simple Auditory Reaction Times According to the Phase of the Cardiac Cycle in Which the Stimuli Were Presented

(Young adult subjects, aged 20-30 years)[1]

	P	QRS	T	T-P
Men (N = 31):				
Mean	.1418	.1502	.1487	.1481
S.D.	.023	.0276	.035	.0275
Women (N = 25):				
Mean	.1482	.1568	.1574	.1546
S.D.	.0199	.0283	.0287	.0295

[1]Mixed-model analyses of variance were carried out separately for males and females and for the combined groups; the Hotelling T^2 statistics were significant at nearly the .10 level in each of the separate analyses (16) and at the .01 level for the combined sexes. The differences in mean reaction times to stimuli presented at QRS and P phases were tested by the Scheffé Multiple Comparison Procedure (44); significance obtained at the .05 level for males and at the .10 level for females, and at the .005 level in the combined analysis.

The statistical consultation and assistance of Dr. Donald F. Morrison are gratefully acknowledged.

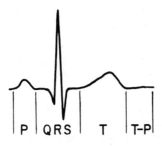

Fig. 28.—Representation of the cardiac cycle by a normal electrocardiogram. Vertical lines arbitrarily divide the cycle into the four intervals used for the analysis of the reaction time. Letters are those conventionally used to designate the principal deflections of the EKG.

Birren: Strangely enough, the older subjects, although showing slower reaction times, do not show this phenomenon. The results may suggest that the older brain may not show moment-to-moment differences in peak expectancy as do the young.

Fremont-Smith: What about the total difference in the alerting time, regardless of the cycle, between the older and the young?

Birren: The difference in simple reaction time between young and old was about 100 millisec. The work of Botwinick (20) suggests that it is more difficult to establish an alert expectancy and to maintain it in the older person.

Sacher: Is this done with a prior warning signal?

Birren: Yes.

Sacher: How is it affected by the duration of wait? Is that an age-dependent character?

Birren: That could be. However, we used a fixed 2-sec rest and a 1-sec regular warning interval, which would, I think, give an optimum set of circumstances for it to appear. There is some work to be published soon by Enoch Calloway III of Langley-Porter Clinic suggesting that there is a relationship between peak excitability of the cortex in relation to the cardiac cycle. What is implied is a phase relation between excitability of the cortex and the cardiac cycle.

Quastler: What was the absolute length of the reaction time?

Birren: Very small. About 150 to 160 millisec is the average reaction time in the young subject. The difference between the QRS and P would be of the order of 9 millisec. That is the same order one gets for different phases of the electroencephalogram and reaction time.

Fremont-Smith: This might not in any way be secondary to greater circulation resulting from the cardiac cycle, but more likely to be part of the same mechanism that produces the cardiac cycle.

Birren: Calloway had measurements of pulse wave. The change in response time seems to antecede the arrival at the brain of the pulse wave itself. Thus it is probably not a circulatory finding.

Fremont-Smith: The capillary flow is pretty steady. The pulse wave is practically gone by the time blood gets into the capillaries where the oxygen is delivered.

Birren: I think this is a neurophysiological rather than a circulatory phenomenon.

Quimby: The cardiac cycle doesn't originate in the cortex. I don't understand this at all.

Fremont-Smith: It originates in the nervous system and can be reflected to the cortex and, at the same time, to the heart.

Quimby: The heart can be made to beat all by itself.

Fremont-Smith: Of course, but it doesn't beat all by itself in the organism.

Birren: I don't see why activity initiated at the baroreceptors couldn't be modulating the excitability of the cortex of the brain. I am not suggesting that the cortex is driving the heart cycle but that there is a kind of phase relationship here.

Simms: Could it be in the ear, where the cycle of pulsation could affect the sensitivity to sound?

Birren: Except there these changes in response time occur prior to the arrival of the pulse wave at the ear. Calloway put a recorder on the ear lobe, I recall, and these changes occur much earlier and do not seem to be based on the arrival of increased blood flow.

Fenn: It could be due to the previous cardiac cycle. But it seems to me that so many things stand between the initiation of the beat in the pacemaker of the heart and the arrival of a wave that the time of arrival would vary among different persons. It seems most improbable that a correlation of minimum reaction time with the same point in the cardiac cycle among different individuals could be explained by anything as remote as that.

Birren: Let me say we have run 100 observations on each of 56 young adult subjects, 31 men and 25 women, and we get the same result for both men and women. Now the finding is replicated, I gather, in the work of Calloway. I rather believe this association is real, although it may not necessarily occur in all individuals. Some of our subjects don't show the association. This may then relate to Lacey's work (33), in which those individuals who show cardiac variability are the ones that show fastest reaction time. These are the people who are prone to respond quickly. This almost suggests a kind of typology. I don't mean this literally, but it is conceivable that, as Lacey puts it, there is a stabile type and a labile type. The very people who show these fluctuations are the ones who can respond quickly. This would seem, at least, to be related to our age data. The older people do not show much cardiac variability and generally they are slower.

Fry: Was there sinus arrhythmia in the young but not in the old subjects?

Birren: No, not in our subjects, I believe. Let me go on to another set of data. In Table 7 are correlations between age, education, and the eleven tests in the Wechsler Adult Intelligence Scale (18).

The point I want to make is that the information items here are very trivially related to chronological age, but highly related to educational level.

The second component is highly related to age, 0.67, and this is only over the age range of 25 to 64 years. Note that age is particularly related to the digit-symbol test. The digit-symbol test shows the largest loading on the second or "aging" component. In other studies of older adults, it also shows a close relation to reaction time (19).

What one sees, then, in the performance of a mental test, is an influence of accumulated information that is positively related to age. That is, one sees an increment of information with advancing age. At the same time, one sees a decrement in the speed of behavior. The loss of speed seems relatively smaller in its influence, perhaps more specific in its action. In advancing age, one is faced with a larger mass of stored information and a reduced speed of recognition and selection of appropriate responses.

This means that the point of maximization of function or behavior occurs as a joint function of at least these two components of the intellect: the speed of processing information and the amount of stored information.

Fremont-Smith: Do you have any information on the speed of recognition, which is different from the speed of alerting?

Birren: There was a study by Bronson Price (38) at Stanford many years ago. The tachistoscopically presented material was recognized somewhat more slowly by older adults.

The next set of data shows the effects of health as well as age upon mental test performance (Fig. 29).

Figure 30 was prepared by plotting the horizontal dashed line at the expected level of performance in young adult subjects (15). The tests were standardized to give a mean performance level of 10 in young adults. Along the abscissa are

TABLE 7

WAIS Correlation Matrix: 11 Subtests and Age and Education

N = 933 native-born white males and females, aged 25-64

(Decimal points omitted)

	1	2	3	4	5	6	7	8	9	10	11	12
1 Information												
2 Comprehension	67											
3 Arithmetic	62	54										
4 Similarities	66	60	51									
5 Digit span	47	39	51	41								
6 Vocabulary	81	72	58	68	45							
7 Digit symbol	47	40	41	49	45	49						
8 Picture completion	60	54	46	56	42	57	50					
9 Block design	49	45	48	50	39	46	50	61				
10 Picture arrangement	51	49	43	50	42	52	52	59	54			
11 Object assembly	41	38	37	41	31	40	46	51	59	46		
12 Age	-07	-08	-08	-19	-19	-02	-46	-28	-32	-37	-28	
13 Education	66	52	49	55	43	62	57	48	44	49	40	-29

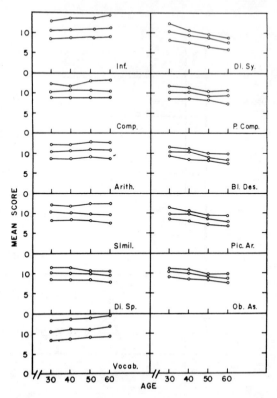

Fig. 29.—Mean scores on the WAIS subtests as a function of age and education. Upper curves for education 13 years and above; middle curves for 8-12 years; and lower curves for less than 8 years. Age intervals are 25-34, 35-44, 45-54, and 55-64 years.

the names of the subtests, comprehension, information, vocabulary, etc. A sample of superior healthy men all over the age of 65 that we studied showed significantly higher over-all performance on verbal tests than their young counterparts. But their mean scores on the 5 performance items were lower than the younger men's scores. So I think this set of data requires differentiating concepts. With advancing age, one has an increasing store of information and, simultaneously, a change in a speed factor.

According to the physicians who examined them, a subgroup of 20 men out of the total group of 47 may have had subclinical or asymptomatic disease. It is interesting that these groups do not differ so much on the digit-symbol test as they do on the information or verbal items.

What I am suggesting is that disease—particularly vas-

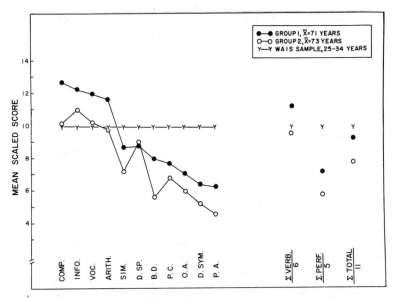

Fig. 30.—Comparison of subtest scores of the WAIS for three groups of subjects: young adult standardization group and groups I and II of the present study. The expected mean value for young adults (25-34 years) is 10 on each subtest.

cular disease—may lead to cortical damage, which in turn results in a loss of stored information. If the integrity of the nervous system is maintained, one should show a continually increasing amount of stored information, but this will not necessarily influence the reduction of speed of response with age.

A point I would like to raise in closing is this: how does the human deal with his increasing amount of information as he advances in age? From college age to age 60, one's vocabulary, in a group such as this, might go from 20,000 to 40,000 words out of a possible several hundred thousand words in the English language. If one is going to maintain communication at a conventional rate of speed, and this is one thing group behavior puts pressure on us to do, one has to communicate within normal time limits. It would seem to me that we either have to group our verbal associations in larger and larger units or concepts—our communication could become more redundant because we are dealing with larger series of associations—or go to another level, that is, increasing abstraction.

I think our behavior here is a way of trying to cope with the additional information that we acquire with age and because of which we are forced to higher levels of abstraction in order to maintain effective behavior in communication. In those individuals who are not disposed in this way, who operate with non-abstract concepts, communication perhaps becomes more redundant with age, that is, it has less information.

Jarvik: You tested a younger group of men as well, didn't you? Where would their information level be, on the same scale?

Birren: Absolutely flat, or equal among the subtests.

Jarvik: It was not superior to the older men in terms of education?

Birren: I think that our older men were not too different from the standardization sample.

Jarvik: I thought they were a superior group.

Birren: Superior in health but not necessarily greatly superior, say, in educational level: 20 had grade school or less; 11 high school; and 16 some college.

Jarvik: We have been engaged in a study of aging twins, including their intellectual competence, which ties in well with Dr. Birren's discussion. When we started, the twins were at least 60 years old and we have followed them for a period of about 12 years. They were tested at intervals, more or less irregularly, for a maximum number of four tests, most of them participating in three test sessions (25). Originally, there were 134 twin pairs, all of the same sex; that is, the two partners were of the same sex. These included 88 one-egg and 46 two-egg pairs.

First, from the genetic point of view, we found that the intellectual similarity which had been demonstrated for school-age twins persisted in the upper age groups, so that the differences in the test scores of one-egg twin partners were smaller than those for two-egg twins. The difference between the zygosity groups was consistent for all of the subtests.

We then analyzed the time changes—what changes occur in a given individual with advancing age. We found exactly what Dr. Birren has referred to: the most marked changes with time were seen on tests involving speed and motor co-ordination, that is, the digit-symbol substitution test and the simple paper-and-pencil tapping test. We tried to determine whether the decline on the digit-symbol test was purely due to deficits in speed of motor co-ordination. The answer was no, according to factor analysis carried out in collaboration with the late Professor I. Lorge. The hand-eye co-ordination factor did not account for all of the loss on this particular test.

Instead, the digit-symbol substitution test showed a positive relation also to the verbal factor (27).

In general, our longitudinal data agreed with the cross-sectional data, in that all tests showed a decline with advancing age, but of far lesser degree than would have been suspected from cross-sectional studies. Moreover, not all people declined. Some showed an increase in score during the follow-up period, some maintained unchanged scores, and some showed a decrease in score. A decrease in score occurred oftener than either an increase or a lack of change, accounting for the net loss in mean scores.

Subsequently, we analyzed the scores of persons who had at least three testings during the dozen years or so, in terms of having increased, remained unchanged, or decreased with time (Fig. 31). A very small percentage of subjects showed an increase on the tapping or the digit-symbol test, which are speeded tests of motor co-ordination; but more than 20% showed an increase in vocabulary score with advancing age, although they were between 60 and 80 years of age at the time of the first testing.

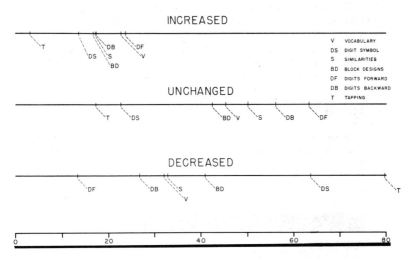

Fig. 31

Since our subjects were not all of the same age at the time of first testing, ranging from 60 years up, we wondered whether the older twins showed a decrease in score and the younger ones an increase. We have found no evidence for this (24).

Since we did not find any relationship between increase,

decrease, or unchanged scores with chronological age, we tried to find out if, for any given test, there was a relationship between change in score and survival. For this purpose we borrowed from clinical medicine the concept of 5-year survival. Unsatisfactory in many respects, it is the best we could find. Thus we examined the scores of those twins who had survived for 5 years or more after the last test, and those who had died within a 5-year period after the last test. We omitted the middle group, those still alive but for whom less than 5 years had elapsed since the last testing.

We examined each test separately for differences between the 5-year survivors and those who died within the 5-year period—the deceased group. We found that on the vocabulary test the survivors tended to show an increase rather than a decrease in score, while on the similarities and digit-symbol tests the "critical loss" represented an annual rate of decline exceeding 10 and 2%, respectively. These are purely empirical, retrospective figures which we derived from the data rather than having predetermined them.

When we plot "critical loss" for subjects alive 5 years after the last testing or dead within that period, we find that a critical loss was shown on one test or none by 22 out of 23 of the survivors, whereas only 4 of the 11 deceased fell into the same category (Fig. 32). Critical loss on two or all three of the tests was shown by 7 of the 11 deceased, and by only 1 of the 23 survivors. We postulated, therefore, that there may be

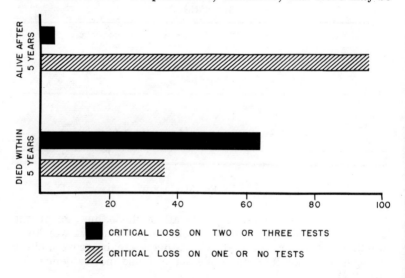

Fig. 32

a relationship between the rate of change on a psychological test, such as the digit-symbol substitution test, and some cerebral dysfunction. The change on these psychological tests may precede clinical symptoms, and that may be the reason for group differences in survival related to specific psychometric performance.

Sacher: Do you attribute this relation of test score and subsequent survival to the mental ability of the subjects or to the rate of deterioration of the mental ability of the given age groups? These results do not say that more intelligent people live longer, but rather that people of advanced age who are losing ability at a lesser rate have a greater probability of surviving through the inter-test interval.

Jarvik: We don't know. I should have mentioned this before and I am glad you have given me the opportunity to do so now. Originally, we found that people with the higher initial scores on most of the subtests tended to live longer than those with lower scores (26, 27). The question then arose of whether intelligence and life span are related, in the sense that people who start out being brighter also live longer. Or, is the relationship due to the fact that, when they entered our study at age 60 and over, the ones who had declined less appeared to be brighter, and their longer life could be related to relative lack of decline rather than initial difference in endowment. I don't think we have the final answer yet. First of all, there are differences from test to test. Only a few of the tests give us this specific decline associated with low survival. I think the best way would be to try to get data on people at younger ages and follow them for prolonged periods. There should be some data available, for instance, from the army: take a top-scoring group and lower-scoring group from the First World War, and see what their survival has been. That might give us an answer.

What we are doing here is purely speculative. Also, the conclusions we have drawn should be verified by prospective studies.

Brues: It is an intriguing idea that if a man was more intelligent when he was drafted into the army, he may be more likely still to be alive many years later. Obviously there is a great deal of information filed away. I suppose very few people have missed having an intelligence test of some sort at one time or another. Is there no current information bearing on that?

Jarvik: Dr. Owens (40) has followed a group for about 20 years now, but he has not completed the latest analyses. The first follow-up reports were compiled when the subjects were around the age of 40, and they failed to show the expected decline in intelligence. The curves based on cross-sectional studies had predicted that a demonstrable decline in intelligence would have occurred. By now, these ex-soldiers are close to the age of 60 and they are being followed and retested.

Brues: The problem we are concerned with is the extent to which aging leads to dullness, and the extent to which dullness leads to aging.

Fremont-Smith: I think it is also very interesting, and entirely appropriate, to look for the earliest changes of deterioration in the most complex functions. These are the psychological functions, and therefore, one would expect the changes in the central nervous system to show up first. I am delighted to see this come out. I think it is quite important to balance this possibility—of studying aging in terms of behavioral science—against the idea that the best things are going to be found in terms of millivolts, milliseconds, and milliequivalents. We should now be looking at milli-behavioral-units, also.

Atwood: It might be a nice idea to invent tests that are based on commonly accepted signs of aging. For example, I think everyone recognizes that with increasing age he becomes more prolix and more forgetful.

Fremont-Smith: Others recognize it.

Atwood: At least by simply asking people, "What do you think is going wrong with you?" one could probably arrive at a set of criteria that would be pertinent to the problem.

Quastler: We have finally heard today that one performance improves with age, and that is the vocabulary test. We are too much fascinated with degeneration with age.

Fremont-Smith: I agree with you. (Laughter)

Atwood: It must be a mistake. I don't see how anyone's vocabulary increases.

Quastler: There are other things that go up. As men grow older they can grow more coarse hair on the shoulders and out of the ears. What's wrong with that? Sure, we grow less hair on top of our heads, and this is considered more important than hair on the shoulders—but this value judgment may not be universally accepted.

Birren: I wonder if I can add a little note at this point about the output of a complex system being a rather sensitive

indication of change. I would like to underscore this and, perhaps, get Dr. Jarvik's reaction to it. Frequently, the psychologists regard behavior as being remote from the basic
changes. If one has a small change at a synapse, it might be
unobservable at the present time with the electron microscope or with chemical measurements. However, if we measure the output of a long chain of elements, we may see behavioral differences much earlier than a biological alteration can
be seen by the morphologist or the neurochemist. So, in a
sense, behavior can be a more sensitive indicator of underlying physiological change.

Jarvik: I agree. I also think that Dr. Atwood's idea of de-
vising special tests is a good one. Tests have been designed in
the past to measure the intelligence of school children, which
means to measure the potential educability of young children.
This is not really a valid concept when applied to adults, and
particularly to the older age group. If we could devise tests
for the older person, then it would be advisable to concentrate
upon specific functions instead of operating in terms of a
global intelligence.

Fremont-Smith: Would you agree that the global function may not even be sound with respect to school children?

Jarvik: I guess there is a good deal of discussion on that.

Sacher: Dr. Birren's remark about misfiring synapses
raises the question of loss of nervous tissue with age. My
reading of the literature leaves me with the impression that
it is still an equivocal point whether loss of nervous tissue is
a uniform characteristic of aging or a sequel to other patho-
logic changes.

Fremont-Smith: This reminds me of a question I wanted
to have raised, and that is: Are the signs and symptoms of decrepitude or failing with old age due to the loss of cells, which
we know takes place in most body systems, or are they due to
the still present, malfunctioning cells which, I suspect, are
very much larger in number than the cells that are lost?

Atwood: I don't see that there is anything equivocal about
the loss of nervous tissue. Data have been published on the
number of fibers in a ventral root and the number of cells in a
dorsal root ganglion that decrease with age (22a). The brain
weight, corrected for fluid differences, decreases (2a). I think
one can't ignore the reality of decrease in number of neuronal
elements with age.

Fremont-Smith: Are the symptoms and signs due to the

decrease in number, or to cells that haven't yet decreased in number but are malfunctioning and will continue to malfunction for another 4, 5, or 10 years?

Atwood: One could reasonably surmise that a decrease in number would inevitably affect the function.

Fremont-Smith: Patients with general paresis have marked atrophy of the frontal lobe, yet they may have remissions. Therefore, the symptoms they showed when they didn't have remission could not be due primarily to the loss of cells or to the frontal lobe atrophy; they are much more likely to be due to the cells that have not yet atrophied, that are, perhaps, at the point of being the next group to atrophy.

Brues: Also, could not some sort of base line be used for testing particular functions, such as the effects of removing substantial parts of the brain? I don't know whether that has been used as a sort of qualitative comparison for the particular changes that are being associated with aging.

I have another thought: It seems to me it would be important to look at these particular changes in the light of what might be called an atrophying of the will that occurs in people. I have heard it suggested that, for instance, the loss of memory for recent events represents a striving of the individual to contemplate or recapture an earlier time in his life, and so on. How many of these things might relate to that?

I should assume that the tests we were talking about are probably selected so as to be fairly free from content that might be psychogenically motivating.

Birren: In our data we would want to control volitional differences as much as possible, although it would still be a component. I did not elaborate on some of the data, such as the finding of a negative correlation between speed of response and hypertension. In individuals that have a somewhat elevated blood pressure, an association may be found between still higher blood pressure and increasing slowness of response. Therefore, it could conceivably be possible that if an individual did something about his hypertension, either by controlling the tempo of his life or by taking medication, his reaction time would be improved. Walter Spieth at the Federal Aviation Agency told me that some men they studied who had hypertension and were on hypotensive drugs were, indeed, faster in psychomotor speed than non-treated hypertensives.[*]

Fremont-Smith: I am very much interested in the ques-

_____
[*] Personal communication.

tion about loss of recent memory that you raised, Dr. Brues. As far as I know, all disease processes which interfere with memory interfere, primarily, with the most recent memory.

When a young person or a child gets a retrograde amnesia from a concussion, there is always the loss of the most recent memory. As the memory returns, or as recovery from aphasia takes place, that is, the return of capacity for speech, the first language learned comes back first. There was a very famous case of a man who had been born in Russia, lived in Germany, came over to this country, and learned English. He had concussion and aphasia, and his English was very much delayed in returning. This is a general law of the loss of memory and of the return of memory—the loss is always greatest for the most recent events. In fact, events that took place just before the injury may never again be remembered.

There is only one exception to this, as far as I know, and that is psychogenic loss of memory. Here one encounters the fugue states, and so forth, where a whole period of past memory may be blocked out. I think one can almost say that the longer a memory—whatever a memory is—resides in the brain, the less vulnerable it is.

Ehret: I think that James Miller's studies (39) on measures of performance in terms of information input overload and as a function of level of complexity are pertinent here. The channel capacity in bits per second was measured in different systems at cell, organ, individual, group, and social-organization levels. In every case, as one ascended the scale to higher complexity, overload came with fewer bits per time; that is, the larger the number of components, the lower the channel capacity, and the slower the channel. Now let's go a step further and consider group performance, as in an artillery gun crew, as a function of group age. At first the untrained crew would perform poorly, but in time they would improve with training (age). Then, carried to its limits in time, first one crew member then another would become less efficient; consequently crew efficiency would decrease, and the group as a unit would become senescent.

Birren: What I was suggesting, perhaps unclearly, is that at a conference like this we are faced with an information load and, like the gun crew or any other crew, we have to handle it within a certain time limit.

I believe we partly relieve the cognitive strain we feel in situations of this sort by forming new concepts. Thus the unit of information changes, and this is unlike physical systems. We can now, in a sense, improve our effectiveness by regrouping previous things under a superordinating concept. This is how we come out on top of the information load. I don't know an analogy of this in a physical system.

Sacher: Does this bear any relationship to the problem that is presented by the results of Lehman (34) on productivity and creativity as a function of age? He produces evidence, unfortunately contrary to Dr. Owens' (40), that these reach a peak by various kinds of objective measures—such as number of papers published or number of citations of the man's work in the literature of his subject—quite early in life. Yet one feels that the men in question have not by any means exhausted their potential. I wonder if, in effect, they have disappeared into larger organization groups. The individual man can no longer process the larger amount of information or complexity, and he moves up into and is part of an organization in which his contribution is no less important, but in which his personal recognition is decreased.

Atwood: He becomes a dean.

Fremont-Smith: There is a value judgment in the criteria selected there, papers published, etc., which I think can hardly be justified. One would have to use much better criteria of creativity than such grossly oversimplified functions.

Birren: One thing that should be mentioned is that as a person improves his performance, he tends to focus on critical elements of the task. Someone learning a new sport has to take on a mass of information. The skilled athletic performer, by contrast, only attends to the critical elements in the situation. Thus he is actually, in a sense, handling less information by focusing on critical elements, perhaps even as we do here. But this is almost equal, in my terms, to forming an abstraction or concept.

Ehret: I had a somewhat more pragmatic intention. It was related to Dr. Atwood's question about the sort of tests that would be useful for different populations over the country and of relative pertinence to one another. One should like to know if there are some systems, subsystems, components in the whole organism, which show information overload as a function of age and others which do not.

Atwood: In a recent paper, Ashby and Riquet (3) pointed out several inevitable features common to both biological and physical systems that handle information. They try to answer the question of how to avoid overwriting—overwriting being the wiping out of a piece of information in a certain address by another piece of information. There are only two ways of doing this, whether the system is a computer or a brain. One is to have information about the storage problem, so that one knows where the assigned addresses are or where there are storage locations that are no longer needed. The second way is to have just so many addresses that the chance of overwriting is small. They speculate that brains operate on the latter principle if they are adaptable ones, such as ours; possibly on the former principle if they are like spiders that always spin the same kind of web. Our brains are really big just to provide enough addresses so we don't overwrite in a problem.

Fremont-Smith: What does "overwrite" mean? There is no writing involved.

Atwood: An item of information is stored in a certain memory location, and in the subsequent course of the problem, it has to be brought out again and used. If, meanwhile, some other data have been stored in memory, one item may have gone to the occupied address and wiped out what was there previously. If a brain works this way, one consequence is that the dropping out of elements will have the effect of slowing it down. So the test of time needed for performance of computations, or something of this sort, would be a very good one. It would show there were fewer elements.

Lansing: We did make some reference to Lehmann's (34) work on age of maximum contribution. You may have been a little unfair, Dr. Fremont-Smith, in bringing up the matter of proper value judgment in the criteria used for measuring accomplishment. I thought Lehmann carefully avoided the hazard of using the volume, the mass of productivity. Rather, he used the maximal contribution of the individual as measured by the judgment of peers in the field. Major effort was made, if I am not mistaken, to avoid this pitfall of superficial value judgments.

It still remains impressive to me, though I don't like it, that maximal contribution is effected very early in life. I would much rather it was in midlife.

Atwood: Doesn't it make a difference what field is involved?

Lansing: Yes.

Fremont-Smith: Also, how wise. Many Nobel prize winners were not cited until they won the prize. Their work was so different from what was expected, people didn't like it because it interfered with their preconceptions.

Lansing: In all the fields we have referred to, the age of maximum contribution, whatever maximal contributions properly are, was quite early in life. Mathematics was much earlier than chemistry, and so on. It was either in the late 20's or 30's, and not in the 40's or 50's.

REFERENCES

1. Anderson, E. C., and W. H. Langham. 1959. Average potassium concentration of the human body as a function of age. Science 130: 713-14.

2. Andrew, W., N. W. Shock, C. H. Barrows, and M. Yiengst. 1959. Correlation of age changes in histological and chemical characteristics in some tissues of the rat. J. Gerontol. 14: 405-14.

2a. Appel, F. W., and E. M. Appel. 1942. Intracranial variation in the weight of the human brain. Human Biol. 14: 48-68 and 235-50.

3. Ashby, W. R., and J. Riguet. 1961. The avoidance of over-writing in self-organizing systems. J. Theoret. Biol. 1: 431-39.

4. Barrows, C. H., and L. M. Roeder. 1961. Effect of age on protein synthesis in rats. J. Gerontol. 16: 321-25.

5. Berg, B. N. 1956. Muscular dystrophy in aging rats. J. Gerontol. 11: 134-39.

6. Berg, B. N. 1960. Nutrition and longevity in the rat. I. Food intake in relation to size, health and fertility. J. Nutrition 71: 242-54.

7. Berg, B. N., and C. R. Harmison. 1955. Blood pressure and heart size in aging rats. J. Gerontol. 10: 416-19.

8. Berg, B. N., and C. R. Harmison. 1957. Growth, disease, and aging in the rat. J. Gerontol. 12: 370-77.

9. Berg, B. N., and H. S. Simms. 1960. Nutrition and longevity in the rat. II. Longevity and onset of disease with different levels of food intake. J. Nutrition 71: 255-63.

10. Berg, B. N., and H. S. Simms. 1961. Nutrition and longevity in the rat. III. Food restriction beyond 800 days. J. Nutrition 74: 23-32.

11. Berg, B. N., A. Wolf, and H. S. Simms. 1962. Degenerative lesions of spinal roots and peripheral nerves in aging rats. Gerontologia 6: 72-80.

12. Berg, B. N., A. Wolf, and H. S. Simms. 1962. Nutrition and longevity in the rat. IV. Food restriction and the radiculoneuropathy of aging rats. J. Nutrition 77: 439-42.

13. Birren, J. E. 1962. Age differences in learning a two-choice water maze by rats. J. Gerontol. 17: 207-13.

14. Birren, J. E., W. R. Allen, and H. G. Landau. 1954. The relation of

problem length in simple addition to time required, probability of
success, and age. J. Gerontol. 9: 150-61.

15. Birren, J. E., R. N. Butler, S. W. Greenhouse, L. Sokoloff, and M. R.
Yarrow. 1963. Human aging: a biological and behavioral study.
United States Public Health Service Publication No. 986. Washington,
D.C.: Government Printing Office.

16. Birren, J. E., P. V. Cardon, Jr., and S. L. Phillips. 1963. Reaction
time as a function of the cardiac cycle in young adults. Science 140:
195-96.

17. Birren, J. E., and H. Kay. 1958. Swimming speed of the albino rat.
I. Age and sex differences. J. Gerontol. 13: 374-77.

18. Birren, J. E., and D. F. Morrison. 1961. Analysis of the WAIS subtests in relation to age and education. J. Gerontol. 16: 363-69.

19. Birren, J. E., K. F. Riegel, and D. F. Morrison. 1962. Age differences in response speed as a function of controlled variations of
stimulus conditions: evidence of a general speed factor. Gerontologia
6: 1-18.

20. Botwinick, J. 1959. Drives, expectancies, and emotions. In J. E.
Birren (ed.), Handbook of aging and the individual: psychological and
biological aspects, pp. 739-68. Chicago: Univ. of Chicago Press.

21. Everitt, A. V. 1955. The loss in weight of ageing rats. Australas.
J. Med. Technol. 1: 41-45.

22. Everitt, A. V. 1957. The senescent loss of body weight in male rats.
J. Gerontol. 12: 382-87.

22a. Gardner, E. 1940. Decrease in human neurones with age. Anat.
Rec. 77: 529-36.

23. Goldspink, G. 1962. Studies on postembryonic growth and development of skeletal muscle. Proc. Roy. Irish Acad. 62 B: 135-50.

24. Jarvik, L. F., and A. Falek. 1963. Intellectual stability and survival
in the aged. J. Gerontol. 18: 173-76.

25. Jarvik, L. F., F. J. Kallmann, and A. Falek. 1962. Intellectual
changes in aged twins. J. Gerontol. 17: 289-94.

26. Jarvik, L. F., F. J. Kallmann, A. Falek, and M. M. Klaber. 1957.
Changing intellectual functions in senescent twins. Acta Genet. Statist. Med. 7: 421-30.

27. Jarvik, L. F., F. J. Kallmann, I. Lorge, and A. Falek. 1962. Longitudinal study of intellectual changes in senescent twins. In C. Tibbitts
and W. Donohue (eds.), Aging around the world: social and psychological aspects of aging, pp. 839-59. New York: Columbia Univ. Press.

28. Jerome, E. A. 1959. Age and learning—experimental studies. In J. E.

Birren (ed.), Handbook of aging and the individual: psychological and biological aspects, pp. 655-99. Chicago: Univ. of Chicago Press.

29. Johnson, H. D., L. D. Kintner, and H. H. Kibler. 1963. Effects of 48 F (8.9 C) and 83 F (28.4 C) on longevity and pathology of male rats. J. Gerontol. 18: 29-36.

30. Kay, H., and J. E. Birren. 1958. Swimming speed of the albino rat. II. Fatigue, practice, and drug effects on age and sex differences. J. Gerontol. 13: 378-85.

31. Kibler, H. H., H. D. Silsby, and H. D. Johnson. 1963. Metabolic trends and life span of rats living at 9C and 28C. J. Gerontol. 18: 235-39.

32. Kimball, A. W. 1958. Disease incidence estimation in populations subject to multiple causes of death. Bull. Inst. Internat. Statist. 36: 193-204.

33. Lacey, J. I., and B. C. Lacey. 1958. Relationship of resting autonomic activity to motor impulsivity. Res. Pub. Assoc. Res. Nerv. Ment. Dis. 36: 144-209.

34. Lehman, H. C. 1953. Age and achievement. Princeton: Princeton Univ. Press.

35. Lindop, P. J. 1961. Growth rate, lifespan and causes of death in SAS/4 mice. Gerontologia 5: 193-208.

36. McCay, C. M., M. F. Crowell, and L. A. Maynard. 1935. The effect of retarded growth upon the length of the life span and upon ultimate body size. J. Nutrition 10: 63-79.

37. McCay, C. M., L. A. Maynard, G. Sperling, and L. L. Barnes. 1939. Retarded growth, life span, ultimate body size and age changes in the albino rat after feeding diets restricted in calories. J. Nutrition 18: 1-13.

38. Miles, W. R. 1942. Psychological aspects of aging. In E. V. Cowdry (ed.), Problems of ageing (2d ed.), pp. 756-84. Baltimore: Williams and Wilkins.

39. Miller, J. G. 1962. Information input overload. In M. C. Yovits, G. T. Jacobi, and G. D. Goldstein (eds.), Self-organizing systems, pp. 61-78. Washington, D.C.: Spartan Books.

40. Owens, W. A., Jr. 1953. Age and mental abilities: a longitudinal study. Genet. Psychol. Monogr. 48: 3-54.

41. Richter, C. P. 1957. On the phenomenon of sudden deaths in animals and man. Psychosomatic Med. 19: 191-98.

42. Rockstein, M., and K. F. Brandt. 1961. Changes in phosphorus metabolism of the gastrocnemius muscle in aging white rats. Proc. Soc. Exper. Biol. Med. 107: 377-80.

43. Ross, M. H. 1959. Protein, calories and life expectancy. Fed. Proc. 18: 1190-1207.

44. Scheffé, H. 1959. The analysis of variance. New York: John Wiley.

45. Selye, H. 1950. Physiology and pathology of exposure to stress. Montreal: Acta.

46. Simms, H. S. 1946. Logarithmic increase in mortality as a manifestation of aging. J. Gerontol. 1: 13-26.

47. Simms, H. S., and B. N. Berg. 1957. Longevity and the onset of lesions in male rats. J. Gerontol. 12: 244-52.

48. Simms, H. S., and B. N. Berg. 1962. Longevity in relation to lesion onset. Geriatrics 17: 235-42.

49. Simms, H. S., B. N. Berg, and D. F. Davies. 1959. Onset of disease and the longevity of rat and man. In G. E. W. Wolstenholme and M. O'Connor (eds.), Ciba Foundation Colloquia on Ageing. 5. The lifespan of animals, pp. 72-79. Boston: Little, Brown.

50. Simms, H. S., B. N. Berg, and C. A. Slanetz. 1963. Uniform and favorable conditions for experimental rats. Laboratory Animal Care 13: 517-24.

51. Sokolov, E. N. 1960. Neuronal models and the orienting reflex. In M. A. B. Brazier (ed.), The central nervous system and behavior: Transactions of the Third Conference, pp. 187-276. New York: Josiah Macy, Jr., Foundation.

52. Spraragen, S. C., V. P. Bond, and L. K. Dahl. 1962. DNA synthesizing cells in rabbit heart tissue after cholesterol feeding. Circ. Res. 11: 982-86.

53. Swick, R. W., and D. T. Handa. 1956. The distribution of fixed carbon in amino acids. J. Biol. Chem. 218: 577-85.

54. Verzár, F. 1963. Lectures in experimental gerontology. Springfield, Ill.: Charles C Thomas.

55. Whipple, G. H. 1926. The hemoglobin of striated muscle. I. Variations due to age and exercise. Am. J. Physiol. 76: 693-707.

56. Yiengst, M. J., C. H. Barrows, and N. W. Shock. 1959. Age changes in the chemical composition of muscle and liver in the rat. J. Gerontol. 14: 400-404.

Changes in Structure and Performance of Cells and Tissues with Age

PART II

Barrows: I thought we would discuss some of the biochemical changes that we think occur in cells as a function of age. There is probably little doubt that there is a loss of cells with aging.

The work I shall report is done with rats. We do not have the elegant setup described by Dr. Simms, and we find 50% mortality in our animals at about 24 months. It is possible in some experiments to get 29-month-old survivors. Most of our studies are carried out on 24- to 27-month-old rats and 12-month-old rats.

The younger animals are certainly out of the growth phase. I think some of the earlier studies in cellular metabolism are complicated by the fact that comparisons were made between young, growing animals and senescent ones. I have been accused of not being interested in growth because of my criticism of this kind of study. The difficulty lies in deciding whether the differences observed are changes that occur during growth or senescence. Nevertheless there is good reason to believe that what happens during growth may have an impact on longevity. In some studies we did use young, growing animals.

We have used the McCollum strain of rat, so called because Dr. McCollum started it originally, back in 1924. Any time a friend had a nice rat, he would send it to McCollum to be incorporated into the colony. The McCollum rat has been used in various nutritional studies over many years.

Brues: Are they white rats?

152

Barrows: White, black, as well as others. We have also used the Sprague-Dawley strain obtained from Bethesda. On one occasion we were fortunate enough to obtain some 34-month- and 12-month-old wild rats from Dr. J. B. Calhoun.[*] We have not found any large strain differences. We have not routinely been able to have morphological examinations carried out on the animals. Occasionally, we have collaborated and consulted Dr. Warren Andrew,[†] Dr. Katherine Snell,[‡] and Dr. Donald Mach.

In general, we find the age changes in muscle tissue to be a loss of fibers. We do not see the striking changes in the kidney observed by Dr. Simms. Generally, we see a small infiltration of lymphocytes, at randomly distributed foci, but not to any large extent. We may find what I think the morphologists call colloid in the tubules, which probably is protein since we know the rat normally excretes protein in the urine and that there is an increase in the amount excreted with age.

Fremont-Smith: Do you find necrotic glomeruli that disappear?

Barrows: I have never seen them.

Fremont-Smith: In the human, as I understand, the newborn baby already has some necrotic glomeruli and it goes on progressively.

Barrows: This we did not see.

Fremont-Smith: Did you look for it?

Barrows: We have looked at tissue on three or four different series, but we do not do it routinely.

Fremont-Smith: Was a fairly careful search made through the kidney?

Barrows: Usually a segment through the middle of the kidney is fixed and then the morphologist can work in this area.

Fremont-Smith: That is a single section?

Barrows: Yes.

---

[*] Calhoun, J. B., Present address: Research Branch, National Institute of Mental Health, Bethesda, Maryland.

[†] Andrew, W., Present address: Department of Anatomy, Indiana University School of Medicine, Indianapolis 7, Indiana.

[‡] Snell, K. C., Present address: National Cancer Institute, Bethesda, Maryland.

Fremont-Smith: By law of chance, it will vary and it could easily be missed.

Barrows: We could miss it. We rarely ever see anything in the liver of these animals. The presence of large nuclei has been described, but their appearance is not very frequent. Even the people who see them will admit to this.

Lansing: When you say the large nuclei, are you referring to the polyploids?

Barrows: Yes, the giant ones, so to speak. Dr. Joseph Falzone (14) has isolated the nuclei. I think the frequency he found was 0.06% in senescent animals.

Brues: These nuclei are extraordinarily large. The rat liver normally contains huge superoctoploid nuclei.

Barrows: Their dimensions are greater than 15 μ.

Lansing: These go beyond the octoploids and the tetraploids.

Barrows: As we isolate the nuclei, I think almost 70% are tetraploid and 30% diploid, so that the frequency of the larger ones, at least by size estimations, is rather small.

Table 8 illustrates the magnitude of the basic change we find. The greatest change in loss of cells occurs in muscle tissue. We find, generally, some loss in the body weights of the senescent animals; the liver weight does not change very much.

TABLE 8

Effect of Age on Body Weight, Liver Weight, and Muscle Mass of the Hind Limb of Male Rats

	Young	Old	$P_{diff.}$
Body weight (g)	469 ± 19.6	433 ± 8.2	NS
Liver weight (g)	13.34 ± 0.82	13.05 ± 0.52	NS
Percentage of liver weight to body weight	2.85 ± 0.13	3.02 ± 0.13	NS
Muscle mass (g)	28.05 ± 2.01	18.45 ± 1.83	.003
Percentage of muscle mass to body weight	5.87 ± 0.33	4.23 ± 0.31	.002

Lansing: Didn't somebody say earlier that liver changes dramatically?

Barrows: Yes, Dr. Cottier said that about the mouse, I believe.

Cottier: Yes, in mice of our strain, more than 30 months old.

Lansing: Then the rat, in this respect, is quite different from the mouse.

Barrows: Don't forget, these are 24- to 27-month-old animals. I have no way of knowing what would happen in a 32- or 33-month-old rat. There was no difference in the liver weight of the 34-month-old wild rat as compared with a 21-month-old. In the 34-month-old wild rats, the gastrocnemius weight was only 45% of the weight of that of the 12-month-old animal (4).

Fremont-Smith: The body weight hasn't changed, but the muscle weight has. What is replacing the muscle to make up the body weight?

Barrows: Body weight has gone down.

Fremont-Smith: Not enough to account for the muscle. I gather there is a discrepancy between the loss in muscle mass—and maybe I am quite wrong—and the very slight loss of body weight.

Barrows: In this particular experiment, let us assume there is a 10 g loss in the muscle mass of a hind limb. In a rat this represents quite a lot of muscle mass. There is about a 40 g loss in body weight in these particular animals.

Keys: Are you saying, in effect, that the muscle mass elsewhere must be maintained?

Barrows: I don't know whether that occurs.

Keys: If other muscles are behaving this way, Dr. Fremont-Smith's question is pertinent. Either the muscle you measured is peculiar among muscles in the rat or it is similar to them. If it is similar to other muscle, there is some more weight recovery.

Fremont-Smith: Do you think there is enough room in the 40 g so it doesn't have to be replaced with water or fat or connective tissue?

Keys: I don't know about rats, but the muscle loss in people is about 50%.

Barrows: If one measures the body water in humans, there is, on the average, about a 15 to 20% loss of total body water. Assuming this is muscle, it is of this order of magnitude.

<u>Fremont-Smith</u>: Did you measure body water in the rats?

<u>Barrows</u>: No, we have not.

I would now like to discuss some biochemical studies we have done in these animals. Back in 1956 we reviewed the literature on cellular metabolism (3) and found a couple of points that looked interesting. One was that if one excised the liver or kidney and measured the oxygen uptake of kidney slices there did, indeed, seem to be a loss in oxygen uptake per unit wet weight with age. This more or less agreed with the drop in so-called BMR per unit surface area that one finds in man. Thus it all seemed to hold together. Most of the studies, however, were done on the young, growing rat and the question arose as to whether or not the weight of the tissue is a valid index of the number of cells.

At about the same time Dr. Shock (48) initiated studies which employed antipyrine space as an index of total body water. If the BMR was based on total water, an estimation of the total number of cells in man, the age difference was not observed. We wondered whether or not the age difference in tissue respiration was merely a reflection of the cells being crowded closer together in the young, growing animal. In order to study the effect of age on tissue respiration we had to have some index of the number of cells in the slices tested. We decided to use the concentration of DNA as the index of the number of cells. This, of course, depends on the fact that the DNA per nucleus is constant with age.

The first study we carried out with Dr. Falzone was the determination of the DNA content of nuclei isolated from the livers of young and old rats (Table 9).

TABLE 9

Age Comparison of Mean DNA per Nucleus in Rat Liver

(Values in $\mu\mu$g followed by standard error of the mean)

	Young	Old
Females	11.8 ± 0.43	12.6 ± 0.44
Males	11.9 ± 0.42	11.9 ± 0.53

We did not find any difference in the mean DNA per nucleus. We felt that our use of DNA as an index of the number of cells in these preparations was valid.

In the first studies we simply determined the oxygen uptake of slices of liver and kidney of young and old rats and based the values on the concentration of DNA in the individual slices.

The oxygen uptake of liver slices tends to be lower in the old animals. However, no statistical difference was observed. A similar pattern is observed in the concentration of DNA (Table 10). The decrement in the oxygen uptake of kidney slices was found to be statistically lower in the old animals. This decrease was about 10% and was approximately equal to the decrease in the concentration of DNA, so we feel that the oxygen uptake of cells does not change with age. The age-associated decrease in endogenous oxygen uptake previously described is due, I believe, to the use of growing animals, where the cellular density of the tissue is high, and to the use of poor indices of cell numbers.

TABLE 10

Effect of Age on Respiration of Liver and Kidney of Female Rats

	Young	Old	$P_{diff.}$	$\frac{\text{Young - old}}{\text{Young}}$ x 100
Liver				
Endogenous oxygen uptake (mm³O_2/100 mg wet wt./hr.)	114 ± 6	94 ± 10	NS	--
Desoxyribose nucleic acid (μg/100 mg wet wt.)	325 ± 9	306 ± 6	NS	--
Kidney				
Endogenous oxygen uptake (mm³O_2/100 mg wet wt./hr.)	378 ± 7	344 ± 10	.01	11
Desoxyribose nucleic acid (μg/100 mg wet wt.)	395 ± 6	366 ± 6	.01	8

At this time, data also became available on the concentration of various enzymes during the life span of both animals and man. I refer to the experiments by Kirk (11) on aortic tissue of men, by Zorzoli (55) on the liver of mice, and by Lightbody (32) on the liver of rats. A plot of the concentrations of these enzymes as a function of age indicated, in general, an increasing concentration during growth, a stable concentration during adulthood, and a decreasing concentration during senescence.

In the rat, stability is attained at approximately 4 to 6 months. However, Kirk (27, 28, 29) has shown that in humans the concentration of β-glucuronidase increases until the fifth or sixth decade. I would not associate this with growth.

On the other hand, the concentration of alkaline phosphatase of liver and plasma was found to decrease during early life, remain stable during adulthood, and increase during senescence.

Being naive, I thought that looked fine. If that were so, maybe one could discover the basic mechanism controlling the enzyme concentrations and how it is affected by age.

Sacher: Did the alkaline phosphatase go down from birth onward?

Barrows: The youngest animals employed by Zorzoli were 1 month old. In the experiments of Clark and Shock (9), the youngest individual was a 1-year-old infant.

So, our first study was simply an excursion, to see whether there was any truth to the concept that something went wrong with the regulatory mechanism.

In Table 11 is presented the data on the changes in the concentration of enzymes in the liver and kidneys of 1-, 3-1/2-, 12-, and 24-month-old rats. As you see, the concentration of succinoxidase in the liver increases during the early part of life, is stable during adulthood, and tends to be lower in the oldest animals. This same pattern is observed with pyrophosphatase, cholinesterase, and D-amino oxidase. Essentially the same pattern is observed in kidney. In all these data, the only statistical change is the decrement of succinoxidase in kidney in senescent animals. In Table 12 the concentrations of the other enzymes are presented. As you see, the alkaline phosphatase did decrease during growth. We were unable to demonstrate the increased concentration associated with senescence as suggested in earlier studies. The changes in the concentrations of acid phosphatase and the cathepsin with age were not similar to those exhibited by alkaline phosphatase.

Tyler: These are all on a wet-weight basis?

Barrows: Yes. The changes in the concentration of DNA are shown in Table 12.

Tyler: I am still trying to puzzle out the results. What were your conclusions with regard to DNA? There is this reduction in liver size that occurs with age, which most people seem to agree about. Is that right, and is this a reduction in cell number?

Barrows: On a gross-weight basis, we do not find reduction in liver size with age. The concentration of DNA (per gram wet weight of liver tissue) tends in some studies to drop perhaps only 10%. This is the most we have ever been able to find.

Tyler: I was referring to the over-all reduction in liver size with age. Was there agreement about this earlier today?

TABLE 11

Effect of Age on Various Enzymes of the Livers and Kidneys of Female Rats

(Enzymatic activities expressed per 100 mg wet wt./hr.)

Age (Mo.)	N	Succinoxidase: mm^3O_2 consumed	Pyrophosphatase: μg P liberated	Cholinesterase: mm^3CO_2 evolved	D-amino acid oxidase: mm^3O_2 consumed
Liver					
I	10	1,758 ± 44	9,180 ± 640	47.4 ± 4.6	47.3 ± 6.5
3.5	10	2,152 ± 84	14,440 ± 490	63.8 ± 9.8	58.2 ± 6.3
12	10	2,212 ± 40	13,290 ± 450	108.6 ± 11.8	81.5 ± 5.7
24	10	1,870 ± 34	13,420 ± 500	120.0 ± 5.4	78.3 ± 4.0
Kidney					
1	10	2,936 ± 128	2,980 ± 140		
3.5	10	4,172 ± 148	5,190 ± 190		
12	10	3,944 ± 144	5,130 ± 190		
24	10	3,448 ± 144	5,540 ± 310		

TABLE 12

Effect of Age on Various Enzymes of the Livers and Kidneys of Female Rats
(Enzymatic activities expressed per 100 mg wet wt./hr.)

Age (Mo.)	N	Alkaline phosphatase: μg P liberated	Acid phosphatase: μg P liberated	Cathepsin: μg tyrosine liberated	Desoxyribose nucleic acid: μg
Liver					
1	10	390 ± 17	550 ± 24	640 ± 49	323 ± 7.0
3.5	10	270 ± 9	560 ± 63	640 ± 37	378 ± 11.2
12	10	280 ± 15	520 ± 20	680 ± 43	392 ± 14.5
24	10	270 ± 82	520 ± 29	1,080 ± 58	368 ± 8.0
Kidney					
1	10	6,080 ± 360		1,010 ± 100	544 ± 21.0
3.5	10	7,780 ± 540		1,440 ± 60	424 ± 25.6
12	10	6,580 ± 620		1,290 ± 40	439 ± 11.3
24	10	6,360 ± 548		1,780 ± 100	394 ± 14.0

Barrows: Dr. Cottier said his experience has been that the liver weight decreases in old mice.

Fremont-Smith: Is there any information on other species? Do we know anything about man's liver weight with age?

Barrows: I do not know. The kidney weight in man decreases markedly in senescence. How much of this is complicated by inanition due to closing off of the renal arteries, I think, is anybody's guess. To continue, the alkaline phosphatase didn't change in senescent animals, whereas the cathepsin increased markedly in old animals. There is about a 50% increase per cell. In this particular series, it is also true in kidney. We do not always find the increase in kidney consistently as we do in the liver. We have repeated this in five groups of animals of different strains and have found it four out of five times. One time we did not find it, but that time we had received some animals from the outside, whose age could very well be questioned. But the general concept that I thought we could use as a working model does not seem acceptable. I think it is much too complicated; things are going in too many directions to try to make any generalizations regarding enzyme changes.

Jarvik: I am a bit puzzled. In dealing with DNA of tissues, wouldn't one expect a higher value for liver, with polyploid cells, than for kidney? Or are there more cells in kidney tissue?

Barrows: In a growing animal, I am not sure DNA in the liver can really be used as an index of cell numbers, because the frequency of binucleate cells decreases quite precipitously during the early growth phase, while at the same time the degree of polyploidy increases. So, up to 3-1/2 months, the DNA in liver is a nebulous thing in terms of cell number; after cessation of growth it is valid.

Jarvik: Would you say there are fewer cells per gram of tissue in liver than in kidney, to explain your finding of very similar values for the DNA content in diploidy and in polyploidy?

Barrows: That can be calculated on the basis that the DNA content of liver is 11 $\mu\mu$g and that of kidney is 66 $\mu\mu$g.

Brues: I would be just as willing, or more willing, in view of what we know about how enzymes are made, to consider that the amount of DNA is a good basis, as to quibble about how many cells the DNA is in.

Barrows: If one compares the same tissue in adult animals, it is a reasonable index.

Cottier: When you saw round-cell infiltrates in the kidney, did you correct for their DNA content?

Barrows: No.

Cottier: Were there any round-cell infiltrates in the liver?

Barrows: We have not seen them. We see them in the kidney, but never to any large extent. It is a localized phenomenon. Fifteen, 20, or 30 may be gathered in one little area, and that is about it.

Brues: That is a very important point. I would like to modify my remark and include consideration of the different sorts of cell in the liver. If the relative numbers of the various types of cells shift, that is important.

Barrows: Here, again, we don't see any big differences. Throughout all of these studies, decreases in DNA per unit wet weight is about 10%. It is never very much larger than that. The increased cathepsin found in old animals is interesting, for, as you all know, it is an intracellular proteolytic enzyme. I can suggest only one explanation for the cathepsin in the cell: we know that the amino acid composition of cells is pretty small relative to the total protein content, and it may be that when the cell is breaking down one kind of enzyme or protein to build up another, the availability of the amino acids is brought about by this proteolytic enzyme. The marked increase of cathepsin in the liver of senescent animals suggests that there may be differences in the rate of protein degradation. Therefore, it was of interest to determine whether age-associated differences in protein synthesis could be demonstrated. We did this by the depletion-repletion method, which is simply feeding the animals a protein-free diet, which, of course, produces marked changes in the enzyme concentrations. The animals were then refed and the concentrations of the enzymes determined at two points during the refeeding period.

Figure 33 shows the results. There are a number of interesting points. One is that the enzymes that increased during growth are those that decreased during the feeding of a protein-free diet. On the other hand, those enzymes that did not increase during growth changed very little during the experimental procedure. It is intriguing that one can categorize the enzymes under these two conditions.

There are no major age differences in either the rate of

loss of the enzymes or the recovery, with the possible exception of the D-amino acid oxidase. This difference, however, is between the young, growing animals and the adult ones. Thus, these data offer no evidence that there is impairment in protein synthesis by the liver cell under these experimental conditions.

Figure 34 shows the data obtained on the kidney. The decreases in the enzyme concentrations in the kidney are not as great as those seen in the liver. The alkaline phosphatase, for some unknown reason, decreased. There is no evidence of impairment in the synthetic capacity of old kidney cells under these circumstances.

Since it can be argued that this experimental procedure does not measure protein synthesis in normal animals, studies employing radioactive materials were initiated. In these studies, radioactive methionine was injected into 12- and 24-month-old rats, and we measured the rate of disappearance of activity. I am not really sure we did this experiment wisely, because we killed after 1 week, 2 weeks, 3 weeks, and 4 weeks.

We found large individual variability in this study. I am not quite sure that it would not have been better to employ fewer animals at a given time and use more time points.

Table 13 presents the slopes of the lines describing the disappearance of the isotope from the proteins of the various tissues. Although there is, on the average, an increase of approximately 28% in the slope of the line obtained in the livers of the old as compared with the young rats, this difference was not found to be statistically significant. No other age-associated differences are apparent.

Quastler: Did you check primary uptake?

Barrows: We were afraid we would get more variability in the upswing than we would in the downswing. Here, again, perhaps we were wrong; I don't know. Incidentally, the work was carried out in conjunction with the experiments on mitochondrial turnover carried out by Fletcher and Sanadi (17).

The next point I wish to discuss regards the greater decrease in the concentration of succinoxidase than cellular loss. Some of our earlier studies indicate that this decrement also occurred when cytochrome C oxidase and succinic dehydrogenase were measured in kidney homogenates.

Since these enzymatic activities are believed to be associated with mitochondria, the results suggest that aging is accompanied by either (a), a uniform reduction in the activities of these enzymes per mitochondrion, or (b), a loss of mitochondria from kidney cells. The present study was an attempt to determine which of these alternatives is more likely. Thus

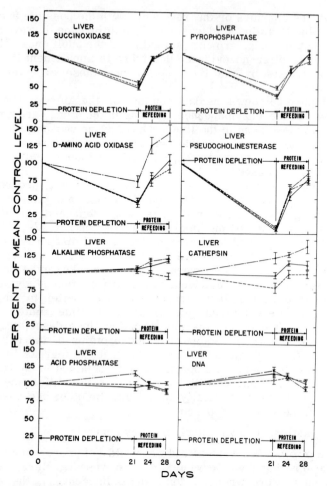

Figs. 33 and 34.—The mean enzymatic activities for the depleted, 3-day repleted, and 7-day repleted animals are expressed as the percentage of the mean enzymatic activity of the normal animals of corresponding age. The standard errors of the means are expressed as the percentages of the adjusted means and are represented by the vertical bars. (———·——— = 3.5-month-old animals, --- = 12-month-old animals, ——— = 24-month-old animals.)

the succinoxidase activities of whole homogenates as well as isolated mitochondria of liver and kidney cortex were measured in young (12-14 months) and old (24-27 months) rats of both sexes. Another metabolic system associated with mitochondria—succinate-stimulated oxidative phosphorylation—was measured in whole homogenates to determine whether an

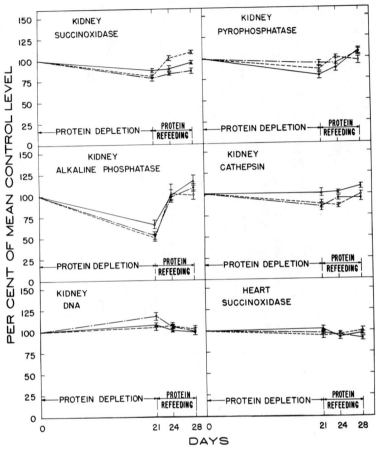

Fig. 34.

age-related decrement occurred in kidney cortex or in liver. The concentrations of DNA and protein nitrogen in the homogenates as well as the protein nitrogen contents of the mitochondrial preparations were determined.

A significant age-related decrease (11%) in the activities of succinoxidase of homogenates prepared from kidney cortical tissue of both male and female rats was observed (Table 14). Similar age-dependent decreases in the rates of succinate-stimulated oxidative phosphorylation of these homogenates were also found. In contrast, the concentration of DNA and protein nitrogen per unit wet weight did not decrease in the kidney tissue of the old rats. No age-dependent decrements in the succinoxidase activity, based on the protein nitrogen con-

TABLE 13

Rate of Disappearance of Radioactivity from Various Tissues of Young and Old Rats Following Administration of S^{35}-Labeled Methionine

Age	N	Liver k*	Kidney k	Heart k	Muscle k
			Experiment 1		
Old (24 mo.)	11	.298 ± .080	.299 ± .029	.162 ± .024	.034 ± .031
Young (12 mo.)	10	.226 ± .041	.279 ± .027	.122 ± .022	.040 ± .029
			Experiment 2		
Old (24 mo.)	9	.291 ± .010	.228 ± .062	.116 ± .022	.057 ± .028
Young (12 mo.)	13	.237 ± .056	.227 ± .042	.115 ± .017	.014 ± .020

*k from equation, log S. A. = kt + b, where S. A. = cpm/mg benzidine sulfate and t = time in weeks.

TABLE 14

The Effect of Age on Succinate-stimulated Metabolism of Whole Homogenates and Mitochondria from Kidneys of the Rat

	Females				Males			
	Young	Old	$P_{diff.}$	$\frac{Young - old}{Young} \times 100$	Young	Old	$P_{diff.}$	$\frac{Young - old}{Young} \times 100$
Whole homogenates								
N	13	11			10	13		
Succinoxidase (mm^3O_2/100 mg wet wt./hr.)	3,472 ± 56	3,096 ± 112	.01	11	3,292 ± 116	2,932 ± 88	.01	11
Oxidative phosphorylation O(μatoms/150 mg wet wt./20 min.)	11.4 ± 0.25	10.3 ± 0.26	.01	11	11.9 ± 0.20	10.6 ± 0.36	.01	11
P(μmoles/150 mg wet wt./20 min.)	19.1 ± 0.31	17.0 ± 0.94	.05	10	22.0 ± 0.92	18.7 ± 0.68	.01	15
P/O	1.7 ± 0.04	1.7 ± 0.08	NS	0	1.8 ± 0.06	1.9 ± 0.04	NS	-1
Desoxyribose nucleic acid (μg/100 mg wet wt.)	366 ± 6.0	356 ± 7.5	NS	3	355 ± 8.4	359 ± 6.0	NS	-2
Protein nitrogen (mg/100 mg wet wt.)	2.52 ± 0.024	2.44 ± 0.045	NS	5	2.57 ± 0.037	2.47 ± 0.036	NS	4
Mitochondria								
Succinoxidase (mm^3O_2/mg PN/hr.)	4,014 ± 106.8	4,077 ± 93.5	NS	-2	3,902 ± 68.0	3,726 ± 90.0	NS	4
Protein nitrogen (μg/cc (OD 320 m = 0.100))	47.2 ± 1.40	47.6 ± 1.44	NS	-1	51.6 ± 0.84	49.2 ± 1.06	NS	4

tent of mitochondria isolated from kidney cortical tissue, were established. Comparisons of the protein nitrogen content of mitochondria from young and old rats, based on the turbidimetric estimation of the number of particles within the suspension, also failed to demonstrate any differences.

The data of this experiment agree with our previous report that a decrement in the concentration of succinoxidase relative to that of DNA per unit wet weight is found in the kidney but not in the liver of senescent rats. The magnitude of this decrement, 11%, is approximately equal to that previously observed. In this experiment, the rates of oxidative phosphorylation decreased in kidney homogenates by approximately the same per cent as the concentration of succinoxidase. The evidence that these changes represent a loss of mitochondria rather than changes in the enzyme concentrations per mitochondrion is found in the lack of an age difference in the concentration of succinoxidase per unit of mitochondrial protein nitrogen.

We interpret these data to mean there are 10 to 15% fewer mitochondria per cell in the kidneys of old rats. One question that still remains is whether these data mean that of 100 cells, 90 have a full complement of mitochondria and 10 have practically none, and that the latter are in the process of dying. The answer to this question lies in the hands of the histochemist.

Our next series of studies was stimulated by some of the earlier work Dr. Shock (37) did on human subjects. In the following experiment, the physiological responsiveness of tubule cells to vasopressin* was determined in men of different ages. Maximum diuresis was effected by the oral administration of water during a pre-experimental period, and by intravenous infusion of dextrose to which was added inulin prior to the administration of Pitressin. The results of this experiment are shown in Figure 35. The ratio of the inulin concentration in urine to that in plasma is plotted against time. During maximum water diuresis, most of the material filtered by the glomeruli passes on through the tubules and appears in the urine, so that the urine-to-plasma ratio of inulin is relatively low. Following the administration of Pitressin, there is a pronounced increase in the urine-plasma ratio for inulin, indicating an increase in the amount of water reabsorbed by the tubules. The response in the old individuals was considerably less than in the young.

These data indicate that the tubule cells in the older individual show a reduced responsiveness to a physiological

---

*"Pitressin," Parke, Davis and Company.

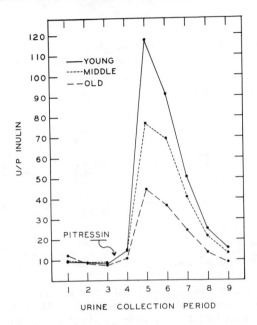

Fig. 35.—Mean values of U/P inulin ratio for each of 3 age groups before and after the intravenous administration of Pitressin. Urine collection periods 1-9 represent 9 consecutive 12-minute periods. Pitressin was administered immediately after the conclusion of period 3.

stimulus for increased osmotic work. In order to pursue this idea further, we used the technique described by Cross and Taggart (10), which measures the ability of kidney slices to concentrate p-amino hippurate (PAH). Differences in the concentration of enzymes or in metabolic rates are more readily demonstrated under conditions which insure maximum initial rates of reaction, namely, high levels of substrate. Therefore, in the present study, a system employing high concentrations of PAH (200 μg/ml) in the medium was used. In addition, for purposes of comparison, a modification of the system described by Cross and Taggart (10) was included, which employed a low concentration of PAH (4 μg/ml).

In the first series of studies, we kept the concentration in the medium low, so that a small number of moles, S, would pass across the membrane, but one would expect a high concentration gradient, S/M.

The results are shown in Table 15. Under this set of circumstances, we did not find an age difference in the kidney slices of these rats. DNA, in this case, dropped about 10%; so the PAH per DNA does not change.

TABLE 15

Accumulation of PAH (S/M) by Kidney Slices of Rats of Different Ages

Age (Mo.)	N	S/M[*]	S[*]	DNA mg/g	PAH/DNA µg/mg
2-3.5 (Mn = 2.7)	13	8.12 ±0.27	32.3 ±1.0	3.94 ±0.11	8.26 ±0.53
12-15 (Mn = 13.5)	12	8.18 ±0.25	31.7 ±0.9	3.82 ±0.07	8.59 ±0.27
26-33 (Mn = 28)	13	7.97 ±0.33	31.1 ±1.3	3.61 ±0.07	8.59 ±0.22
Significance of differences					
Young vs. adult		NS	NS	NS	NS
Adult vs. senescent		NS	NS	< .05	NS
Young vs. senescent		NS	NS	.02	NS

[*]S = µg PAH/g tissue, and M = µg PAH/ml medium.

Preliminary studies indicated that one can get more PAH in the slice by increasing the concentration. Maximal PAH accumulation was found to be brought about by 200 µg/ml in the medium. The rate of PAH accumulation, expressed as S - M, is shown in Figure 36. For the first 30 min, initial maximal rates are observed; between 30 and 60 min the S - M value is stable. After 60 min, there may be a decrease in the S - M.

In the next series of studies, we measured the initial rate of PAH uptake and also the peak rate. The results are shown in Table 16.

In 15 min, the initial rates of these reactions, as expressed by the amount of PAH actively transported, are not different at the three ages tested. DNA drops a little and PAH per DNA does not. If the reaction is allowed to continue for 60 min, a rather large age difference becomes apparent (Table 17). This decrease exceeds the drop in DNA; so that would imply that the amount of PAH actively transported per cell is quite different. One can calculate the amount of work done in this system since the S and the M are known.

In terms of work done, there is roughly a 50% decrease in the ability to perform osmotic work in this system.

Atwood: Doesn't the PAH come out of the slice again?

Barrows: It does. If the slice is taken out of the system, put in saline and left there for an unusually long time, there will be run-out.

Atwood: Since the initial rates are not different, it is

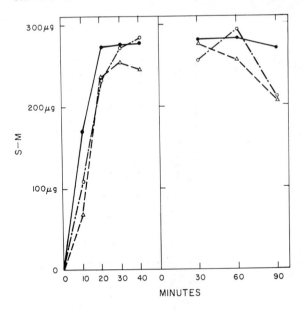

Fig. 36.—Accumulation of PAH by rat-kidney slices expressed as S-M following various times of incubation in a medium containing 200 μg PAH/cc. The curves represent data obtained from six individual animals. Three animals were used to determine PAH uptake during the early part of the curve and three for the latter part of the curve.

necessary to find out why the final level is different. This could be explained by the fact that PAH runs out more rapidly in the old cell.

Barrows: That is true. Difference in run-out could be one explanation. The amount of run-out is a function of available energy. For instance, run-out can be increased by putting in 2,4-dinitrophenol. It may be that there is a difference in the stability of the mitochondria.

It may well be, also, that there is some limiting factor in the PAH-uptake mechanism itself. We don't know, but we are still working on it.

Generally, I think the point is that one can demonstrate differences in metabolic systems at the cellular level as a function of age. This can be shown in the succinoxidase data, in loss of mitochondria per cell in the PAH system, and also in the cathepsin system.

Atwood: Still, if the lesser accumulation of PAH is due to run-out, then the same amount of work could have been done, but one would calculate that less was done. If the kidney slice just pumps the PAH around in a circle, it has to do just as much work.

TABLE 16

Effect of Age on the Accumulation of PAH by Kidney Slices of Female Rats

(M = 200 μg PAH/cc; t = 15 minutes)

Age (Mo.)	N	S	S - M	S/M	DNA* (mg/g)	Work min. (Cal x 10^{-7}/g)	$\frac{Work\ min.}{DNA}$	S - M/DNA
2-3.5 (Mn = 2.7)	10	383.3 ± 11.3	186.8 ± 9.2	1.89 ± 0.05	4.33 ± 0.11	77.5 ± 5.4	18.0 ± 1.4	42.7 ± 2.6
12-15 (Mn = 13.5)	10	382.1 ± 10.5	178.6 ± 11.0	1.88 ± 0.05	4.03 ± 0.06	76.6 ± 5.3	19.0 ± 1.3	44.1 ± 2.3
26-33 (Mn = 28.0)	9	372.8 ± 12.2	169.2 ± 11.5	1.82 ± 0.05	3.86 ± 0.14	71.2 ± 5.6	18.5 ± 1.7	44.0 ± 2.5

*Young vs. adult, $P_{diff.} < .05$, and young vs. senescent, $P_{diff.} = .01$.

TABLE 17

Effect of Age on the Accumulation of PAH by Kidney Slices of Female Rats

(M = 200 μg PAH/ml; t = 60 minutes)

Age (Mo.)	N	S	S - M	S/M	DNA (mg/g)	$Work_{min.}$ (Cal x 10^{-7}/g)	$\dfrac{Work_{min.}}{DNA}$	S - M/DNA
2-3.5 (Av = 2.7)	10	481.4 ± 8.8	273.0 ± 8.8	2.41 ± 0.05	4.11 ± 0.09	127.7 ± 5.2	37.4 ± 1.9	66.9 ± 3.2
12-15 (Av = 13.5)	10	433.0 ± 14.4	224.4 ± 13.4	2.07 ± 0.06	3.91 ± 0.05	100.4 ± 7.3	30.8 ± 2.3	57.5 ± 3.4
26-33 (Av = 28.0)	9	376.1 ± 14.8	164.9 ± 13.7	1.77 ± 0.06	3.77 ± 0.08	68.6 ± 6.6	22.2 ± 2.3	46.0 ± 3.8
Significance of differences								
Young vs. adult		.01	<.01	<.001	.05	.005	.05	.05
Adult vs. senescent		.01	<.01	<.005	NS	.005	.02	.01
Young vs. senescent		<.001	<.001	<.001	.01	<.001	<.001	<.001

<u>Barrows</u>: How do you envision a run-out—a passive run-out?

<u>Atwood</u>: I don't know what it is like. Is the membrane full of holes? Do the tubules fill up in the lumen?

<u>Barrows</u>: We don't know where the PAH is in the system. That is one of the major binds. Run-out can be effected by inhibiting the energy production. If that is the case, the limitation on the old rat is maintaining this energy level for the same period of time.

<u>Atwood</u>: When the PAH diffuses into the slice, structural differences between young and old may prevent it from encountering the same amount of cell surface.

<u>Barrows</u>: This is not seen initially, Dr. Atwood.

<u>Brues</u>: I am not quite sure I understand the argument here. Is it that it takes work to get the PAH into the cell, and work to keep it in, and that the first kind of work is being done equally well, and the second kind not so well by the older tissue? Is that the point?

<u>Barrows</u>: I am not quite sure whether these are two discrete systems or whether this is an equilibrium kind of situation.

<u>Steinbach</u>: You may well be dealing with some sort of active uptake mechanism, and some sort of a leak. What is in the tissue depends upon a balance between the pump and a leak, and the metabolic inhibitor could conceivably affect either. It would be nice if it could be done on an influx-outflux basis. We wouldn't have the particular argument that is going on now. On the basis of net changes, it probably can't be really settled.

<u>Barrows</u>: I would like to discuss one or two things that may perhaps be of further interest. One is something that Dr. Simms talked about earlier—the experimental increase in life span through dietary manipulation.

My understanding is that most people who have studied experimental increase in life span feel that one is simply speeding up or retarding the normal physiological and biochemical processes in the organism. When one increases the life span, it is like taking a rubber band or an accordion and opening it way out. When one shortens the life span, one has, essentially, squeezed it all together.

Our first study was designed to test this concept on the basis of changes in the enzyme concentrations as a function of age during the growth phase.

We have said that enzymes may increase or decrease

during growth. It seems that if one is doing nothing but extending the life span by retarding the growth processes, the enzymes that increase in the normal rats should increase at a slower rate in the retarded ones, whereas those that decrease should do so at a lower rate. This would give credence to the opinion that the normal physiological process is slowed down.

Dr. Ross (44) has done an experiment similar to those of Dr. Simms (5) and Dr. McCay (35), but he used various diets. The only data available are for a comparison of laboratory animals fed Purina Chow ad lib with a group of animals fed an 8% casein diet ad lib. These later animals, as I said earlier, will select less food and grow more slowly, but their life span will be increased approximately 50%.

Dr. Ross did, indeed, measure the activity of various enzymes in the liver at various ages in the two groups of animals. His results indicated that during early life, the liver has a lower ATPase activity in restricted rats than in the animals fed ad lib. The activity of alkaline phosphatase in liver of restricted rats was higher than in the controls. Thus these data indicate that the restricted rats were similar to chronologically younger animals.

However, as we showed in the protein-free feeding study, the enzymes that increase during growth decrease markedly during protein-free feeding. Ross has shown that under this experimental condition, the alkaline phosphatase activity increases. So under conditions of poor protein nutrition one would expect the changes described by Ross (45). There are two variables here. One is the protein content of the diet, and the other is the amount of food consumed. For these reasons, in our experiment we used the method of Drs. Simms and Berg (5); that is, we gave a less-than-adequate diet to young, growing animals.

The design of the experiment was this: we would feed the ad lib rats and measure the daily intake; 2 days later we would feed half that amount of food to the restricted rats. We had another group which we restricted throughout the total growth period; then we released them and let them eat all they wanted.

The daily food intake of the animals fed ad lib increased from 9 g at weaning to 22 g within 6 weeks and was essentially constant thereafter (Fig. 37). The intake of the restricted rats was, by experimental design, one-half that of the controls. The food consumption of the released animals following the return to ad libitum feeding increased rapidly to that of the controls.

The growth curves of the animals are shown in Figure 38. A typical growth curve for animals fed ad libitum was obtained from the control group. The mean body weight of the

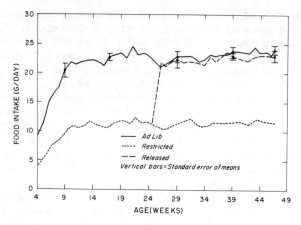

Fig. 37.—Food consumption of ad libitum, restricted, and released rats.

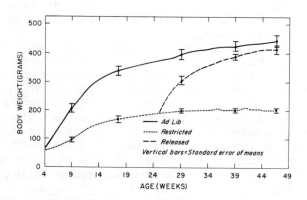

Fig. 38.—Growth curves of ad libitum, restricted, and released rats.

restricted rats increased to approximately 200 g and remained relatively constant thereafter. The body weight of the released animals increased rapidly after food was offered ad libitum and was not significantly different from that of the controls at the time of sacrifice.

Reduced dietary intake had no effect on the activities of D-amino acid oxidase and alkaline phosphatase of liver (Fig. 39). The activities of these enzymes in the tissues of released animals were also the same as those of the controls. However, a significantly higher succinoxidase activity was observed in restricted compared with ad libitum–fed rats. This change due

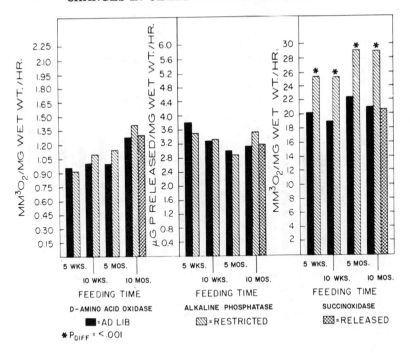

Fig. 39.—Effects of reduced dietary intake on enzymatic activities in the livers of male rats.

to restriction was reversible since the activity returned to normal after ad libitum feeding.

D-amino acid oxidase activity of kidney tissue was not altered by reduced dietary intake (Fig. 40). In contrast to liver, however, the activity of succinoxidase in kidney remained unchanged following restriction. On the other hand, a marked increase in alkaline phosphatase activity was found in restricted compared with normal animals. Similar to the results obtained on liver tissue, the enzymatic activities in the kidneys of released rats were the same as those of the controls. The livers and kidneys of the animals fed for 5 or 10 months were also analyzed for the activities of pyrophosphatase and cathepsin and the concentrations of DNA and protein nitrogen. Except for a small (10%) increase in the concentration of protein nitrogen of liver, no effects of dietary restriction were found in any of these tissue components.

Lansing: All on the wet-weight basis?

Barrows: Yes.

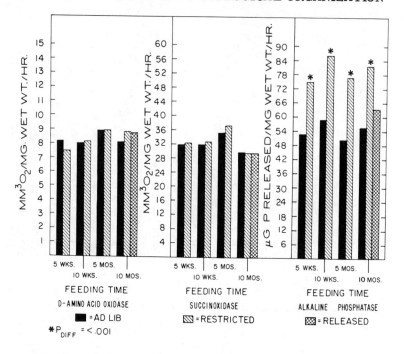

Fig. 40.—Effects of reduced dietary intake on enzymatic activities in the kidneys of male rats.

Lansing: Wouldn't it be more meaningful if the data were plotted as enzyme activity per cell, or per unit DNA?

Barrows: We had the DNA data. There is no difference in the 5- and the 10-month-old. I did not determine DNA on the young, growing animals because, as I said, I don't know what it means. There is some slight increase in the DNA, about 6 or 7%, at 5 months and 10 months. Basically, these data are based per cell or DNA.

In addition to the enzymes I have mentioned, we did five or six others at 5 and 10 months, and they did not differ from the controls. These data imply to me that there are biochemical differences in rats whose life expectancy is increased through dietary manipulation, but they are not necessarily those of chronologically younger animals. So I feel these data do not support the concept of simple retardation of normal physiological and biochemical changes.

Simms: This morning I pointed out that five diseases, and there are actually more, are affected by underfeeding. If Dr. Barrows' concept is right, that would mean that the changes in these two enzymes might be responsible for the delayed onset of lesions of five or six different types of disease. Do you think that is possible? There must be some common factor between at least six diseases that is influenced, on the one hand, by underfeeding and, on the other hand, by sex. The females have similar delay in onset of the same diseases. Obviously, there is some underlying factor. Perhaps it is change in enzyme activities.

Barrows: I would like to think that differences in the activity of the enzymes was the basis for the increased longevity.

The choice of our next series of experiments may not have been wise. The rationale was essentially this: if the increased life span is not due simply to a retardation of the normal physiological processes, and if there is no evidence for an irreversible change in young, growing animals exposed throughout the growth period to dietary restriction, it may be thought that adult animals should respond to reduced dietary intake, both in pattern of enzyme changes and increase in life span.

In these studies, the food consumption of 12-month-old rats was measured over a period of 2 to 3 weeks. Following this period, the animals were fed 50% of their daily intake. They lost approximately 33% of their body weight within 6 to 8 weeks; the body weight stabilized thereafter. We sacrificed the animals and examined the livers and kidneys for the activities of various enzymes. The only differences observed were, again, the increased succinoxidase of liver and alkaline phosphatase of kidney. We concluded that adult animals respond to this type of diet restriction in the same manner as young, growing ones. Unfortunately, I do not have the answer to the question, "Will these animals live longer?" We are doing this study now. It is hoped that this experiment will answer the question of whether an adult organism has the capacity to respond to an experimental condition which will increase the life span in a growing animal.

We have recently attempted to repeat the classical work of Dr. Lansing (31), using the rotifer. Our data at present are only in the preliminary stage; so the results should be considered tentative. We have failed to demonstrate any difference in life span of 5- or 10-day orthoclones. However, by the eighth generation, the life span of the 15-day orthoclones is approximately 50% of the parent generation (parent life span 32.3 ± 0.9 days at 25° C).

Quimby: What is the variable?

Barrows: The age of the mother when the eggs are col-

lected. There is a shortening of life span if the eggs are selected from old parents.

I felt that such experimental data had been interpreted as
indicating an increase in the rate of change in normal physiological and biochemical function which decrease the life span
of the organism.

Lansing: I don't remember anybody proposing that.

Barrows: I believe that Rudzinska (46) explains her data
on the effect of overfeeding of Tokophrya infusionum in this
way.

Lansing: I don't think it is a generally accepted concept.
Nor do I think we should set up a straw man in order to knock
him down.

Barrows: To my mind, the man was set up. I think you
said that this was accelerated aging.

Lansing: I said shortened life span; this I know. I don't
know about accelerated aging.

Barrows: At any rate, our rationale was that the short-
lived rotifers ought to lay as many eggs as the normal one,
but in the course of a shorter length of time. This is not the
case, because we found that the old clones do not lay as many
eggs; the egg production is about half.

There is one other thing I would like to bring out. It is
well known that if rotifers, as well as other organisms, are
subjected to reduced temperature they will live longer. I was
trying to determine whether old organisms can respond to an
experimental condition that will increase the life span of a
young organism. In this study we put the rotifers, at different
periods in their lives, in the cold at a temperature of 6° C. We
did this when they were 6, 12, 18, and 24 days old. The life
span of the parent is about 30 days.

Transfer of the rotifers to the cold at 6 or 12 days almost
tripled the life span. The life span of those transferred on the
eighteenth day was approximately doubled. The oldest rotifers
experienced only a slight increase of life span as a result of
transfer to the cold.

Fremont-Smith: They were put in the cold and kept there?

Barrows: And kept there. We are also doing the reverse
order. They can be started in the cold and taken out. I would
like to see whether one can equate the life spans of these various groups of rotifers in terms of the concept of rate of living.

This suggests to me that it is possible to take an adult,

perhaps even an old organism, and experimentally increase its life span by some of these techniques.

Lansing: What was the mean number of eggs laid during the life span?

Barrows: It was 29.

Quimby: Are you just reducing the metabolic rate?

Barrows: I would like to be able to decide whether that is so or not. Everybody says: "Sure, you are increasing the life span just by virtue of the Q_{10} of 2."

Quimby: Exactly!

Barrows: The metabolic data aren't in; so I can't calculate the Q_{10}. It seems to me that by manipulating temperature in this order, and also in the reverse order, where they are started in the cold and taken out at different times, one should be able to see whether or not there is a constant rate. I feel it is not going to be constant.

Simms: I think it is analogous to the studies of Loeb and Northrop (33) when they subjected Drosophila to cold. The lower the temperature, the longer they lived.

Barrows: That is a slightly different kind of manipulation. They put the Drosophila in at a certain temperature until they died. One can calculate the Q_{10} on this basis. I don't think that the old idea about the Q_{10} of 2 or 1.5 is going to stick, but I can't prove it yet.

Sacher: After you exposed them at 6° C, all groups seemed to go on from that point in about the same way; the rate of death seemed to be roughly the same. To really examine this point we would have to normalize the curves so they could be compared. It is hard to scale with the eye and stretch and raise.

Barrows: As I pointed out, the experiment is still in progress and we do not as yet have the definitive results.

Sacher: Your result is somewhat different from that obtained by Maynard Smith (34) in which several days of exposure to high temperature was followed by transfer to low temperature and no residual effect of the high-temperature exposure was detectable.

Barrows: In a recent paper Strehler (52) showed a residual effect.

Quimby: To go back to your prognostication about the

animals that were put on the 50% reduced diet—were they young or adult animals? It doesn't look as if they are going to live any longer.

Barrows: These were 20 months old. They do not look as if they will respond. This may be similar to the rotifer, in that the old organisms do not respond as well as the young.

Quimby: How many are left of the younger group that are on the reduced rations?

Barrows: We keep adding to it. We can't obtain 60 24-month-old rats on the same day; so we have to keep putting them in as we get them. We plan to have 60 on the ad lib and 60 on the restricted diet at both ages.

Lansing: Can you tell us something about the characteristics of the species of rotifers you worked with?

Barrows: This colony was established by Dr. Donald Malkoff,* who was a graduate student in your laboratory. Dr. Malkoff was asked to establish the same rotifers you had employed, namely, Philodina citrina. Thus far, we have not obtained an independent opinion as to whether this is or is not Philodina citrina.

Lansing: P. citrina lives 24 days at 18° C; your species lives 30 days at 25° C. There is a tremendous discrepancy here. I suspect you are dealing with another species. It makes no great difference; all that matters is that you get the general result.

Atwood: What is the cause of death in rotifers?

Barrows: I will have to refer that question to Dr. Lansing.

Lansing: No one really knows. Under controlled, standardized conditions, after the vitellarium has exhausted its eggs, there is about a 20% gross decline in activity, measured, for example, by decreasing ciliary beat, and almost simultaneous death in the whole population. It is possible that some exotic disease exists in the rotifer population that decimates it with mathematical regularity at a particular moment in the life span. It is also very likely that we are dealing with a true, endogenous aging mechanism, with the animals dying of aging or senescence relatively free, so far as we know, of exogenous lethal factors. But it would be foolish of me to make a cate-

---

*Malkoff, D. B. Present address: Department of Neurology, University of Michigan Medical Center, Ann Arbor, Michigan.

gorical statement that there are absolutely no viral diseases in the rotifer. I don't know that. The cultures are essentially sterile. The few bacteria that do drop in are immediately metabolized; they are used as food by the rotifer. It is a self-purging system.

It appears from the life history of the organism under standardized conditions that we are dealing with endogenous senescence. The experimental manipulations that we can effect through selection for maternal age probably further establish that we are dealing with senescence, rather than with a complex pattern of exogenous factors operating to kill off a population. Pushing to the extreme, one really doesn't know. The burden of proof is on the investigator who wants to establish that this is an endogenous system.

Fremont-Smith: How narrow is the range of time for the simultaneous death of the whole colony?

Lansing: That depends on the particular conditions being used. With Philodina citrina in isolation culture at 18° C, and with maternal age, which is a major variable, controlled, 24 hours will determine the decimation of the population.

Quimby: When you speak of decimating the population, do you mean it dies all at once?

Lansing: We have, essentially, a rectangular survival curve.

Quimby: How big is the population? Thousands?

Lansing: No, this is done in hundreds.

Quimby: Most populations of microorganisms die exponentially, no matter how they are killed.

Lansing: These are not microorganisms; they are multicellular and they are grown in isolation culture. It is literally impossible to work with thousands of rotifers. Each one must be manipulated, each one must be transferred daily to maintain isolation cultures. Records are maintained of the fecundity. At the peak of my career, the most I could handle was about 1,000 to 1,500 rotifers a day.

Barrows: We now have techniques available that measure four or five different enzymes in rotifers. We hope that such data will lead to the biochemical mechanisms which regulate the life span of the species.

Atwood: Have you tried chelating agents such as EDTA, to see if they help the rotifers stay alive?

184 AGING AND LEVELS OF BIOLOGICAL ORGANIZATION

Barrows: No, we haven't.

Atwood: It probably wouldn't work. (Laughter)

Birren: The issue seems related to the complexity of the organism. We use low temperature in the rat as a noxious condition. While low temperature in the smaller organism favors survival, in the rat it is an unfavorable condition. There is now a study under way in our laboratory on the rat, but from the reverse point of view—the amount of work an old animal will do to get heat from its environment.* So that a favorable condition at one level of organism complexity is unfavorable at another.

A question occurs to me, Dr. Barrows, which concerns the possible relationship of your studies to what Dr. Simms sees in the kidney. He is studying the kidney in the rat morphologically; you are studying it enzymatically. Are you measuring aspects of the same changes he has seen?

Barrows: In normal animals there is a decrease in the enzyme succinoxidase.

Birren: You reject kidneys that would, perhaps, show lesions?

Barrows: Grossly, yes. We do not make a routine histological examination on each kidney. I am sure that the concentration of DNA would be markedly reduced in the kidneys Dr. Simms has referred to.

Birren: Doesn't he find degeneration in almost 100% of animals by 2 years?

Barrows: We just don't see it.

Steinbach: Does the kidney show the alkaline phosphatase decrease?

Barrows: Not as uniformly as the succinoxidase.

Steinbach: Is it your idea those represent enzymes of the major functions of those two tissues?

Barrows: Yes.

Steinbach: What is your explanation?

Barrows: I don't know. We wondered whether the increase in the activity of the enzymes in restricted rats was associated with structural changes within the cells. Experiments carried out in collaboration with Dr. Falzone (14) failed

---

*Dr. Leonard Jakubczak, Research Fellow, Section on Aging, National Institute of Mental Health: Research in progress.

to show any difference in the distribution of alkaline phosphatase determined histochemically. Nevertheless, a high correlation between the activity of the enzyme determined histochemically and biochemically was observed.

Recently we have shown that there is a relationship between the degree of dietary restriction and the increment in the succinoxidase of liver in the growing rat. For example, the succinoxidase activity of livers of animals restricted 75%, 50%, and 25%, was increased 65%, 35%, and 22%, respectively over that of the control animals. On the other hand, in the case of alkaline phosphatase we found that 25% restriction did not produce a significant increment, but 50% and 75% restriction did. The response was the same in the last two groups.

Now we will be able to manipulate animals with different patterns of enzymes and correlate this with longevity.

Steinbach: To see whether the pattern of an enzyme concerned is elevated on restricted diet, could we get someone to enunciate a mathematical theory to prove that restriction must necessarily increase what has to be done by the organism?

Barrows: What concerns me is the apparent inability thus far to correlate the degree of dietary restriction with the increase of life span. Thus, it becomes necessary to determine whether intercorrelations exist between (a) degree of diet restriction, and (b) patterns of enzymatic activity and longevity.

Steinbach: Isn't it true that when yeast or some microorganisms are starved, one sees relative increases in a number of the enzymes?

Atwood: Yes. A number of enzymes are repressed by glucose, for example.

Fremont-Smith: This is the opposite. There is an increase if they are starved.

Atwood: When the glucose is taken away, enzyme synthesis goes up.

Barrows: There are some interesting observations regarding the exposure of Drosophila to reduced temperatures during the various stages of development, beginning as of a certain stage.

I believe that the data of Alpatov and Pearl (1) showed that flies reared through the larval period at 18° C exhibited longer mean life spans than those reared at 25° C. This was the case whether the flies were kept during the adult period at 18, 25, or 28° C.

Sacher: Has anybody correlated the phosphatase levels with rate of weight gain? I seem to recall the rule is that alkaline phosphatase level diminishes about as growth rate does.

Barrows: Yes, it is the general rule that alkaline phosphatase of liver decreases during growth. However, I know of no data which has attempted to correlate changes in the growth rate with changes in enzymatic activity during growth.

Fremont-Smith: Isn't it true, in many studies of the area in which we are feeling our way, that there is a tendency at first to make a cross-species generalization? We have been doing this right across the board here. But isn't it also our experience that, as we learn more and more, although there still may remain common denominators, there will be many highly species-specific factors? We shouldn't be too distressed when we don't find the correlations cutting across. I feel quite sure we will reach a point where we will have to be species-specific in the area of aging, especially when moving from vertebrates to invertebrates, or to single-cell organisms.

Barrows: With regard to temperature, on the other hand, it seems that if an increase in life span can be induced by reducing the temperature in one species, one likes to hope the same thing can be done in another.

Fremont-Smith: By all means. It might not be the same mechanism.

Barrows: It may not be the same but one would like to think it was.

Fenn: If a mammal is exposed to low temperature, his rate of oxygen consumption is increased, which is just the reverse of what occurs with other organisms.

Fremont-Smith: According to Audrey Smith (45, 50), who froze rats and hamsters, the oxygen utilization was reduced.

Fenn: If the animal is simply exposed to a cold room, then Dr. Barrows' experiment has not been duplicated. The basis of his work, it seems to me, is the general idea that we consume just so much oxygen before we die, and if it is consumed more slowly we will live longer. Of course, this explains some other things, too. Large mammals have a smaller rate of oxygen consumption per gram and they live longer, and females have a smaller rate of oxygen consumption than males (per unit of surface area but, perhaps, not per gram of fat-free body mass), and they live longer. This is the oxygen theory of aging which I should like to bring up for discussion.

Simms: Northrop (33) said it is a question of the amount of carbon dioxide produced. (Laughter)

Barrows: This fits in with the rate-of-living concept. I think that is what you are saying.

I don't know of anyone, for instance, who has exposed rats to cold temperature, measured their oxygen consumption, and shown that the short-lived, cold-exposed rat has equivalent oxygen consumption to the normal animal. Kibler (26) has published some data on this recently.

Sacher: Loren Carlson and his colleagues (8) did such an experiment. They followed the survival of rats kept either in a cold or a normal ambient temperature, and either in the presence or absence of a small daily dose of gamma rays. They measured metabolic rates at intervals throughout life. Food consumption was doubled at 5° C and longevity was halved, as compared with 26° C. However, at elevated temperature (35° C), food consumption was diminished (as was metabolic rate) and longevity was, nevertheless, reduced.

Steinbach: Is it respectable to hold the theory that you have enunciated, Dr. Fenn? It is a lot of fun to multiply life span by metabolic rates and be amazed at the constancy.

Fenn: I think it is a respectable subject for discussion although oxygen is certainly not the only factor involved. There is a good deal to be said for oxygen theory, and I am sure there is a lot that can be said against it.

Atwood: What can be said for it?

Fenn: There is the accumulation of oxidized products, pigments that are oxidized, lipid materials, and there is the toxicity of oxygen itself. Over a certain range at least. The higher the oxygen tension, the sooner a person dies. There is the possibility that we actually have more oxygen now than we are able to compete with, that it is somewhat toxic for us, even at our present level. You see, life originated in an anaerobic environment, but evolved into plants that produce oxygen and animals that use oxygen. In order to protect itself against the toxicity of oxygen, a living cell must build up some antioxygen defenses. Vitamin E is an antioxygen defense, as is glutathione, I suppose. So perhaps in our present environment we don't have as much antioxygen defense as we need to live as long as Methuselah.

Atwood: According to theory, since the oxygen tension can be raised, this would be expected to accelerate senescence in a rather natural way. I don't think that happens.

Fenn: I am not sure. Who has actually done the experiment?

Brues: It is well established that oxygen is toxic to an animal being irradiated in terms of everything we know about, including life-span effects.

Fenn: It is toxic to any living animal at a sufficiently high level. Another possibility is that oxygen does this by forming free radicals in the normal stages of the univalent oxidation. In the oxidation by one electron at a time, free radicals are formed, according to Michaelis (36), and these may be responsible for oxidizing lipids and producing accumulation of pigment or other debris in the cell. It is possible that the toxicity of oxygen is due to the accumulation of free radicals in extra quantity, just as radiation is toxic because of the formation of free radicals. If a higher rate of oxygen consumption produced more free radicals (which has not, perhaps, been very well demonstrated), this would also shorten life by the same mechanism.

Ehret: One of the effects of oxygen in the irradiated organism is actually to scavenge the free radicals produced by radiation, producing in them another radical (13).

Fenn: On the other hand, the absence of oxygen protects against irradiation, and the presence of high oxygen intensifies the effects. I think it is also true that simultaneous radiation increases the toxicity of oxygen, which might indicate that through this free radical mechanism there is some common effect. This is the theory of a former colleague, Dr. Rebeca Gerschman (18), who used to work in my laboratory and was very enthusiastic about the oxygen theory of aging. I don't think this theory has been proved, but I think it is good enough to test further.

Birren: What has the diet-restriction theory proved?

Fenn: Diet restriction limits the amount of oxidation which goes along certain channels where more oxidized products or free radicals might accumulate than elsewhere. It might be that for such a reason it prolongs life. I don't know.

Lindop: David Harman (23) is working on the role of free radicals in spontaneous aging, by giving antioxidants to mice. In his analysis of the results, there is a 20% life-lengthening in the animals to which he has given these. The numbers used, however, were small and the variance large.

Fenn: It may make a difference where the test is made and what other conflicting and confusing factors may be present. Oxygen can hardly be the only factor of importance.

Storer: We have one bit of preliminary data bearing on this point. Certainly, between species a very attractive hypothesis is that a low metabolic rate leads to greater longevity. Within a species, and specifically within mice, we have measured metabolic rates in 20 or 25 inbred strains. The life tables are not yet complete on these strains, but it does not appear that there is any relationship between metabolic rate and longevity. There are undoubtedly other factors involved.

Sacher: The relation of length of life to basal metabolic rate is not a consequence of the oxygen hypothesis. Metabolic rate (cal/kg day) varies by a factor of 50 from the smallest to the largest homeotherms, and life span varies inversely by almost the same factor. For these data to accord with the oxygen hypothesis, it would be necessary to show a corresponding difference in oxygen tension of the tissues. I think that in fact the tensions are about the same, but the transport rates change in proportion to metabolic rate.

Fenn: There is a lot of truth in that. The tension would be higher in some parts of the lungs if a high-oxygen mixture is being breathed, but it does not go up as much in the other tissues.

Fremont-Smith: Isn't there also a concept that free radicals may precipitate the induction of cancer?

Fenn: Yes.

Fremont-Smith: This would not be opposed to the oxygen theory.

Brues: Before we leave the matter of enzymes, I would like to ask Dr. Quastler to present an interesting communication that may point out a connection between genetics and enzymes which may not have been apparent from the discussion so far.

Quastler: I'll report on work done by Wulff et al. (53); it concerns uptake of a radioactive tracer—tritiated cytidine—into RNA. A number of kinds of cells were tested. In some tissues (dorsal root ganglia, liver, kidney, mature intestinal epithelium), the uptake was considerably higher in old animals than in young ones; in others (muscle, Purkinje cells, pyramidal nuclei) there was a slight increase, or no change. In either case, the ratio of cytidine uptake to content of RNA in the tissue increases considerably with age. The following explanation was proposed: as somatic mutations accumulate, there will be production of faulty messenger RNA which is presumably unstable and won't result in production of very effective enzymes. However, lack of effective enzymes results in de-repression and increased production of messenger RNA and protein (which would correspond to the increased uptake). As long as the cell can compensate by increase in quantity for loss in quality, enzyme activity levels will remain normal.

Fry: Does that mean that there was more defective RNA in liver cells of old animals?

Quastler: That is the interpretation.

Barrows: I heard Dr. Wulff (54) present these data in Miami. It is indeed quite striking. We have shown that one sometimes sees an increase in the concentration of RNA in livers of old rats (4). It represents perhaps a 10 or 15% increase.

In regard to the protein, I wonder whether the high cathepsin activity I showed in Table 12 does not support Wulff; it may be a way of getting rid of the bad molecules. When we go to other tissues, I am not quite sure we are in as good a position. I don't think anyone has ever shown increased RNA in kidney of old rats. As I recall, Dr. Wulff's increases were in kidney, liver, and cardiac muscle.

Lansing: Are we talking about labeling of RNA or analysis?

Quastler: Labeling, that is, uptake.

Lansing: You are talking about increased turnover rather than increase in total amount?

Barrows: I am saying that if a lot of these errors are being made, one would expect to see a net increase. This may not necessarily be so if the rate of turnover is high.

Lansing: I want to make sure I know what Wulff did.

Quastler: Tritiated cytidine is injected and the uptake measured autoradiographically, by grain count. The grain count is a rough measure of the rate of RNA synthesis, and this is greatly increased in some kinds of cells in old mice—which agrees nicely with small increases in RNA and increase in cathepsins.

Lansing: This is done by means of radioautography?

Quastler: Right.

Lansing: Is there any particular distribution of the labeling?

Quastler: Autoradiographs of RNA-labeled cells, soon after injection, always show the label in the nucleus. About 2 hours after injection, label appears in the cytoplasm, and within about 6 hours, it is all over the cytoplasm.

Lansing: Originating in the nucleolus?

Quastler: In the nucleus, around the chromosomes; concentration around the nucleolus occurs later.

Lansing: And is then generally distributed?

Quastler: Cytoplasmic labeling comes after nuclear and nucleolar labeling. This time sequence agrees with the general idea that messenger RNA is laid down on the DNA matrix in the chromosome, possibly stored in the nucleolus and transported into the cytoplasm.

Cottier: Actually, Drs. Feinendegen and Bond (16) at Brookhaven have shown autoradiographically that, in cultured cells (HeLa-S_3), nuclear RNA is associated with the chromosomal surface rather than the core.

Dr. Quastler, is there a possibility that at least a small part of this increased labeling intensity may be due to another metabolic situation, in the sense that, per unit RNA formed, more labeled cytidine is incorporated?

Quastler: Yes, but it would have to be a large difference to explain a factor of more than 2.

Cottier: That is why I say a small fraction.

Quastler: Sure. We know that cytidine feeds into a large pool, and we don't know what changes of the pool occur with age.

Jarvik: Is this true of all cells?

Quastler: No.

Jarvik: Which ones do not show the increased uptake?

Quastler: Purkinje cells and some other nerve cells and striated muscle.

Ehret: Is there a possible time-of-day effect? If there were time-of-day changes in synthesis in the cell populations that were represented, one might deduce there was an increased performance in cytidine utilization by RNA, whereas one would really be looking at a different phase of RNA synthesis in the cells.

Quastler: Old and young mice were injected at the same time; thus there would have to be a differential effect caused by the time of day. Incidentally, under ordinary laboratory conditions, mice are not as strictly phased as in Halberg's laboratory, and the daily rhythms are not nearly as pronounced as he finds them.

Ehret: If the reaction course includes a spurt, it may be difficult to catch even in strictly phased animals. But in non-dividing populations of Paramecium, in the absence of DNA synthesis, there are circadian oscillations in the turnover of RNA. It is rather slight but significant (12).

Fry: The number of cells in mitosis and the number in synthesis, in the intestines of mice, as assessed by the number of cells that take up injected tritiated thymidine, is greater at 2:00 A.M. or 4:00 A.M., and the same pattern is observed for different age groups—young, middle-aged, and old animals. There is a quantitative difference but exactly the same time relationship in the day, in the three age groups.

Ehret: If it turns out that all mitotic and performance indices match, then I am satisfied. But this I strongly doubt. As I recall, Halberg showed certain correlations in mitotic indices of different tissues which, though not necessarily age correlated, were definitely not in phase synchrony with one another (20, 21).

Quastler: I don't think mitotic indices vary by more than a factor of 2. As I said before, Halberg's animals are strictly phased. They live in a room that nobody enters, and where food and water are given automatically. They are undisturbed for 2 weeks before the experiment. Under ordinary conditions, mice are bothered at various times of the day because somebody will wander into the animal room; some will eat, some won't, some will move around a lot, and some very little—under those conditions, phases are not as nicely expressed as in Halberg's material, and time-of-day effects are not as large.

Brues: Dr. Storer, will you present your material?

Storer: This summarizes an attempt to estimate the mean homeostatic level for genotypes and populations as a function of age.* Our methodology is as follows: we work with strains of mice which have been inbred for so many generations that for all practical purposes they are homozygous at all gene loci.

---

*The research reported was supported in part by the United States Atomic Energy Commission under contract AT (30-1)-2313, and by research grant RH-71 from the Division of Radiological Health, Bureau of State Services, Public Health Service.

The actual level of residual heterozygosity can be calculated. It is negligible for these strains. In effect, then, we have identical twins except that we have very large numbers of these genetically identical individuals. Because, within a strain, there is no residual genetic variability or genetic variance, any variability in phenotype such as body weight or response to stress is due to differences between individuals in their responses to their environment, both prenatal and postnatal. This is called environmental variance.

All individuals within a strain, or a species for that matter, tend to resist environmental forces that would lead to major displacements or changes in morphology or physiology. These buffering and restorative forces which tend to hold the individual within the narrow limits of what is normal or close to average for the strain or species can be considered the homeostatic mechanisms.

If a number of inbred strains are maintained in an approximately common environment, and one strain shows a greater environmental variance than another with respect to some measurable characteristic, then it should follow that the strain or genotype showing a large variance has less efficient homeostasis than a strain showing a small variance. By this line of reasoning, the environmental variance is inversely related to the adequacy of the homeostasis and is its estimator for a genotype or a population.

For this reason, if in a genetically uniform population the variance with respect to a number of measurable characteristics increases with increasing age, it follows that the level or adequacy of homeostasis is declining.

What we have done is to measure various characteristics as a function of age and calculate the variance around the mean values. Like Dr. Barrows, we have looked at mean values for a number of measurements and find these particularly unrewarding. Mean values don't seem to change very much with age, but variance does.

We first noticed this increase in variance in some studies done for different reasons. We were measuring how long mice would live under a daily exposure to 100 r of X ray. This was a longitudinal study in that a single cohort of mice was set up and samples of animals tested at various ages. The results are shown in Figure 41. We have plotted the variance and survival time as a function of age in months.

Figure 42 shows the same sort of result in a horizontal study. We took the animals off the shelf, ran them through the test procedure, and calculated the variance. It can be seen that the variance increases at quite a remarkable rate. At this point we decided to estimate variance in a number of other systems.

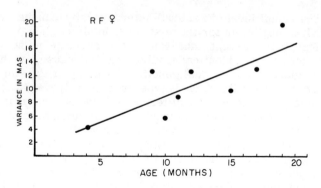

Fig. 41.—Change in variance in survival time under exposure to 100 r per day (MAS) as a function of age in RF/J female mice.

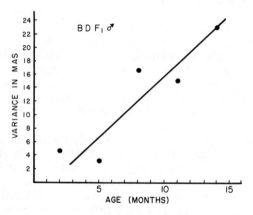

Fig. 42.—Change in variance in survival time under 100 r per day (MAS) as a function of age in BDF_1/J male mice.

Table 18 shows the variance in body weight as a function of age for an inbred strain of mice. We used a logarithmic transformation because body weight is apparently log normal. Also, this procedure avoids the problem of the variance being dependent on the mean. Variance in body weight increased remarkably from 4 months up to 16 months of age.

Table 19 shows another study in which we estimated variance. This time we used the toxicity of single exposures to X rays. From the slope of the regression line relating dose to response at each age, it was possible to estimate the variance of the subpopulation. With the exception of the first two values, which ideally should be reversed, the variance increased greatly as a function of increasing age. This again was a hori-

TABLE 18

Body Weight of C57BL/6J Male Mice at Various Ages

Age (Mo.)	No. of mice	Mean ± S. E.[*]	Variance
4	50	1.4797 ± .00653	.00213
6	50	1.5225 ± .00778	.00303
8	54	1.5447 ± .00889	.00427
11	75	1.5617 ± .00912	.00624
13	53	1.6331 ± .01179	.00737
16	50	1.6376 ± .01323	.00873

[*]Standard error.

TABLE 19

Acute Lethal Response to X Rays in C57BL/6J Male Mice at Various Ages

Age (Mo.)	No. of mice	LD_{50} ± S. E.	Variance
5	44	788 ± 22 r	6,762
6	57	774 ± 16 r	4,653
8	69	820 ± 22 r	7,525
10	88	776 ± 22 r	16,849
12	65	774 ± 27 r	18,867
14	88	845 ± 29 r	25,016
17	50	707 ± 39 r	40,128

zontal study. All these animals were run at the same time.

Table 20 shows the results for studies of pentobarbital toxicity. In this case we used a logarithmic transformation of doses. Again there appears to be a general trend upward in the variance. As before, these variances were estimative of the dose-response curve.

We next studied hematocrits in a strain of mice ranging in age from 5 to 17 months (Table 21). In this particular strain of mice there is appreciable mortality by 17 months and the variance in the hematocrit increased dramatically at this point. We felt that this might introduce a bias for the following reason: we hadn't selected the animals. If they happened to be moribund when we took them from their cages we still included them. If an animal is moribund and anemic, this fact contributes disproportionately to the variance in the hematocrit. To avoid this bias, we arbitrarily rejected values of less

TABLE 20

Toxicity of Sodium Pentobarbital (mg/kg) at Various Ages in C57BL/6J Male Mice (log Transformation of Dose)

Age (Mo.)	No. of mice	$LD_{50} \pm$ S. E.	Variance
6	40	2.0837 ± .01615	.00292
8	39	2.0614 ± .02020	.00685
10	42	2.0991 ± .01706	.00435
13	54	2.0628 ± .02313	.01107

TABLE 21

Hematocrit (%) at Various Ages in C57BL/6J Male Mice

Age (Mo.)	No. of mice	Mean ± S. E.	Variance
5	47	47.15 ± 0.321%	4.837
10	45	45.56 ± 0.361%	5.840
14	46	45.32 ± 0.455%	9.530 (6.300)[*]
17	50	45.48 ± 0.599%	17.946 (7.515)[*]

[*]Values recalculated after arbitrary exclusion of hematocrit values less than 40%. See text.

than 40 for the hematocrit and recalculated the variances. The recalculated values are shown in parentheses. Despite this arbitrary correction, there was still a progressive increase in variance with increasing age.

Table 22 shows the results of some tests on the osmotic fragility of erythrocytes from mice of various ages. The tests were run by placing the cells in tubes containing various concentrations of saline, and determining the extent of hemolysis.

TABLE 22

Osmotic Fragility of Erythrocytes from C57BL/6J Male Mice at Various Ages

Age (Mo.)	No. of mice	ED_{50}[*] ± S. E.	Variance
3	19	.493 ± .0026%	.000129
10	18	.502 ± .0028%	.000149
16	19	.502 ± .0034%	.000216

[*]ED_{50} is the mean concentration of saline (%) required to lyse 50% of the erythrocytes.

For each mouse we calculated the concentration of saline which lysed 50% of the cells. From the individual ED_{50} values we calculated a mean which did not change very much with increasing age. The variance, however, did increase for the three age groups tested.

Figure 43 shows a plot of the results of four of the measurements discussed. We normalized the variance to a "factor of change in variance," taking first the measurement in the youngest mice as unity and plotting the other values as the

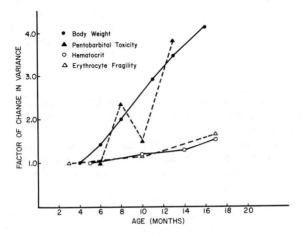

Fig. 43.—Factor of change in variance for a number of measurements as a function of age in C57BL/6J male mice.

factor of change. It can be seen from this plot that variance in body weight apparently increases in linear fashion. Variance in pentobarbital toxicity does not increase in quite such a smooth fashion, but nevertheless increases with age. Variance in the hematocrit and erythrocyte fragility measurements didn't increase nearly so much but certainly showed an upward trend. I think this is not surprising because very great changes in the hematocrit or erythrocyte fragility are not tolerated by the animal. If too great a change occurs, the animal is removed from the population by dying out. On the other hand, big variations are permissible in body weight or in resistance to pentobarbital.

Table 23 summarizes the measurements discussed and shows coefficients of correlation between age and variance. All the coefficients are positive and quite high. The double asterisks indicate significance at the 1% level of probability and the single asterisks indicate significance at the 5% level. Two of the correlation coefficients were not significant at the 5%

TABLE 23

Correlation and Regression Coefficients Relating Variance and Age for 5
Characteristics in C57BL/6J Male Mice

Measurement	N	Coefficient of correlation	Regression coefficient ± S. E. (Variance on age)
Body weight	6	+.988[**]	+.0560 ± .00432[**]
Hematocrit	4	+.974[*]	+.2084 ± .03374[*]
Pentobarbital toxicity	4	+.835	+.099 ± .04654
X-ray toxicity	7	+.966[**]	+2.795 ± .3351 (x 10^3)[**]
Erythrocyte fragility	3	+.940	+0.659 ± .2371 (x 10^{-4})

[*]P <.05.
[**]P <.01.

level. This is not surprising since the number of points where
measurements were made were relatively small, namely, only
three and four.

Included in Table 23 are the regression coefficients.
Their significance levels are of course identical to those of
the correlation coefficients, by virtue of the mathematical relationships between the two.

If our hypothesis is correct, and variance estimates the
mean homeostatic level in a population, and if, further, the
mean homeostatic level is important in maintaining life, then
there should be some relationship between the rate of change
in variance and the longevity of the animals. This was the next
point we examined.

In the course of some experiments on the effect of irradiation on longevity, we set up some populations of mice and assigned treatment levels of irradiation at random within the
cages. Included, of course, were unirradiated control mice.
Through an error, one of the replications set out didn't receive its scheduled X-ray treatment. This error inadvertently
provided us with a population of control mice caged with irradiated mice and a population of control mice caged with other
controls. We measured the body weights of these animals at
frequent intervals for a number of months and calculated the
variance in body weight as a function of age. The variances for
each population were, of course, not independent, since measurements were made repeatedly on the same animals, but this
objection is probably not serious.

The results are summarized in Figure 44. I should like to
emphasize again that all these data are for control mice. The
open circles show the variance in body weight with age for
control mice caged with other controls, and the solid circles

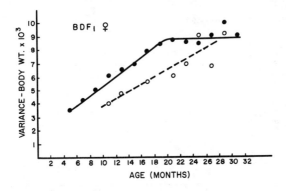

Fig. 44.—Change in variance in body weight as a function of age in two populations of control BDF$_1$/J female mice maintained under dissimilar environmental conditions.

are for controls caged with irradiated mice. It can be seen that the variance increased more rapidly in the controls caged with irradiated than in the controls caged with controls. The life tables are not complete for these two groups of animals, but it appears that the cages containing irradiated mice provided a less favorable environment than the cages containing only control mice. This conclusion is based on the fact that it appears that the control animals housed with the irradiated animals will show a shorter longevity than the other group. This difference appears to have been predicted by the rate of change in variance in body weight as a function of age, inasmuch as the shorter-lived group showed a more rapid rate of increase in variance. For a single strain of animals, then, it appears that changes in variance may predict longevity.

Of course this is really not an adequate test of our hypothesis; so I would like to present some entirely preliminary data on rate of change in variance for a number of inbred strains having known differences in longevity. These data are all for female mice. According to our hypothesis, the short-lived strains should show a more rapid increase in variance than the long-lived strains. We are in the process of determining variance in a number of characteristics, but I will confine my remarks to changes in the variance in body weight.

Figures 45, 46, and 47 show plots of variance in body weight as a function of age for strains SJL/J, 129/J, and C57BL/6J respectively. It can be seen that in all cases the variance increased considerably with increasing age.

In Figure 48 we have plotted the regression lines for the six inbred strains on which we have a reasonable amount of data. The actual data points have been omitted in the interest

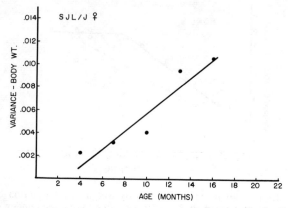

Fig. 45.—Change in variance in body weight as a function of age in SJL/J female mice.

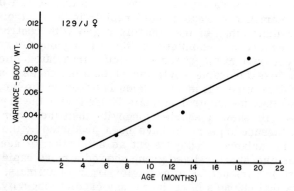

Fig. 46.—Change in variance in body weight as a function of age in 129/J female mice.

of clarity. It can be seen that all six strains show a positive slope to the regression line and that there are differences between some of these slopes and differences in intercepts. According to our hypothesis, those strains which show a steep slope and/or a high intercept value should be the short-lived strains. Unfortunately for any critical test of the hypothesis, we apparently made a poor selection of strains. We do know that the A/J strain is short-lived. This fact agrees nicely with the change in variance. We also know that the 129/J strain is long-lived, and that C57BL/6J is intermediate between the two. For these three strains, then, there is good agreement between the data and the hypothesis. The SJL/J strain appears to be a vigorous one, but unfortunately does not have a long

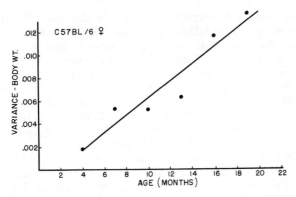

Fig. 47.—Change in variance in body weight as a function of age in C57BL/6J female mice.

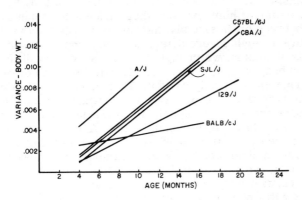

Fig. 48.—Regression of variance in body weight on age in six strains of female mice.

life span because of a high incidence of reticulum sarcoma relatively early in life. Similarly, the CBA/J mice are not particularly long lived because of a very high incidence of mammary carcinoma in the females. For these five strains, then, there is reasonable agreement between prediction and observation. The one real difficulty in the study is presented by the BALB/cJ strain. In our hands this is a short-lived strain but its variance increases at a much slower rate than that for any of the other strains. We wonder whether in our laboratory there is some unidentified unfavorable environment factor for this strain, because other people using it, particularly Henry Kohn (30) in San Francisco, get much longer survival times than we do in these animals.

To summarize to this point, we would like to suggest that

202 AGING AND LEVELS OF BIOLOGICAL ORGANIZATION

variance measurements may estimate the homeostatic level for a genotype or population and that homeostasis may decline with age. Animals with dissimilar longevity may show characteristic differences in the rate of increase in variance. We postulate that longevity is genetically controlled by a determination of the initial level of homeostasis or functional capacity of the integrative systems and its rate of decline.

We next looked for possible differences between these strains which might account for the differences in rate of increase in variance. Sacher (47) and others have pointed out that there is a relationship between brain size and longevity. Sacher has suggested that this may result from the fact that the central nervous system is probably of critical importance in the total integrative system for maintaining homeostasis. For this reason, if brain size is important in maintaining homeostasis, and if these changes in variance in body weight actually estimate homeostasis, there should be some relationship between brain size and the rate of increase in variance.

Brain weights were determined on samples of mice from the six strains shown in Figure 48. These strains differ somewhat in body weight; so we simply calculated the brain weight in terms of the body weight. This gives us a brain/body-weight ratio which is probably the critical parameter. Table 24 shows the slope constants for variance in body weight on age, and the brain/body-weight ratios. A rank order correlation yielded a coefficient of -0.89, which is significant at the 5% level. In other words, those strains which showed a high brain/body-weight ratio showed a slow rate of increase in variance with age, and those which showed a low brain/body-weight ratio showed a rapid increase in variance with age. This finding suggests that the amount of body mass serviced per unit of mass of brain is indeed of importance, in terms of homeostatic capability.

TABLE 24

Slope Constants for Variance in Body Weight As a Function of Age and Brain/Body-Weight Ratios for Six Strains of Female Mice

Strain	Slope constant S^2 (body wt.) on age	Brain wt./body wt.
BALB/cJ	1.66×10^{-4}	.0207
129/J	4.80×10^{-4}	.0199
C57BL/6J	7.55×10^{-4}	.0204
SJL/J	7.62×10^{-4}	.0187
CBA/J	7.68×10^{-4}	.0122
A/J	8.00×10^{-4}	.0148

Note: Rank correlation = -0.89 and P = .05.

Since it appears that the level of homeostasis in specific genotypes or in populations declines with increasing age, it should follow that an individual within a population should also show a progressive decline in homeostatic ability. Ideally, then, we should measure variance in individual animals as a function of age. A major difficulty with this approach is that the measurement itself may cause enough of a disturbance so that the induced disturbance overshadows normal fluctuations within the animal. There are, however, a few methods of approach available, and one that we have chosen for further study is the measurement of the distribution of red-cell sizes in animals as a function of age. Just before I left the laboratory, we measured these distributions on five young and five old mice. I do not yet have the computations for this pilot run, but a plot of the data indicates that older animals do indeed show a wider distribution of red-cell sizes than the young animals. This finding, if it stands up under further testing, tends to support the hypothesis of an increasing variability within an individual with increasing age.

Brues: In the case of many biochemical reactions that have developed through the course of evolution, an increase in variance in any direction may take one away from the optimum condition, and therefore be what one might call deleterious to those individuals who have crossed the line, as illustrated in Figure 49. But I am thinking about something that might be different, namely, resistance to toxins, poisons, X ray,

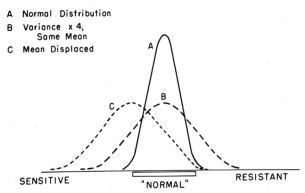

Fig. 49.—Contrast between effect of increasing variance of a variable, (1) where the normal value represents an optimal physiological condition (so that a deviation in either direction is deleterious) or (2) where it represents sensitivity to a toxic agent (so that a deviation in one direction is advantageous). Line under curve A: optimum range of variable (case 1) or normal range of sensitivity (case 2). Solid curve: Variance in young individual. Broken curves: Hypothetical variance in senile individual.

and so on. When the variance increases in this situation, does it always increase in the direction of making the animal more sensitive, or might it sometimes make it less sensitive than the young one?

Storer: It is difficult for me to visualize, particularly with X-ray toxicity and pentobarbital toxicity, that some of the older animals are hyper-resistant. I think the increased variance must mean that more of them are relatively sensitive. I do not see any mechanism for hyper-resistance, but from the data we have so far collected it isn't possible to rule it out.

Keys: On some of the characteristics, you made the point at the outset that the mean value didn't indicate very much.

Storer: That is right.

Keys: Therefore, either your analysis is improperly applied, or there must be a distribution similar on both sides, with both hyper- and hyposensitive cells in equal proportion.

Storer: For these two measurements, that is correct. Certainly body weight can be high or low, and hematocrits may go up or down. For evaluating resistance to these toxins, I agree this may be the wrong analysis. Data were simply not adequate to say whether or not we had hyper-resistance.

Brues: That still would not rule out the possibility that the older animals which varied one way and another, especially if they did it cyclically, might have a bigger chance of falling off the precipice in their fluctuations toward sensitivity to the environment.

Storer: Not only does it not rule it out, I think it supports the concept.

Fremont-Smith: I like the concept of aging being related to breakdown in homeostatic capacity. It has intrigued me for some time, although I had no information on it. But wouldn't it be necessary, eventually, to include the hormonal system in the homeostatic setup?

Storer: Yes, I would consider this probably an additional very important aspect of homeostasis. The total integrative system or homeostatic mechanism must include the nervous system, hormonal system, biochemical systems, and so on.

Fremont-Smith: When measuring brain weight, might not something of functional activity of the glands of internal secretion have to be included? I don't know whether it would be weight of those organs or something else.

Storer: I think it would be very interesting to make such functional measurements. The difficulty is that to establish variances with any sort of precision requires a great number of measurements, and for this reason they must be of a simple nature.

Keys: I said earlier I had come along for the ride, so to speak, and to listen. The more I have listened, the more fascinated I have become but, also, the more convinced that my particular line of endeavor in recent years does not have much to do with what we are talking about. If I understand correctly, there is an urge here to find a general, single process of "aging" and to try to explain this process so as to get a unitary theory of aging. So I can't contribute because I don't have enough evidence to convince me there is such a thing.

I work with human beings and human populations, comparing populations and population samples and seeing what happens in follow-up studies over time. I have been known to suggest this has something to do with aging, because I have some support from sources that like to give money for aging studies.

Perhaps all we have done that has any connection with aging is to observe, record, and measure certain variables, some of which are associated with age trends; they tend to change as time goes on. We found that some of these variables are associated with differences in the prevalence and incidence of certain diseases which are also strongly age related. Rather than give actual, numerical data, I propose only to discuss some points of observation that might be of interest.

This week, we began the sixteenth year of detailed examinations of a group of business and professional men, who were set up as a cohort of healthy men originally numbering 281 and aged 45-55. They have been re-examined annually, for the most part with about 95% coverage. So we have data on them from 16 consecutive sets of detailed examinations. Several interesting things have come out of this.

First, let us consider blood pressure, about which little has been said here so far. We and many others have made cross-sectional observations on blood pressure in different populations and subgroups of populations, and observed the sort of thing everyone else had observed—that there is a relationship between blood pressure and age.

We have about 220 men on whom we have full data on at least 12 out of 15 annual examinations' data. We had an unusual opportunity with this group to see what happens over time in individuals about whom a great deal else is known. We found that there is substantially the same kind of age trend found in

cross-sections of populations. The slopes of the individual re-
gressions of blood pressure on age were calculated for each
individual. The distribution of these slopes proves to be nearly normal, that is, gaussian.

Then we asked: Can we find any evidence that there are
basically different kinds of people in this population? It has
been postulated recently by Platt (2), Morris (1), and others,
that people can be classed into two types, those who have a
major age trend in blood pressure and those who do not. We
applied every technique we could think of to analyze the observed characteristic rise of blood pressure, but it proved to
be an almost perfectly normal distribution; only a very few
men out at the far end had hypertensive disease. And we calculated the errors of all these slopes and found the distribution of errors to be normal also. So we found no trace for discrete differences between kinds of men.

Then there is the question of the rise of blood pressure
with age in different populations. We have available data from
11 different populations in Europe, three in Japan, and our own
in the United States, a total of around 12,000 men initially aged
40 to 59 who represent substantially all men of the age in defined geographical areas (38, 39).

So far, we have not been able to find any important differences in the distribution of blood pressure with age when we
compare the several populations. We feel fairly confident
about some technical matters that could disturb the comparisons. Our own international teams made the measurements,
and the technique has been standardized, including our personal bias.

In view of the quite violent polemics in British journals
during the last couple of years (41, 43) about different kinds of
persons within the population who do or do not develop an increase in blood pressure with age, we examined the question
in the same way as J. N. Morris (40), one of the polemicists.
We asked whether the age at death of parents might separate a
population into subpopulations which would differ in respect to
the change of blood pressure with age.

For his purpose, Dr. Morris had data on about 300 men,
including information about whether or not one or both of the
parents had died as early as at age 60 or 65 (40). We had data
of this kind on four different population groups, each representing a "chunk" sample of all men in the geographic area
aged 40-59, with numbers running from over 600 in the smallest to over 900 in the largest.

We also had information on the parents' age at death and
ascribed causes of their deaths, as well as on the age of surviving parents. We did not pay much heed to the ascribed

cause of death, except we could perhaps believe the statement that "Father was killed in the war" or that the mother died in a tuberculosis hospital. We eliminated the relatively very few cases where death had been attributed to violence or to infectious disease, so we had left a somewhat purified group of parents who were dead or alive at given ages. This was better, we thought, than including all causes of death as had been done by Dr. Morris (40).

With this material we made all the comparisons we could think of. The men were classified as to early-mother-death, late-mother-survival, early-father-death, late-father-survival, or both. The curves of the distribution of blood pressure with age were generally completely superimposable; there was no difference with regard to the shape of the curve and no evidence for bimodal distributions.

This is the sort of work I am engaged in. I am not at all sure it has anything to do with aging. I am interested in the causes of disability and death, and the differences among populations in survival up to, one might say, a useful age. "Useful age," of course, is at least 15 or 20 years older than oneself. (Laughter) In total survival we do find great differences between populations, at least for men; we don't know about women.

It is interesting that these population differences in mortality rate do not disclose a single pattern for the major causes of death beyond the age of, say, 40, in most of our populations. The cause of death differs and the biggest differential is coronary heart disease. In citing this difference we are not merely relying on vital statistics. We have been busy going out and counting the bodies ourselves. At the same age, there is a large difference in the incidence of coronary heart disease. It is as great as 20:1 between population groups in Cape Town. A ration of 6:1 at the same age would apply to comparisons between men in eastern Finland with men on the island of Kyushu in Japan. These populations do not differ in some other respects that we think of as related to age. For example, the incidence of neoplasms is similar, although there are some differences in the preferential site.

Another interesting point is with regard to cerebral vascular disease. We satisfied ourselves, at least, that there is a very high incidence of cerebral vascular disease in Japan although the incidence may be about 20% overestimated by the Japanese. When a person of middle age or older is found dead and the doctor doesn't know the cause, he puts down "cerebral vascular," whereas U.S. doctors would put down "coronary." If such death data are examined, the indication is that perhaps "strokes" might be 20% overestimated. Of course, this also means an underestimate of the incidence of coronary heart disease, and we suggest that "coronaries" might be 10% more frequent than the Japanese say. But that is about as much of the reported difference between the U.S. and Japan that can be accounted for in this way. There is no parallel at all among various populations between hypertension and strokes on the one hand, and coronary heart disease on the other.

One conclusion I have drawn from this work is that we should not talk about a generalized process of aging. Most of the major things that kill people, if not rats, seem to involve independent disease situations and pathological developments, or those that are, one might say, "normal," but in time proceed further away from normality to the point where we speak of "disease." Two of the major age-related causes of death— hypertensive disease and complications, and coronary heart disease—seem to have, basically, very different etiologies because, epidemiologically, their frequency distributions cannot be accounted for on any common ground.

Birren: I am puzzled by your position that this work has nothing to do with aging, conceptually. One can reverse this and say it has, in a sense, everything to do with aging, because you obtained a normal distribution of the rates of change in blood pressure. This means you have observed a characteristic of universality; every member of these populations shows a trait which is characteristic of aging, and there is no bimodality or trimodality to indicate a mixture of populations of diseased and non-diseased. I think this comes very close to my concepts of aging. The age-associated change may in turn lead to consequences in the greater likelihood of different diseases, say, cerebral vascular or coronary artery. In any event the data might be interpreted as reflecting aging.

Keys: We can point to blood pressure and say, "Yes, this is age-related." Whether this is, in itself, enough to call it the universal aging process, I would very much doubt. I don't think there is any such thing as a universal aging process. The fact that everybody tends to have an increase in blood pressure with age is true. Individuals differ, but there is no clear line of differentiation between various kinds or classes of people within the population. Therefore, you are correct; this is universal, in that respect. All it means is that no basic support can be found here for the idea of a genetic foundation for the development of increasing blood pressure with age. You may be right; maybe this does concerning aging, I don't know.

Fremont-Smith: Might there not be a genetic factor that was carried right through all related populations? That is what you are saying, isn't it?

Birren: Yes. In the instance of neoplasms, where some people in the population show the trait and some do not, I would think we are justified in using the concept, disease.

Brues: You mentioned that the incidence of cancer is about the same but the site is different. Would this hold true if a generalized term, such as vascular disease, were used?

Keys: No, I think we could say that there are larger differences among populations (6, 25) in the amount of vascular disease of the coronary arteries than there is in other arteries that have been investigated. These differences are highly significant. The work now going on, comparing Japanese, Bantu, and various other populations, indicates that the difference in the aorta is smaller than the difference in the coronary artery, but there is still a very large difference among populations in aortic disease.

Kalimann: What effect did the parental age level have on your findings?

Keys: When we compared men whose parents died early with those whose parents had longer survival, we were testing the idea advanced by Dr. J. N. Morris (40) that the population is made up of two kinds of men genetically different in regard to the tendency to develop hypertension, and that this difference may be revealed by separating the men according to longevity of the parents. The assumption, made by Morris, is that among parents who die at a relatively young age many of the deaths will be due to or associated with hypertension. Accordingly, among men with early parental deaths there would be a concentration of those who carry the hypertensive trait. Morris suggested that this might be indicated by a bimodal distribution of blood pressures for the men with early parental death. But, as I have said, our data cover far more men in much better samples than in Morris's study, and show no such tendency.

Ehret: Some of Dr. Storer's results revive and extend our earlier questions of the possibility that a time-of-day effect has been overlooked. In general, I think we should all agree that recognition and control of the circadian aspects of animal behavior in an experiment are just as important as control of the other fundamental variables including temperature, nutrition, phenotype, and pathogens. Unfortunately, there are no extensive data on its relationship to aging.

In circadian rhythms, the duration of one full cycle is not necessarily precisely the length of a sidereal day but is usually some length of time (say, 22.3 hours), that is, approximately a day's length (circa dies). When a circadian system is driven by a light-dark cycle of 24 hours' duration, it is also diurnally rhythmical. Immediately, a basic paradox occurs to the student of aging: The life-expectancy measure for an organism is different if it is calculated from circadian "days" instead of from sidereal days. What does this mean?

The question should be asked against the background of a rule established by Jurgen Aschoff (2, 42). Consider an animal in continuous darkness for days, undergoing circadian oscillation in its physiological behavior. One of the best ways of resetting the active or inactive phase in such a system is to introduce a shot of light at a particular time. Depending upon the time of application, resetting may be to an earlier or to a later than "normal" time, but, as in resetting a mechanical time piece, the fundamental period dictated by its "escapement" is not changed.

Aschoff's rule states that if we have, instead of continuous darkness, continuous light under constant conditions, the characteristic cycle length for the circadian is different. It is different systematically in this fashion: for a day-active animal, such as a bird, as the irradiance increases, the circadian increases; for a night-active animal, like a mouse, as the irradiance increases, the circadian decreases.

Corollary questions arising from Aschoff's rule can also be asked. When we repeatedly alter, reset, or stress the circadian, does this influence the organism's longevity? If so, then can stress be minimized and longevity increased by regulated light levels (or by other phase-shifting stimuli) appropriate to the individual's unique circadian?

Reflecting back upon our earlier discussion, I think it is just as important to ask with reference to each experiment, "How was the circadian controlled?" as it is to expect that it was, along with the other physical variables. I pointed out, with reference to Dr. Quastler's comments about Wulff's (53) experiment, an equally plausible interpretation that there is no difference in inherent RNA synthesis capacity between the young and old rats, but rather a phase shift in the one for the time of peak synthesis. The expected empirical results are the same; only time-course data can resolve the challenge.

Dr. Simms's experiments referred to the influence of underfeeding. The food was always given in the morning. These nocturnal animals now became morning feeders. It is well known that psychological factors can override the potent influence of light as a resetting factor. So there are at least two variables to explain the increased longevity: (a) underfeeding, and (b) a phase-shifted or stressed circadian.

Dr. Storer's results—and his own interpretations may be

the correct ones—nevertheless remind me of some equally valid alternative ones. Consider, for example, Arne Sollberger's (51) measures of glycogen levels in the chicken. These clearly suggested a diurnal rhythmicity of the mean values, but even more striking than the means was the rhythmicity shown by their variances.

If, then, one makes a measurement and sees that the variance has increased, can one validly conclude that homeostasis is collapsing? Couldn't this represent a form of homeostasis like Sollberger's; that is, to be consistently variable at a particular time of day from day to day? And might the treatment not have resulted in a phase shift from a plateau of low variance to a transition region in which the variance is normally high?

Quastler: Is there any evidence of change of circadian rhythms with age?

Ehret: I don't know of any, but then I don't know of any systematic searches for this. There are some quantum jumps, if you will, in which an animal behaving with a very characteristic circadian for a long period of time suddenly switches over to another. Some measurements have been made on arctic animals (42) in which the animal appears to be active around the clock, but when the measures are viewed over a very long period of time, one sees patterns that cross each other, as if there were several control systems causing the animal to have his onset of running time. One interpretation is that it is like having several alarm clocks each on its own schedule. Each day, the first clock determines one circadian; the second is on another circadian. The running-wheel activity shows a very beautiful pattern of crisscrossing, and of course some of the most bizarre cases of aphasic behavior in humans have been shown in psychotic, although not elderly, adults (19).

Fremont-Smith: Is there any evidence that our days have been getting longer through time? In other words, might the circadian correspond to a day of a previous period in geological history?

Ehret: I am not qualified to say, but there has been speculation along those lines. There also has been speculation along the lines that, with the clock so precise as to be diurnal, the resetting mechanism might be lost; and because of the seasonal transitions we have in time it is of selective value to retain the resetting mechanism. The best way to maintain the resetting mechanism is to use it daily in correcting the circadian to the diurnal time interval.

Atwood: The change in the day length because of tidal friction is known. I think you could look it up in the World Almanac and extrapolate back to find out at what time the circadian evolved.

Storer: I don't think Methuselah can be explained on the basis of changing the length of the day. (Laughter)

Birren: There are so many possible rhythms that we seem to need a term beyond or more embracing than circadian. When functions such as sensory threshold are measured they vary periodically, vary in cycles within minutes. Certainly estrous cycles vary over several days. "Circadian" may not be the proper term here. It seems to me we have to be alert to many cyclical activities. For certain kinds of observations, these are appropriately averaged out. For other considerations, they may become highly relevant. Franz Halberg, who coined the term "circadian," also speaks of ultradian and infradian rhythms. Most investigators also believe that rather than external cosmic signals, magnetic fields, rotation of the earth, or something of that sort determining the cycles (7), the organism is stuck with an internal timekeeper in the form of an assembly-line sequence that takes about a day to complete itself. The sequences may be related to day-length because of the way they are related to the original photosynthetic organism by inheritance. All organisms retain DNA, RNA, protein, and, generally, similar molecular aspects of synthesis; perhaps they retain the larger details of synthesis as well.

Atwood: When you allow normal day and night, then it is exactly 24 hours, is it not?

Ehret: Yes, because the clock is reset.

Fenn: Do organisms have this rhythm from the beginning even if they had never been exposed to light and dark cycles?

Ehret: It is a good question. Janet Harker (22) has shown that in some insects no such rhythm is observed at first until the insect sees light. Then, having been exposed to light, a circadian rhythm of activity is firmly established.

Fenn: It is the effort of the organism to guess how long 24 hours is, when it doesn't have the cue and doesn't see the light. Every time it guesses it is either too short or too long.

Ehret: These may even represent randomized populations of cells, but the mechanism is not really known.

Fenn: If it had never been exposed to light, it isn't guessing; it is inherent.

Ehret: Each cell may be synthesizing on its own circadian, but the whole population of cells, the larva, may appear to be doing as it pleases, free of cycles.

Sacher: Will anything else reset the rhythm, such as temperature shock or non-visible radiation?

Ehret: Yes, the best resetter we found, in fact, was ultraviolet irradiation in protozoa. This is photoreactivable (12). UV resetting is always late, whereas light resetting can be reset for early or late. Recently Karakashian and Hastings (24) found actinomycin D to be effective.

Atwood: It is more than a resetter; it stops the clock. They get one more peak after actinomycin or, if given late in the cycle, two more peaks. Then the rhythm stops, although the organisms live on for a long time.

Quastler: What is the organism?

Atwood: Gonyaulax, a marine dinoflagellate.
Actinomycin attaches to DNA and prevents the DNA-dependent synthesis of RNA. Subsequently this prevents protein synthesis. The rhythm in this organism is observed in its luminescence, which shows circadian peaks. In this case the effect on the clock is distinct from any effect on luminescence itself. The treated organisms continue to luminesce at a constant level.

Fry: Can you start the clock?

Atwood: So far, the actinomycin effect has been irreversible.

REFERENCES

1. Alpatov, W. W., and R. Pearl. 1929. Experimental studies on the duration of life. XII. Influence of temperature during the larval period and adult life on the duration of life of the imago of Drosophila melanogaster. Am. Nat. 63: 37-67.

2. Aschoff, J. 1960. Exogenous and endogenous components in circadian rhythms. Cold Spring Harbor Symp. on Quantitative Biology 25: 11-28.

3. Barrows, C. H., Jr. 1956. Cellular metabolism and aging. Fed. Proc. 15: 954-59.

4. Barrows, C. H., Jr., L. M. Roeder, and J. A. Falzone. 1962. Effect of age on the activities of enzymes and the concentrations of nucleic acids in the tissues of female wild rats. J. Gerontol. 17: 144-47.

5. Berg, B. N., and H. S. Simms. 1960. Nutrition and longevity in the

rat. II. Longevity and onset of disease with different levels of food intake. J. Nutr. 71: 255-63.

6. Bronte-Steward, B., A. Keys, and J. F. Brock. 1955. Serum-cholesterol, diet, and coronary heart disease. Lancet 2: 1103-8.

7. Brown, F. A. 1962. Biological clocks. In W. Auffenberg (ed.), Biological Sciences Curriculum Series (American Institute of Biological Sciences) Pamphlet No. 2, pp. 1-36. Boston: D. C. Heath.

8. Carlson, L. D., and B. H. Jackson. 1959. The combined effects of ionizing radiation and high temperature on the longevity of the Sprague-Dawley rat. Radiation Res. 11: 509-19.

9. Clark, L. C., Jr., E. I. Beck, and N. W. Shock. 1951. Serum alkaline phosphatase in middle and old age. J. Gerontol. 6: 7-12.

10. Cross, R. J., and J. V. Taggart. 1950. Renal tubular transport: Accumulation of p-amino-hippurate by rabbit kidney slices. Am. J. Physiol. 161: 181-90.

11. Dyrbye, M., and J. E. Kirk. 1956. The beta-glucuronidase activity of aortic and pulmonary artery tissue in individuals of various ages. J. Gerontol. 11: 33-37.

12. Ehret, C. F. 1960. Action spectra and nucleic acid metabolism in circadian rhythms at the cellular level. Cold Spring Harbor Symp. on Quantitative Biology 25: 149-58.

13. Ehret, C. F., B. Smaller, E. L. Powers, and R. B. Webb. 1960. Thermal annealment and nitric oxide effects on free radicals in X-irradiated cells. Science 132 : 1768-69.

14. Falzone, J. A., Jr., and C. H. Barrows, Jr. 1963. The effect of dietary restriction on the activity and histochemical distribution of renal alkaline phosphatase in male rats. J. Gerontol. 18: 240-45.

15. Falzone, J. A., Jr., C. H. Barrows, Jr., and N. W. Shock. 1959. Age and polyploidy of rat liver nuclei as measured by volume and DNA content. J. Gerontol. 14: 2-8.

16. Feinendegen, L. E., and V. P. Bond. 1963. Observations on nuclear RNA during mitosis in human cancer cells in culture (HeLa-S3) studied with tritiated cytidine. Exper. Cell Res. 30: 393-404.

17. Fletcher, M. J., and D. R. Sanadi. 1961. Turnover of liver mitochondrial components in adult and senescent rats. J. Gerontol. 16: 255-57.

18. Gerschman, R., D. L. Gilbert, S. W. Nye, P. Dwyer, and W. O. Fenn. 1954. Oxygen poisoning and X-irradiation: a mechanism in common. Science 119: 623-26.

19. Halberg, F. 1960. Temporal coordination of physiologic function. Cold Spring Harbor Symp. on Quantitative Biology 25: 289-310.

20. Halberg, F., M. J. Frantz, and J. J. Bittner. 1957. Phase differences

between 24-hour rhythms in cortical adrenal mitoses and blood eosinophils in the mouse. Anat. Rec. 129: 349-56.

21. Halberg, F., E. Halberg, C. P. Barnum, and J. J. Bittner. 1959. Physiologic 24-hour periodicity in human beings and mice, the lighting regimen and daily routine. In: R. B. Withrow (ed.), Photoperiodism and related phenomena in plants and animals, pp. 803-78. AAAS Publ. No. 55.

22. Harker, J. E. 1958. Diurnal rhythms in the animal kingdom. Biol. Rev. Cambridge Philos. Soc. 33: 1-52.

23. Harman, D. 1962. Role of free radicals in mutation, cancer, aging, and the maintenance of life. Radiation Res. 16: 752-63.

24. Karakashian, M., and J. W. Hastings. 1962. The inhibition of a biological clock by Actinomycin D. Proc. Nat. Acad. Sci. 48: 2130-37.

25. Keys, A., N. Kimjra, A. Kusukawa, B. Bronte-Stewart, N. P. Larsen, and M. H. Keys. 1958. Lessons from serum cholesterol studies in Japan, Hawaii, and Los Angeles. Ann. Int. Med. 48: 83-94.

26. Kibler, H. H., H. D. Silsby, and H. D. Johnson. 1963. Metabolic trends and life span of rats living at 9 C and 28 C. J. Gerontol. 18: 235-39.

27. Kirk, J. E. 1961. The aconitase activity of arterial tissue in individuals of various ages. J. Gerontol. 16: 25-28.

28. Kirk, J. E. 1962. The glycogen phosphorylase activity of arterial tissue in individuals of various ages. J. Gerontol. 17: 154-57.

29. Kirk, J. E., J. R. Matzke, N. Brandstrup, and I. Wang. 1958. The lactic dehydrogenase, malic dehydrogenase, and phosphoglucoisomerose activities of coronary artery tissue in individuals of various ages. J. Gerontol. 13: 24-26.

30. Kohn, H. I., and P. H. Guttman. 1963. Age at exposure and the late effects of X rays. Survival and tumor incidence in CAF1 mice irradiated at 1 to 2 years of age. Radiation Res. 18: 348-73.

31. Lansing, A. I. 1947. A transmissible, cumulative, and reversible factor in aging. J. Gerontol. 2: 228-39.

32. Lightbody, H. D. 1938. Variations associated with age in the concentration of arginase in the livers of white rats. J. Biol. Chem. 124: 169-78.

33. Loeb, J., and J. H. Northrop. 1917. On the influence of food and temperature upon the duration of life. J. Biol. Chem. 32: 103-21.

34. Maynard Smith, J. 1962. Review lectures on senescence. I. The causes of ageing. Proc. Roy. Soc. (London) Ser. B 157: 115-27.

35. McCay, C. M., L. A. Maynard, G. Sperling, and L. L. Barnes. 1939. Retarded growth, life span, ultimate body size and age changes in the

albino rat after feeding diets restricted in calories. J. Nutrition 18: 1-13.

36. Michaelis, L. 1946. Fundamentals of oxidation and respiration. Am. Sci. 34: 573-96.

37. Miller, J. H., and N. W. Shock. 1953. Age differences in the renal tubular response to antidiuretic hormone. J. Gerontol. 8: 446-50.

38. Morris, J. N. 1960. Epidemiology and cardiovascular disease of middle age, I. Mod. Conc. Cardiovasc. Dis. 29: 625-32.

39. Morris, J. N. 1961. Epidemiology and cardiovascular disease of middle age, II. Mod. Conc. Cardiovasc. Dis. 30: 633-38.

40. Morrison, S. L., and J. N. Morris. 1960. Nature of essential hypertension. Lancet 2: 829-32.

41. Pickering, G. 1961. Relation between genetic and social factors and arterial pressure. Recent Progr. Med. 30: 397-416.

42. Pittendrigh, C. S. 1960. Circadian rhythms and the circadian organization of living systems. Cold Spring Harbor Symp. on Quantitative Biology 25: 159-84.

43. Platt, R. 1961. Essential hypertension. Incidence, course and heredity. Ann. Int. Med. 55: 1-11.

44. Ross, M. H. 1959. Protein, calories and life expectancy. Fed. Proc. 18: 1190-1207.

45. Ross, M. H., and J. O. Ely. 1954. Protein depletion and age. J. Franklin Inst. 258: 241-43.

46. Rudzinska, M. A. 1951. The influence of amount of food on the reproduction rate and longevity of a suctorian (Tokophrya infusionum). Science 113: 10-12.

47. Sacher, G. A. 1959. Relation of lifespan to brain weight in mammals. In G. E. W. Wolstenholme and M. O'Connor (eds.), CIBA Foundation Colloquia on Aging. 5. The lifespan of animals, pp. 115-33. Boston: Little, Brown.

48. Shock, N. W., D. M. Watkin, M. J. Yiengst, A. H. Norris, G. W. Gaffney, R. I. Gregerman, and J. A. Falzone. 1963. Age differences in the water content of the body as related to basal oxygen consumption in males. J. Gerontol. 18: 1-8.

49. Smith, A. U. 1961. Biological effects of freezing and super-cooling. Baltimore: Williams and Wilkins Co.

50. Smith, A. U., and R. K. Andjus. 1956. Resuscitation of hypothermic, super-cooled and frozen mammals. In M. I. Ferrer (ed.), Cold Injury: Transactions of the Fourth Conference, pp. 225-79. New York: Josiah Macy, Jr., Foundation.

51. Sollberger, A. 1955. Diurnal changes in biological variability. Acta Anat. 23: 259-87.

52. Strehler, B. L. 1961. Studies on the comparative physiology of aging. II. On the mechanism of temperature life-shortening in Drosophila melanogaster. J. Gerontol. 16: 2-12.

53. Wulff, V. J., H. Quastler, and F. G. Sherman. 1962. An hypothesis concerning RNA metabolism and aging. Proc. Nat. Acad. Sci. U. S. 48: 1373-75.

54. Wulff, V. J., H. Quastler, and F. G. Sherman. 1962. A possible role of RNA metabolism in the aging process. J. Gerontol. 17: 456.

55. Zorzoli, A. 1955. The influence of age on phosphatase activity in the liver of the mouse. J. Gerontol. 10: 156-64.

Similarities and Differences between Natural and Induced Biological Aging

Brues: A great deal of the best work on aging has been done by people concerned primarily with radiation. Dr. Lindop has done a good share of work having this orientation. We have given this session the special title, "Similarities or differences between natural aging (which we have mainly talked about so far) and radiation-induced aging."

Lindop:[*] Over the past few years, since radiation-induced life shortening was noted, there have been many meetings on radiation-induced aging which have contributed a great deal to the field of both radiation-biology and aging. It might be a good idea to find out whether such a close association will contribute further, or whether we have come to the stage when we must recognize the similarities and differences and then separate into those who are doing radiation research and those who are doing aging research.

There are two main ways I think radiation could be used to study the processes of aging. First, in the study of the long-term effects of radiation, we can try to assess the effects and equate them with the changes we can see as a result of aging. Second—and this the reciprocal of the first—we can use age as a variable in radiation studies.

The study of the long-term effects of radiation really led to the idea of the life-shortening effect of radiation being an expression of premature aging. Because animals died sooner as a result of radiation exposure, and because there were very few data on the causes of death, it was postulated that maybe

---
[*] This work was supported by grants from the British Empire Cancer Campaign, the Medical Research Council, the Medical College, and St. Bartholomew's Hospital, to whom the authors, P. J. Lindop and J. Rotblat, wish to express their sincere thanks.

radiation was accelerating aging. Examination of the survival curves shows that this postulate was quite well justified.

The work I am going to describe dealing with the first question is mainly our own, but many other people have done similar sorts of studies. I don't claim that our study is the ideal one, but it is work which I can explain. The life-span work will be kept to a minimum, and the other aspects of radiation-induced aging will be stressed.

We have tried to control as many of the variables as possible in a population of mice. The only experimental variable we have used is the dose of radiation to which they have been exposed. We have kept the mice under identical conditions as nearly as possible and have irradiated them all at 4 weeks of age which is, in our strain, about 1 week after weaning. Figure 50 shows the survival curves for control SAS/4 mice. In

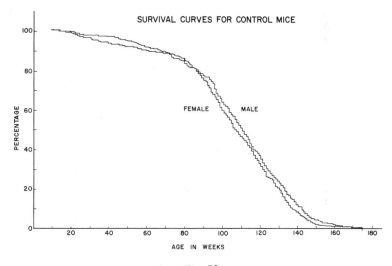

Fig. 50

this strain, the female is shorter-lived than the male. This curve is for mice 8 weeks old at the start. We irradiated them at 4 weeks, and started the life table after the 30-day acute mortality period. The doses have been 50 r and 600 r in single, whole-body exposures. The mice have been kept until they died naturally. Figure 51 shows the effect of a small dose of radiation, 50 r, as a whole-body dose. The life table has shifted to the left, but the general shape of the survival curve is similar in the irradiated and the controls. Other workers have shown similar survival curves (19), and this earlier increase in the force of mortality has been called premature aging.

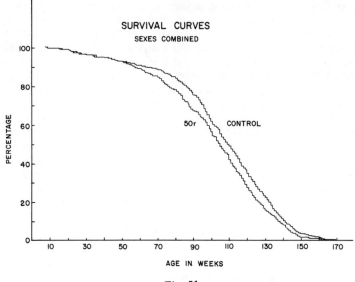

Fig. 51

Lansing: Are we being very fair here? Many of my colleagues here, who are much more learned than I am in this field, have been stressing the likelihood that, to begin with, there is no such thing as aging, that there are many diseases operating late in life that kill individuals, and that, lacking these diseases, there probably would be no aging. We are now simulating the non-existent phenomenon of aging by radiations which, apparently, act by way of shortening life span. Are you suggesting now that aging is any phenomenon that shortens life span?

Lindop: For the present description of aging, I would include any change—morphological, chemical, or functional— which is correlated with increasing age. This is different from senescence. In this case, where there is a straightforward survival curve of a population, its shape is correlated with the age of the population. I am suggesting that, by giving a dose of radiation somewhere at the beginning of life, we bring on at an earlier age changes which normally are associated with age in the control population.

Brues: The fact that the mortality rate is some sort of function of age is not to be denied, and we could leave it, perhaps, on that simple basis. If we want to define aging as narrowly as that, we are on very safe ground.

Lansing: If you elect to make that definition.

Brues: I take it you are thinking of senescence as something more specific, which we don't understand.

Keys: Isn't this a necessary consequence of the fact that a person can only die once? I think that can be established.

Tyler: So far we have only been talking about life span.

Lansing: I think it should be made clear that we are talking about life span and not senescence.

Lindop: The first figures are concerned with the measurement of life span. Figure 51 shows a relatively small displacement of the curves with 50 r of radiation. As the dose is increased the displacement increases.

Keys: If you plotted the age-specific death rate, there would be no difference after that point?

Lindop: In this case the life span can be changed by chopping out a few weeks of early life. This is probably how one would interpret these particular data.

As the dose of radiation increases, the displacement of the curves is even further to the left (Fig. 52). Also, another factor is introduced which was discussed by Dr. Storer earlier: the slope of the curve is increased very little with increasing dose, that is, the variance increases with increasing dose.

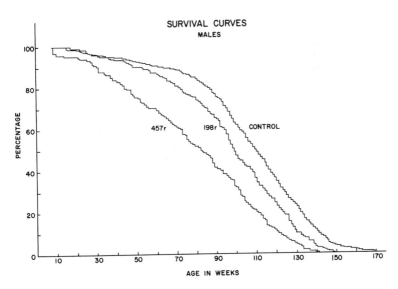

Fig. 52

In our attempts to interpret these data, we have tried to convert the survival curves into something which we can analyze. Most people use the Gompertz function which we find unsatisfactory for our data (11). The survival curve is converted into a straight line by an empirical method of plotting the probit of the survival versus the square of the age (Fig. 53). In this case the data from approximately 90% survival down to about 10% survival are used, and different survival curves give relatively good straight lines, parallel to the control.

Because of this, we feel it is justified to measure the displacement of the line, say, at probit 5, 50% mortality, and use it as a measure of the amount of life shortening being produced by the dose of radiation being given. We have done this in the population and plotted it for each sex against dose in

PLOT OF PROBIT vs. SQUARE OF AGE

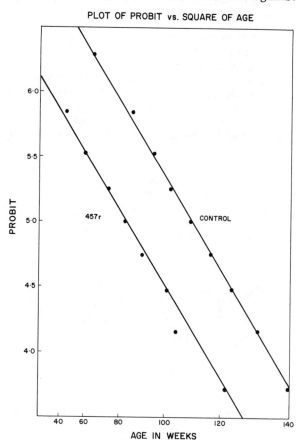

Fig. 53

Figure 54. In the control population, probit 5 is at approximately 110 or 112 weeks in the male and female. Then, with increasing dose, the population dies sooner. In this case, there is a linear relationship with increasing dose. A comparison of ages at 50% survival gives a measure of life shortening.

Keys: Wouldn't you find exactly the same thing if you measured the 5% or 10% probit?

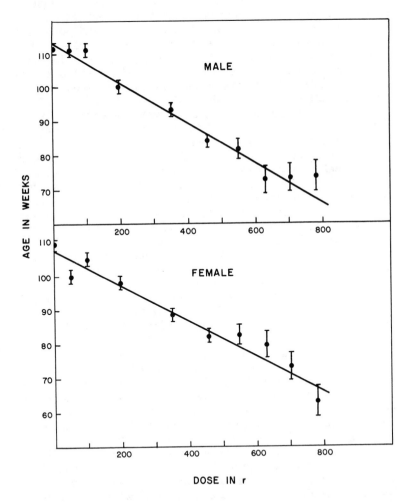

AGE FOR 50% SURVIVAL

Fig. 54

Lindop: Yes. Between 10% and 90% mortality.

Keys: My point is that the differential has been established very early in the picture and, thereafter, all the rest of this is axiomatic. It is a mathematical derivative of the early differential. Isn't that true?

Lindop: Yes. The advantage of a linear plot of this sort is that all the data are used to determine the 50% mortality. We have actually plotted this sort of line for each of the deciles of survival, and the variance increases with increasing deciles, as shown in Figure 55. The divergence of slopes is not very large, but it means a slightly different value if the 5% compared with 50% survival is taken as the end point. By using all the population data, we can get a dose-response relationship for the amount of life shortening, against the dose which the animal received, which is plotted for both sexes in Figure 56. This linear relationship gives, for exposure at 4 weeks old, 5.5 weeks of life shortening per 100 r.

Since the irradiated survival curves are parallel to the control curve, it might be justified to say that natural processes of aging are being imitated. But one needs to know what is going on in these animals to make them die sooner. Death is the final common pathway of many different mechanisms. Just because animals are dying in the right order does not necessarily mean they are dying of the same mechanism. Therefore, we tried to do two more things. One was to measure physiological functions in these animals as they progressed through life, to see if these changed with age and dose in a way similar to the force of mortality effect. Also, we tried to find out what diseases were causing death. For this we did a post-mortem examination on every animal.

We set ourselves criteria beforehand of what we would consider to be a cause of death when two or three pathological conditions were in macroscopic evidence. This has its fallacies, because quite often it is not possible to tell which pathological condition killed an animal. Therefore, by choice of a cause of death, we introduced an arbitrary factor.

On the other hand, if, say, 15 to 20 groupings of causes of death can be classified, as we tried to do, and are studied in populations of about 5,000 mice, even with two or three different examiners using the same criteria, good reproducibility of the distribution of causes of death in the population can be obtained. We felt that this was justified in order to find out whether irradiated animals were dying of the same conditions as the control animals or not, since when we did the post-mortems, we did not know which animal we were examining.

For each type of disease we were able to assess as the

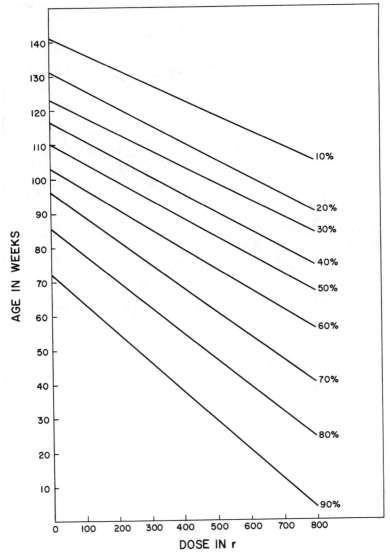

Fig. 55

cause of death, a survival curve was plotted; Figure 57, for
example, shows the curve for leukemia. In the control animals, the earliest onset of leukemia as the cause of death occurred at about 80 weeks. When the dose was increased there

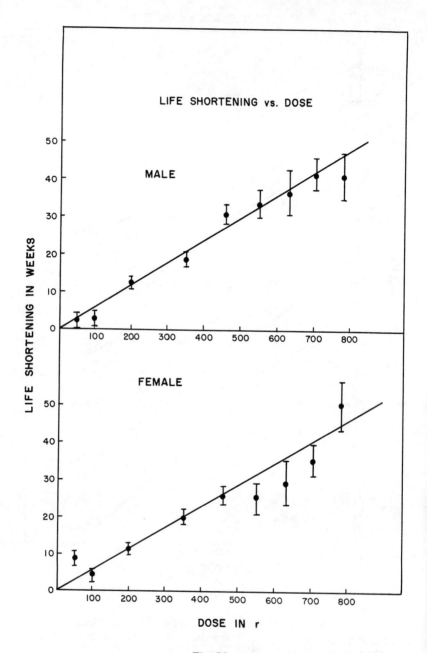

Fig. 56

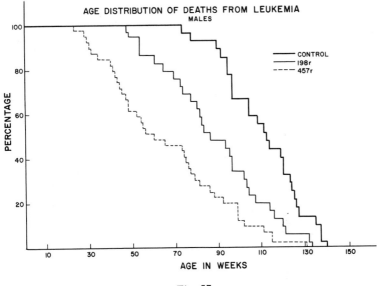

Fig. 57

was displacement of this curve to the left. This is a larger displacement per dose than for all the causes of death combined.

Figure 58 is for all diseases involving the urinary tract, from bladder obstruction to nephrosclerosis. The displacement again increases with increasing dose. In the same way as for the total survival curves, the median age at death for each disease can be examined to see if it has shifted in the same way as the total life span, or whether any particular disease has changed preferentially.

Figure 59 shows the median age at death for all animals. Leukemia has advanced in time more than all causes of death. Certain other tumors, in this case mostly pulmonary tumors, have advanced less.

Keys: The advancement of leukemia depends on the proportion of total deaths that are attributable to it?

Lindop: I would like to put it the other way. Figure 60 shows the incidence of these diseases plotted against the dose. It shows the total incidence in the population that dies, for instance, of leukemia, where there is increasing incidence with increasing dose.

For pulmonary tumors there is a decreasing incidence with increasing dose. Pulmonary tumor is one which was advanced less than all causes.

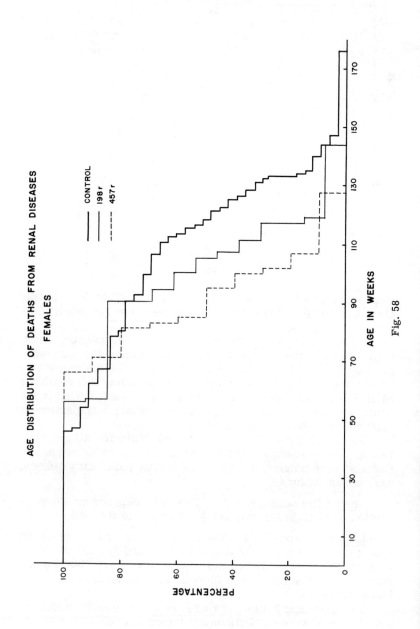

Fig. 58

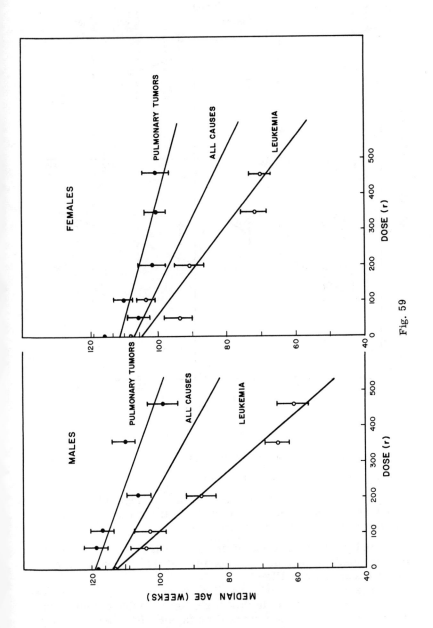

Fig. 59

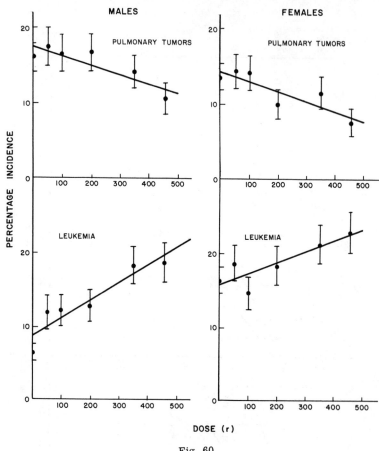

Fig. 60

<u>Simms</u>: Are all ages lumped together?

<u>Lindop</u>: Yes, when 100% dead.

<u>Keys</u>: Does this hark back to the shades of Raymond Pearl who, a long time ago, pointed out that we can only die of one thing at a time? (Laughter)

<u>Lindop</u>: Yes, exactly. If one dies of leukemia, by our arbitrary method one dies too soon to get the things which normally occur later in life.

Because of the relative interdependence of causes of death, it is necessary, in this case, to try to make some form of actuarial correction for the time factor. In other words, if the animals had not died of leukemia, what were the chances of their dying of other diseases? This we have done as a function of dose. It is partly Sacher's method (12, 16) of doing correction for interdependent causes of death, developed by Rotblat (5a). Figure 61 shows the corrected incidence, for instance, of the curves for leukemia and pulmonary tumors taking into account the time at which diseases appeared. With increasing dose, up to about 500 r, in fact, there is no change in the incidence of pulmonary tumors. With increasing dose, up to about 500 r for leukemia, the incidence of the disease is not changed.

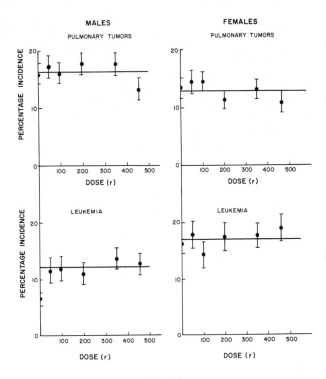

Fig. 61

Because survival curves in the irradiated population are parallel to the control population; because we only find diseases in the irradiated population which occur in the control population; and because, after correcting for time, the incidence of the disease was the same in the irradiated and control populations, we thought that maybe irradiation was, in fact, imitating aging and bringing all diseases on earlier.

What made this particular study difficult to interpret in

terms of imitating aging was that not all diseases were advanced to the same extent; some were advanced much more than others. In fact, some diseases were put out of sequence in the irradiated group compared with the control group. Therefore, we felt there was some indication that irradiation, although producing similar conditions, was not exactly imitating natural aging. Disease, as we have heard in earlier discussions, might not be a manifestation of normal aging.

Because of this, we tried, in serial samples at different times after exposure, to test animals for different physiological functions to see if there was anything we could use as a measure of the aging process. We tried many things but could not find a physiological-function test by which we could discriminate between a 30-week-old and 40-week-old. Whole-body weight was the only thing that seemed to have a group variation with age, and it was quite a useful measure of the function of aging. That is why I disagree with Dr. Berg's suggestion that this was purely a pathological condition. Our mice have been weighed throughout their life spans.

Figure 62 shows the change in body weight observed with increasing age in our control mice as compared with irradi-

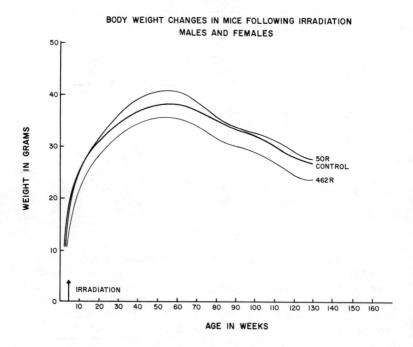

Fig. 62

ated mice. With 470 r, which is a high dose of radiation, there is an initial weight loss after exposure which is maintained throughout life. In fact, they begin the senescent weight drop sooner than the control population. There is some diversion toward the end. If one looked at the weight changes for these high doses just as a function of age, one could again say radiation imitates the process of aging but makes it happen a little sooner. The difficulty is that the lower doses of radiation, anything up to 200 r, will produce an overshoot. In other words, the irradiated mice show the initial acute weight loss which is normal with radiation exposure. After about 15 weeks the lower-dose animals show average weight which is statistically higher than the X rays prove. This obviously is not imitating the natural processes of aging.

Barrows: What is the food intake of the animals?

Lindop: The food intake of the 50 r is no different than the others after the initial loss.

Barrows: Does this mean they are more efficient in the assimilation of food?

Lindop: We have a slightly different interpretation. We tried to determine, first of all, the cause of the weight increase. We put it down to two things: one was skeletal enlargement, the other was an increase in fat tissue. These we determined by specific gravity and X-ray measurements, and the ratio of tibia length to the whole-body weight. We then tested to see if it was due to a thyroid effect by measuring radioiodine uptakes into the thyroid, but it was not of obvious thyroid origin. We then tried to find out if it was an adrenal-cortical effect by testing eosinophil-cell depression in the peripheral blood after a stimulating dose of adrenalin. It was not, apparently, associated with adrenal-cortical function. Nor was it sex-dependent as it was manifested by both the males and the females.

We concluded that the weight increase one gets with low doses is an abnormal, pathological effect and is probably due to some form of pituitary dysfunction. This fits quite well with the distribution of the fat in the animals, which is similar to the fat distribution in humans—in the peritoneal folds and over the shoulder girdle.

Keys: Did you really have to go to all this trouble? It seems to me there is no evidence at all that one can possibly improve digestion and absorption to change efficiency in the calorie/weight relationship. Therefore I assume that these animals became inactive but kept on eating the same food. This is a change in activity, isn't it? It must be.

Lindop: We put mice in a three-point suspended cage to measure total activity, and activity related to body weight. There was apparently no difference in the whole-body activity of these animals. Their food consumption was approximately the same.

Keys: Even the 470 r mouse ate the same food.

Lindop: They all had the weight loss. There was no difference.

Simms: If you will accept Dr. Berg's claim and mine that the healthy rats do not lose weight, then it would appear that the low dosage of radiation may protect against whatever is causing the loss of weight, whereas the high dosage of radiation adds to the effect.

Lindop: Figure 62 shows that the 50-r group begin the weight loss a little sooner than the control mice. In fact, they show the decrease in weight quite well. I don't think that could be the explanation.

We have no evidence that there was any infection in our animals. Since this was surviving population, very few animals were dying. We did do serial killings at this time and found no pathological conditions other than the increased fat. I can't see the interpretation that this can be protection against processes which were not, in fact, present in the control population.

Cottier: For comparable radiation-dose levels we had exactly the same body-weight curves for our mice as Dr. Lindop showed for hers, also with a peak at the age around 300 days. It is wise perhaps to compare mice and rats with some reservations, since the latter continue to grow, in contrast to mice.

Sacher: A pattern similar to that is produced by castration in the male and female, as Korenchevsky (10) has shown in the rat, and as we found recently in the mouse. It is quite well known that doses of the magnitude Dr. Lindop used are sufficient to produce early sterility in the female. There is not a complete cessation of sexual activity in the male but a decrease in sperm production, and presumably some depression of gonadal endocrine activity as well. One can consider this as an example of a pituitary-gonad interaction (7).

Keys: I wouldn't argue in the least about this. The suggestion of endocrine effects is an attempt to get at some detail of the situation which, for the moment, does not concern me. This is mediated in one of two directions: they eat more or exercise less; their efficiency doesn't change. I don't think there is any evidence that the efficiency of calorie conversion from food to adipose tissue is involved here.

Lindop: There is no evidence of altered efficiency. Evidence points to a well-known pituitary dysfunction, that is, a deposition of excess fat, and also an increasing growth after the normal cessation of skeletal growth.

Barrows: What is the possibility that the intestinal flora in these animals has changed?

Lindop: In the acute post-irradiation period the intestinal flora will change. We are talking about changes taking place at least 15 weeks after irradiation. All the normal flora and fauna are back in the bowel by then.

For other physiological functions, we have been unable to find a correlation between the age of the animal and the physiological function or between a physiological function and radiation. Many other people have made similar investigations. For instance, there are changes which take place in interstitial tissue or in collagen in animals with increasing age. Verzar (21) has irradiated animals to see if these changes can be imitated by irradiation, and they cannot.

As for the differences between an irradiated animal and a naturally aging animal, we have to consider the fact that the former does not show the changes in collagen that the latter shows with age. Also, changes in the skin have been demonstrated with increasing age in rats and mice which cannot be seen with increasing doses of radiation. So the skin changes are different from natural aging.

Barrows: As we know from the literature (13), there isn't any real senescent change in the ratio of collagen to hexosamine or in collagen contractility. These changes are basically in the growing phase and not in the senescent phase. I am not quite sure that such criteria should be used as an index of senescence as we know it today.

Recently, Dr. Elden (3) has shown a good senescent change in tail tendon contractibility if he uses 5 M urea.

Keys: Dr. Lindop, I take it you are saying that animals of the same age, irradiated or not, have the same relationship between collagen and elastin. Is that right?

Lindop: Yes.

Keys: What has your comment to do with what Dr. Lindop is saying, Dr. Barrows?

Barrows: I am merely pointing out that many of the changes in collagen are associated with growth, not senescence. Therefore, I think one must be very cautious regarding the use of such criteria as measures of senescence. I am not quite sure whether the changes are meaningful here.

Lansing: I wasn't aware there was a collagen-elastin ratio established in most of the tissues that contain either.

Lindop: This is not my field. I can't take it further than that.

Keys: The relationship between the two is an irrelevant variable, is that right?

Lansing: In my passing familiarity with connective tissues, I have never encountered it.

Birren: I am a curious bystander on these issues. I concluded from past reading that there were two changes: one was in the disappearance of elastic fibers with age, and the other was a change in collagen. I was a little surprised by your comment, Dr. Barrows, that after the age of development collagen did not change. I was told by Verzar that a Hungarian investigator, Banga, has put rats on restricted diets and that the collagen from such rats shows characteristics of relatively young collagen (14). Therefore, to some extent, restricted diet mimics the effects of aging, or is protective against aging. I also understand that a British investigator, Alexander, has done much the same sort of thing, using the hydroxyproline test derived from Verzar's work (22), and found that the collagen changes in irradiated animals are not accelerated.

Barrows: You are referring to the work of Hruza (1). You are right, they are similar to chronologically younger growing animals.

Birren: I will be very surprised if the collagen changes are restricted to the growth phase. It seems to me that several people who have published on this noted continual change in collagen with advancing age.

Barrows: As I have already pointed out, Elden's work (3) does show that a change in collagen occurs after the growth phase. However, I personally feel that most of the data in the literature demonstrate changes associated with growth.

Lindop: The next way radiation can be used in the study of aging is in finding out the use of age as a variable in testing sensitivity to radiation. This is because with radiation the dose being given is known, and it can be a measurable stress. We have tried to determine the sensitivity of mice at different ages, for instance, to the acute effects of radiation.

If the sensitivity to radiation of the mature animal is considered as 1, Figure 63 shows the relative sensitivity to the acute effects of radiation at other ages. The interesting thing here is that there is one period of relative resistance to radiation. That is the 1-day-old. There are two phases when the animal becomes extremely sensitive to radiation: one, around the 3- to 4-week-old age, and the other, when the animal begins to age.

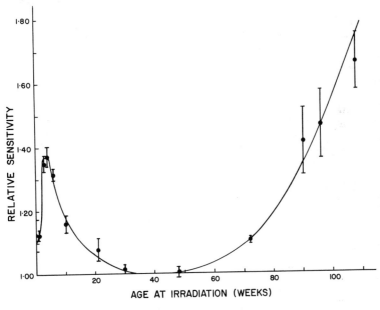

Fig. 63

Keys: What is the measure of sensitivity?

Lindop: The measure in this case is the LD_{50}, the dose to kill 50% of the population within 30 days. This curve is not original in itself but it is one study in which the age change has been followed in the same strain throughout the whole of its life span. Different bits of it fit with most of what other people have found on age changes in sensitivity to the acute effects of radiation. The points which are puzzling radiobiologists—and here they might get help from people studying aging—are the acute sensitivity periods at the 4-week period, around or shortly after weaning, and also at the older ages.

Because long-term studies are also a measure of radiation sensitivity, we wanted to see if, using the life span, there was any age variation in the amount of life shortening which we produced by a given dose of radiation. Figure 64 shows there is. This is the amount of life shortening produced per 100 r of radiation given at these different ages in the animal. To test whether there is a quantitative relationship between the acute effect sensitivity and the long-term effect sensitivity, one can find out the amount of life shortening produced by an LD_{50} dose as shown in Figure 65. Here the life shortening is constant at all ages except for the 1-day-old, which shows a much higher life shortening for the LD_{50} than the other ages.

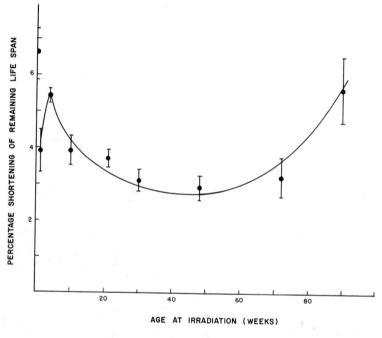

Fig. 64

We have found two useful things. One is that it might be possible to test the sensitivity of the population by using acute effects and, therefore, not have to keep them for the whole development time of long-term radiation. The second is that we have two kinds of radiation damage that vary with age in the same quantitative way.

The problem that has come up about the age variation in sensitivity is in the long-term effect at older ages. In our 4-week-old curve, it was quite obvious there was a linear relationship between the dose of radiation and the amount of life shortening produced; other investigations, in which the ani-

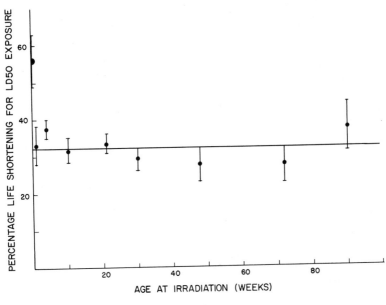

Fig. 65

mals had been older at irradiation, gave indication that if we irradiated at a later age we might not get such a linear relationship. We now have dose-response curves for two more age groups.

Figure 66 shows the life shortening produced in mice as a function of dose for irradiation given at two different ages. It is important to try to find out the cause of the difference in the amount of life shortening produced at different ages. Is it because one particular disease is not appearing, or because the incidence of certain diseases is different when one irradiates at different ages? Other people (8) have found that the incidence of thymic lymphoma, for instance, varies with the age at which the irradiation is given. Therefore we did the same sort of studies on 8- and 30-week-old animals to see the variation with age in the disease patterns obtained.

Figure 67 shows that for leukemia, depending on the age at irradiation, there is a different incidence in relation to dose. For instance, in the 4-week-old and 8-week-old males there is a relatively high incidence. When irradiation is at 30 weeks old, the slope of the increase, with increasing dose, is much lower. In the 30-week-old females, when the natural incidence of leukemia is higher, there is no increase with increasing dose.

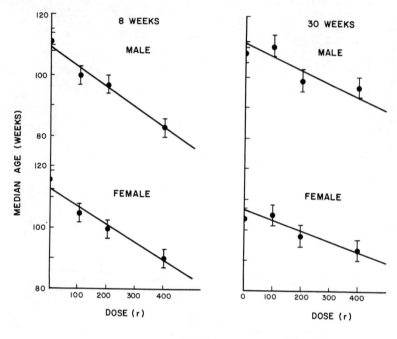

Fig. 66

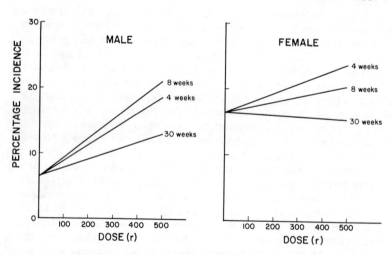

Fig. 67

We think this is interesting because it might give us some idea of the ages for the inception of a particular disease. For instance, if a disease in the control population has a certain age distribution, and we find that by irradiating early in life we can bring it on earlier or increase the incidence, but by irradiating later in life we cannot change the incidence, this might mean that the critical period for the inception, not the final manifestation, of this disease is at the time we gave the stress. In fact, it might be possible to give such a measure of stress as radiation at different times in life and ascertain the critical period for the development of any particular type of disease.

This has been done in the fetal period, for instance, when by giving irradiation at certain stages of fetal development, one can prevent the development of certain organs or certain systems. Perhaps the same sort of study could be done by using stimuli at these different ages of adult life to find out the age of inception of disease. We have evidence, quite by accident, that this might work.

In our own group, the animals in one room—we always run our animals in two completely separate rooms, the same experiments in two separate halves—had Salmonella infection. We started them on terramycin in the diet to try to stop the spread of infection without sacrificing all the animals.

Tyler: Before you go on, may I go back to the thymic lymphomas? What was the interpretation of the decrease with age in incidence of induced thymic lymphomas in the female?

Lindop: If there is a certain age of maximum probability of inducing disease—for example, between 4 and 8 weeks is the period of maximum induction of leukemia—this is the time when the bone marrow is most active and might be influenced by this particular agent. That might also, in part, explain why different radiation fractionation patterns produce different incidences of leukemia, because the hits are at various phases of a cycle of sensitivity of the tissue cells.

Tyler: For the thymus itself, I wondered if this were mainly connected with its involution.

Lindop: The work on age-dependence of thymic lymphomas was done by Kaplan (8). We find age-dependence in all forms of leukemia.

Another thing we know is that the development of leukemia in mice is hormone-dependent. Therefore, at any age, the degree of endocrine development will also influence the possibility of developing the disease.

All the mice that were fed terramycin started to develop

a lesion of chronic glomerulonephritis. When we then irradiated this group of animals, we found we could not further increase the incidence of chronic glomerulonephritis. In other words, once the disease had started it could not be influenced by radiation exposure. We think this would be a useful tool both for the study of long-term effects of radiation and for trying to pick out some of the age changes in disease processes.

Atwood: When you say you couldn't increase the incidence, do you mean the severity?

Lindop: We actually work on an all-or-none principle and do not grade the lesions once they are present histologically.

Storer: Is this nephrosclerosis or true glomerulonephritis?

Lindop: I think it ends up the same way as true glomerulonephritis. It goes through the inflammatory stage and ends up with scarring, as in the sclerosis. I do not think the initial lesion is a sclerosing one.

Lung tumor incidence varied according to the age at which we gave the irradiation (Fig. 68). Histopathologically, the lung tumors induced were identical with those occurring in the control population.

Ovarian tumors (Fig. 69) also vary with age, but this is probably quite obvious because the development of ovarian tumors depends on the hormonal development of the animal. Upton (18) has shown the dependence of the development of ovarian tumors on an intact endocrine system.

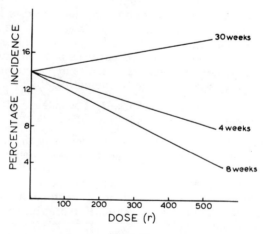

Fig. 68

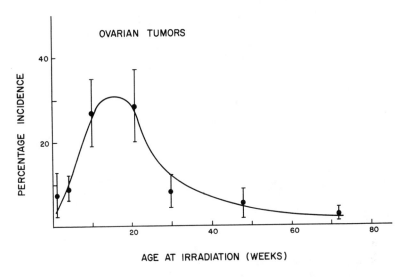

AGE AT IRRADIATION (WEEKS)

Fig. 69

One thing about trying to find a similarity between aging and the long-term effects of radiation is that if we could protect against the long-term effects of radiation we might be able to use these measures to protect against the effects of aging. As most of you know, one of the best methods of protecting against radiation effects is to give the radiation in the absence of oxygen. We have tried to do this in our mice.

Tyler: In Figure 68, does the incidence of lung tumors decrease with dose?

Lindop: In the young age groups the incidence of pulmonary tumors decreases with increasing dose. This might, in part, be due to the increased incidence of leukemia killing them off too soon.

Atwood: That is uncorrected?

Lindop: That is uncorrected.
We tried, first of all, to protect the animals against the acute effects of irradiation by giving them nitrogen to breathe. Figure 70 shows the results obtained in animals irradiated at 1 day old. There is protection against the acute effects by nitrogen and an increase in the radiosensitivity of the animals by giving them oxygen to breathe. It looks, therefore, as if the resistance to the acute effects of radiation seen in the neonatal period might in part be due to hypoxia, neonatal hypoxia being present in the first day after birth.

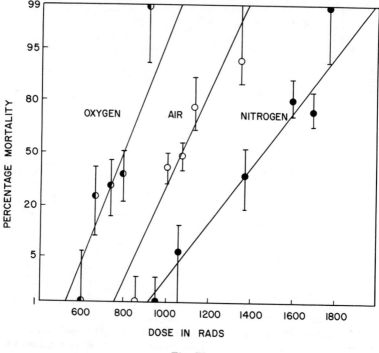

Fig. 70

Figure 71 shows that at the age of 11 weeks, displacement of the nitrogen curve to the right is very much greater than it was for the 1-day-old. This shows that the protection factor is a function of the age of the animal. That might be because of conditions in the animal, such as resting oxygen tension, which might vary with age. If there were a decrease in the resting oxygen tension of the older animals, then removal of oxygen would not give such a large protection factor at the old ages as at young ages. This is what we thought might be happening. The point is that if the animals are given nitrogen to breathe for the same time at different ages, the amount of protection varies according to the age.

The other thing I think is important is that the age variation when the animals are breathing nitrogen is very much larger than when they are breathing air. In other words, it looks as if the presence of oxygen might be masking a very real difference in sensitivity which is present during irradiation in nitrogen. I think, certainly, for future radiation studies, where we want to try to ascertain the age factor in sensitivity, we will do the irradiations in the presence of nitrogen because

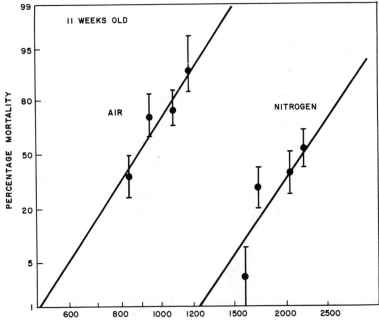

Fig. 71

this gives a larger differential of age sensitivity than irradiation in the presence of oxygen.

Atwood: How do you do that in an animal old enough to need oxygen?

Lindop: We anesthetize the animals with nembutal and then, according to the age, give between 25 and 30 sec of nitrogen, and give the radiation in the last second. We give irradiation at a very high dose rate, and the whole dose can go in within a second. We have about 1% acute deaths from this procedure. The only disadvantage is each animal has to be anesthetized, otherwise they go into convulsion during the rapid hypoxia.

Keys: Do you give 100% nitrogen?

Lindop: Yes.

Quastler: Do you have any explanation for the age-dependence?

Lindop: We thought the oxygen tension was already low at the older ages, so that by withdrawing the oxygen we were not protecting so much.

Keys: Where is the oxygen and how do you know its tension?

Lindop: We have measured the oxygen tension polarographically in tissues we could get a needle into without sacrificing the animal. We found the oxygen tension falls extremely rapidly within the 29 sec but goes nowhere near the extremely low oxygen tension which should be needed for the nearly maximum protection factor of 2.4 to 2.8. Therefore, there must be critical tissue which gets down to oxygen tension at or below the maximum protection level.

Atwood: How do you know what protection to expect?

Lindop: From the work done by Gray (5) and others on cellular systems, the maximum protection anyone has been able to achieve by hypoxia is 3, which can be attained with pO_2 of 10 mm mercury or lower. This has been measured in many cellular systems.

Atwood: In some systems, anoxia lowers the apparent multiplicity number of the survival curve. In such cases the protection factor depends on the survival level chosen for comparison. The conclusion that the oxygen is reduced below the critical level in local regions is perhaps not entirely justified.

Lindop: The protection factor in our case is the ratio of the LD_{50}'s in nitrogen and air in whole animals. From cell systems we can anticipate what is likely to be the protection factor, since nobody, as far as I know, has found a protection factor greater than 3 for simple anoxia.

Atwood: There are lots of them below 3.

Lindop: Yes. I think if we come so close as to get a protection factor of 2.8—which we do at 4 weeks old—on such a measure as whole-body sensitivity we are nearing the maximum protection factor of 3, which I think must mean some critical cells are anoxic.

Atwood: I am not so sure the survival-curve shapes are irrelevant when you obtain a protection factor by comparing LD_{50}'s.

Sacher: It depends upon the number of cellular doses, D_0, that have to be given for a whole-body LD_{50}.

Lindop: There is a fallacy in doing protection curves by comparing effects of a single dose, because if the 50% point is just matched and the slopes in oxygen and nitrogen are different, there is a different protection factor, according to the survival level. The best way to find a protection factor is to do a dose-response curve and then take the ratio of the same effects under the two conditions.

Quastler: Survival or death of the animal depends on survival of a few stem cells which means that at the animal's LD_{50} you are way, way down on the curve of cell survival versus dose.

Keys: What is the confidence level of the ratio of slopes? There must be a tremendous standard error of estimate.

Lindop: For 11-week-olds, the protection factor is 2.45 ± 0.3.

Keys: You haven't given us the standard error of the slope coefficients at all, have you?

Sacher: What you want is not given by the mouse experiment, Dr. Keys. There is only a single parameter, namely, 50% killing, which is achieved by bringing the number of bone-marrow cells down to, say, 1% of the normal value.

Brues: If a mouse can take 2,000 rads it is very far out on the curve of anoxic potential, I would say. It may be unjustified to say there is no oxygen present, but the amount present must be on the basis of what we know in mammalian cytology, that is, small enough to approximate zero.

Lindop: The encouraging thing is that if one can get a good protection factor in a whole animal without reducing the oxygen protection to near zero, our attempts to produce hypoxia in patients might be justifiable. A great deal of work has been done to see if it is. It has heretofore been thought unfeasible.

Tyler: Why is it necessary to use nitrogen at all? Won't animal cells respire at almost the normal rate to very low oxygen tensions and, thereby, very quickly reduce the oxygen tension to pretty low levels by their own activity?

Lindop: The advantage in using nitrogen is that it is an extremely rapid method. Applying a tourniquet to the tissue and allowing it to reduce its oxygen is a long, slow process. We were trying to do it rapidly to diminish possible hypoxic damage to the brain. The fastest way to reduce oxygen tension is to hyperventilate with helium, but helium is much too expensive to use in mice.

Tyler: I think an analysis of diffusion comes in here. I would suppose that one could obtain anoxic conditions for about the same length of time either way.

Lindop: With an arm tourniquet it takes at least 30 to 35 min to reduce the oxygen tension in the muscle to anywhere near the realm of the protective level, and that is much too long. We have studies on larger animals where it takes about 1 min of nitrogen to desaturate the blood of its oxygen supply but not the muscle. I think this is probably the most efficient way of doing it quickly.

Tyler: Perhaps I am wrong here. The whole organism would be calling on reserves of oxygen storage.

Keys: Helium isn't really very expensive and one can approximate the same thing much more quickly than with nitrogen.

Lindop: Helium in our country costs £8/40 ft^3; nitrogen is an industrial gas.

Keys: Why not use hydrogen? The difference between hydrogen and helium in terms of speed, of course, is trivial.

Lindop: We will try using hydrogen.

To return to the discussion of protection factors, two things I think interesting are first that we might have a system by which we can exaggerate an age difference in sensitivity as measured by the acute effects, and second, that when one comes to protection against long-term effects, the protection factor is very much less. For instance, in the 4-week-old, our methods give us a protection factor of about 2.8; if the same animals are followed throughout their remaining life span, the maximum protection is 1.4.

I would like to postulate, and this is sheer conjecture, that for the acute effects we are protecting the bone marrow cells or intestinal epithelium—or anything else concerned with the acute mode of death—but we cannot protect against the lesion, which is the long-term effect of radiation. Possibly this is because with respect to the long-term effects, aging events and ionizing radiations hit the same site. I don't know what the site is. This might well be nonsense, but it is plausible that if the long-term effect of radiation is working in a certain area, and aging is working on the same approximate site, then one would not expect to be able to protect against this particular effect.

We have further evidence that one can protect against relatively acute effects and not against the long-term effects in the protection of the ovary. This shows a very good correlation of function and of radiation sensitivity with age of the animal. Figure 72 shows the correlation of ovarian sensitivity with age (14). It shows the reduction in the reproductive ca-

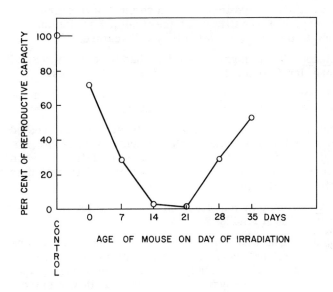

Fig. 72.—Reproductive capacity of mice irradiated at different ages.

pacity of the animal when exposed to a relatively low dose of radiation as a function of age. We have done similar studies on animals irradiated at later ages and in the absence or presence of nitrogen.

Table 25 presents data on mice irradiated at 1 day old and bred at two different times after irradiation. In this case, we cannot give a protection factor because there is no dose-response curve. We can only say there is a measure of protection. This is not shown for breeding at 60 weeks.

TABLE 25

Female Mice Irradiated at 1 Day Old

Dose	Time after exposure (Weeks)	Per cent littered	Average per litter	Per cent surviving to weaning
0 r air or N$_2$	15	75	7.2	91
400 r air	15	8	2.0	100
400 r N$_2$	15	75	5.6	93
800 r N$_2$	15	33	3.5	79
0 r air or N$_2$	60	18	1.0	50
400 r air or N$_2$	60	–	–	–

Atwood: Perhaps this is because the oocytes are in different stages of sensitivity at the time of irradiation, corresponding to the order in which they will mature.

Lindop: That might be so if we had bred at 2 weeks after exposure, but I do not think it holds true at 15 weeks.

Atwood: Do you think that if the oocytes are not matured within a certain time they die, or what?

Lindop: I don't know what it is. What I am interested in is that with increasing age ovarian function falls off. With a dose of irradiation the ovarian function falls off sooner. Therefore, one of the long-term effects of radiation is to shorten the total reproductive life span.

Atwood: is that an effect on the ovary itself, or on the mouse in which it resides?

Lindop: The whole mouse was irradiated. This is one of the good functional changes after radiation exposure which does imitate the aging change, or early ónset of menopause.

The ovary is one system that responds in the same way as whole-body sensitivity, but there are other organs and other systems that respond differently. One that we have recently become interested in is the development of opacity of the lenses, because Kimeldorf (9) has found, for instance, that by giving a certain dose of radiation above a threshold radiation cataracts can be induced. In Arthur Upton's list (17), one of the things that imitated senile changes was the induction of cataracts. We have tried to see whether, in our mice, the induction of cataracts by radiation does imitate the incidence of cataracts in the control population. The first thing we found was that sensitivity to the induction of cataracts has a completely different dependence on age than either whole-body sensitivity or ovarian sensitivity.

The 1-day-old animal is acutely sensitive to the induction of lens opacities; at other ages the incidence of lens opacities cannot be increased very much by the doses we used. This means we have a system that is giving an age-dependent radiation-sensitivity response opposite to the whole-body sensitivity curve.

Figure 73 shows the incidence of lens opacities that occurred in the total population of mice irradiated at 1 day old.

Table 26 shows the sensitivity of the lens at 1 day old in a divided-dose experiment. Here we gave different doses of ir-

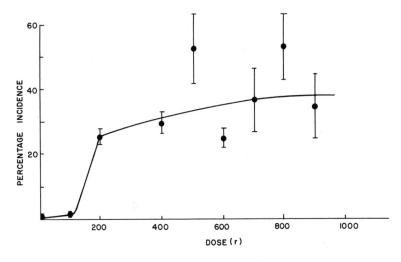

Fig. 73.—Incidence of lens opacities in mice irradiated at one day old

TABLE 26

Lens Opacities in Mice Irradiated at 1 Day and 2 Weeks

Dose at 1 day (r)	Dose at 2 weeks (r)	Number of mice surviving	Number of cataracts at 2 months
0	650-900	90	1
50	650-900	110	0
100	650-900	112	2
200	650-900	83	30

radiation when the animal was 1 day old. We then did the LD_{50} determination when it was 2 weeks old. The number of lens opacities was dependent only on the dose it was given at 1 day old. Although the dose given at 2 weeks old was well over the accepted threshold for this particular lesion, no lens opacities were induced.

Table 27 shows that at 4 weeks old, it is very difficult to induce lens opacities. With increasing dose the induction time is shorter than it is for the unexposed populations.

The other interesting thing about the 1-day-old and opacity induction is that this also can be protected against by giving the animals nitrogen to breathe, as illustrated in Table 28. This cannot be done at any other age.

There is evidence now that this particular radiation le-

TABLE 27

Lens Opacities in Mice Exposed at 30 Days of Age

Dose (r)	Number of mice	Number of lens opacities	Mean induction time (Weeks)
0	854	16	62
50	471	15	33
98	481	15	37
198	457	3	56
350	487	8	42
457	431	13	45
549	103	2	56
630	63	7	39
703	71	0	-
780	29	2	51
Total	3,447	81	

TABLE 28

Incidence of Lens Opacities (Irradiation at 1 Day Old)

Dose	Per cent of incidence
400 r air	28
400 r N_2	5
800 r N_2	34

sion, which has been called one that imitates natural aging, is not similar to natural aging. Also, the induction of lens opacities in the 1-day-old animal is, possibly, a procedure completely different from radiation-induced lens opacities at any other age. It shows what I think is the fallibility of many studies of radiation-induced aging. Just because one sees an end point which can be recognized and is similar to some other end point, one can't really equate the mechanisms. The body can respond to stress and to damage by only a very few manifestations of damage. I believe that many of the radiation-induced changes one sees are of this sort.

One final question concerning life shortening is whether this effect is heritable. If, in accordance with some theories, life shortening is the result of defects accumulated in somatic cells, such defects may also occur in the germ cells and thus be transmitted from generation to generation. These speculations were stimulated by a report in 1957 by W. L. Russell of Oak Ridge that the unirradiated offspring of male mice exposed to a dose of neutrons from a test explosion showed a life shortening of the same amount as animals exposed directly to the radiation. If confirmed, this finding would have far-reaching consequences. Since man has always been exposed to small doses of radiation from the natural background, and if life shortening were transmitted from generation to generation, its effect would gradually accumulate, resulting in a steady decrease in the life span of man throughout history.

We have carried out several long-term experiments during recent years to test Russell's results. A scheme of one such experiment (Fig. 74) consisted in exposing male mice to

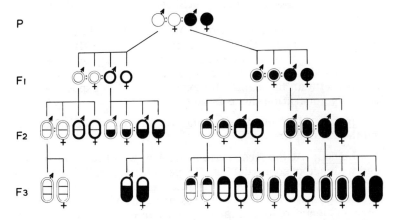

Fig. 74.—Effect of parental irradiation upon offspring: scheme of experiment.

a dose of 350 rads at the age of 4 weeks, mating these mice with unirradiated female mice, then dividing the male offspring into two groups, one being given a single exposure of 350 rads at the same age, the other being kept unexposed. This procedure was repeated down to the F₃ generation. The results of the experiment, which was completed recently, show no evidence of any inheritance of the life-shortening effect (Table 29). The mice coming from parents with a history of exposure to radiation in three generations have the same life span as those from parents without any radiation history. Nor could we detect any change in the sensitivity to radiation as measured by life shortening in mice with different parental history of exposure to radiation. We did demonstrate, however, that the animals from irradiated parents are different from the animals of control parents. With whole-body radiation of over 200 r at 4 weeks old, there is a depression of the body weight maintained throughout life; doses lower than this cause overweight, as mentioned previously. In this experiment,

TABLE 29

Life Spans (in Weeks) of Unirradiated Mice

Exposure history		Male	Female	Exposure history	Male	Female
Parent	C	114	112	C[*]	114	112
F_1	CC	110	121	IC[†]	114	110
F_2	CCC	107	102	IIC	110	112
F_3	CCCC	107	102	IIIC	107	107

[*] C = no paternal exposure.

[†] I = paternal exposure to 350 r at 4 weeks old.

however, as Table 30 shows, 350-rad whole-body radiation at the age of 4 weeks causes a weight deficit in the first generation offspring of irradiated parents of 7.9 g, as compared with unirradiated siblings. The size of this deficit, however, decreases with an increasing history of radiation exposure: thus in the F3 generation there is no deficit.

Jarvik: How many offspring were there in the irradiated and the control groups?

Lindop: At the first mating in 1956, we bred from irradiated males too soon, during the period of greatly decreased fertility. They recovered from this, as one would expect, and so after this we bred at 8 weeks after irradiation. There is some evidence of decreased fertility in the irradiated males. This might be the explanation of the selection in the F2 and F3 generations.

Tyler: Have you tried irradiating the fertilized egg in situ?

Lindop: Glass and Lin (4) have done some work on this.

It is my belief that radiation biology has helped the study of aging a great deal, both by providing good financial support, which is very important, and by bringing some good physical-science approaches to the subject.

TABLE 30

Mean Whole-Body Weight of Male Mice at 50 Weeks of Age

Exposure history	Unirradiated	Irradiated (350 r)	Mean reduction in weight
C	39.2	31.3	7.9
IC	33.7	30.5	3.2
IIC	32.2	30.5	1.7
IIIC	33.8	34.4	-0.2

I also think the radiation biologists could learn—and maybe already have learned—quite a lot by including age as a variable in their particular studies. The time has now come for
us to assess whether we are fooling ourselves by thinking radiation-induced aging is anything like the naturally occurring
disease. The hypothesis has been easy to accept in the past
because we have been equating an unknown with an unknown.

Birren: I appreciate very much Dr. Lindop's very reasonable conclusion here, and I think it leads toward a position
of greater differentiation between radiation effects and the effects of aging.

Being a student of the nervous system, I would have liked
to see her add a fourth category of differentiation: that is the
effects on speed of behavior. One characteristic of older animals is a certain slowing of behavior.

Dr. Herbert Landahl of the University of Chicago visited
us a few years ago and asked what the characteristic change
of aging was, and I said a slowing in behavior. Subsequently,
he irradiated mice and did not produce this characteristic.* I
concluded at that time, perhaps prematurely, that by and large,
the central nervous system is spared injury from chronic,
low-level radiation. Therefore, I regarded radiation as affecting typically the transient tissues, whereas aging is primarily
a characteristic of the relatively stable tissues.

Lindop: Wright and Spink (23) did a similar sort of study,
not on behavior but on loss of neurons in the central nervous
system, and found that the normal loss of neurons in mice
with age is not imitated in irradiated mice.

Fremont-Smith: Soviet studies (5, 20) on acute or chronic radiation effects showed quite striking changes at much
lower dosages than most of the American studies would admit.
They used conditioned reflex as their detection device, which
is a delicate measure of subtle changes in behavior. I have no
way of judging the value of this work, but I think it has been
systematically ignored in this country.

Cottier: I should like to summarize briefly some of the
histopathological differences that appear between natural and
so-called radiation-induced aging. A detailed report on this
study has been published (2).

Swiss mice of an inbred strain (from the Institute of Radiology, University of Bern, Switzerland) of either sex were
given a whole-body X irradiation of 600 rads at the age of 3
months. The irradiated 30-day survivors (479 mice), as well

_____
*Personal communication.

as the untreated controls (669 mice), were divided into three groups: (a) the animals of the first group were killed at regular time intervals throughout their life spans; (b) the second group was allowed to die spontaneously; (c) mice of the third group were killed in a moribund state in order to evaluate pre- and post-mortem changes.

Every mouse was examined macroscopically and 40 to 50 organs per animal were studied histologically. A number of staining procedures and histochemical reactions were applied. Gradual changes were evaluated according to a semiquantitative grading system (2). Radiographs were taken of all mice.

In reviewing some differences in the age-dependent progression of degenerative changes between non-irradiated and irradiated mice, we will restrict ourselves to the comparison of the vascular system, on one hand, and the so-called bradytrophic tissues on the other.

The development of certain vascular alterations was markedly accelerated by whole-body X irradiation. In order

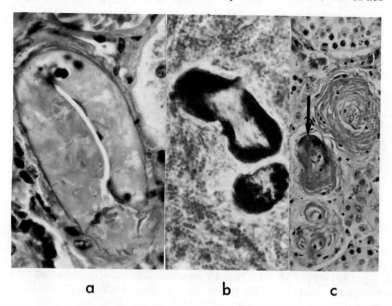

a   b   c

Fig. 75.—Arteriolo-capillary hyalinosis (male mice, killed 18-20 months after whole-body X irradiation with 600 rad).
a) Kidney (hemalum-eosin, enlargement 640:1).
b) Spleen (frozen section, fat red, enlargement 620:1).
c) Testis (↓) (PAS-trichrome, enlargement 260:1).

Figures 75 through 80 are reprinted, by permission, from: Cottier, H. 1961. Strahlenbedingte Lebensverkürzung (Berlin-Göttingen-Heidelberg: Springer Verlag.)

of decreasing degree of acceleration they were as follows. (a) There was an arteriolo-capillary hyalinosis (Fig. 75), characterized by a thickening of the inner layer of the vessel wall by massive deposits of a homogeneous, PAS-positive material rich in lipids. There was no correlation between this change and amyloidosis. (b) Capillary occlusion and focal telangiectasis (Fig. 76) was most marked in females. (c) Deposition of a PAS-positive, lipid-free, homogeneous substance occurred in the intimal layer of arterioles. (d) There was a diffuse thickening of the arteriolar or arterial wall by increased amounts

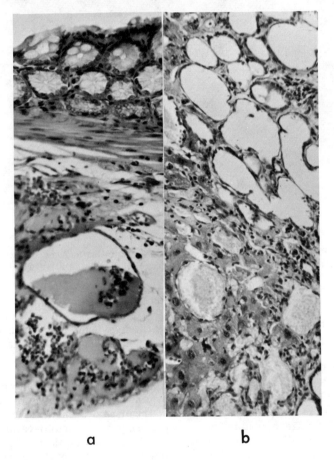

a   b

Fig. 76.—Focal teleangiectasis (female mice, killed 19-20-1/2 months after whole-body X irradiation with 600 rad).
    a) Serosa of colon (hemalum-eosin, enlargement 465:1).
    b) Liver (PAS-trichrome, enlargement 190:1).

of PAS-positive, often lipid-free, intercellular material in the muscular layer. (e) Iron-containing, droplet-like calcifications appeared in the smaller coronary arteries (Fig. 77). (f) Atheroma-like focal thickening of the intimal layer was displayed in medium-sized arteries.

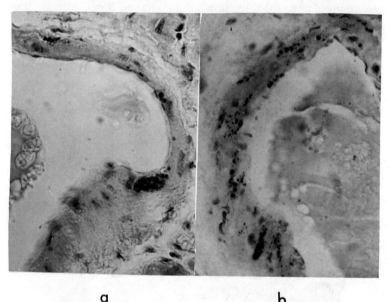

a   b

Fig. 77.—Iron-containing, droplet-like calcifications in the wall of coronary arteries (female mouse, killed 17-1/2 months after whole-body X irradiation with 600 rad).
a) Turnbull reaction, enlargement 425:1.
b) Same reaction, enlargement 285:1.

In contrast to this, the appearance of massive, strandlike calcifications and fatty degeneration of the media in larger arteries was not accelerated appreciably by whole-body X irradiation.

With age the relative number of hemosiderin-containing interstitial cells in various organs increased considerably faster in irradiated than in non-irradiated animals (Fig. 78); this change probably reflects progressive arteriolo-capillary damage with leakage of red cells. In distinction to most of the vascular alterations listed, degenerative changes in so-called bradytrophic tissues were not accelerated detectably by whole-body X irradiation. This holds true particularly for the following age-dependent lesions: (a) calcifications in the intervertebral discs of the tail (Fig. 79); (b) deformities and calci-

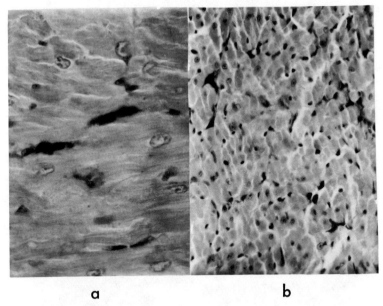

a   b

Fig. 78.—Interstitial hemosiderosis of myocardium (Turnbull reaction, enlargement).
a) 300:1.
b) 700:1.

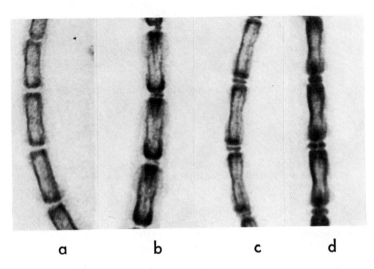

a   b   c   d

Fig. 79.—Various grades of calcification of intervertebral discs of the tail.

fications of the rib cartilage (Fig. 80); (c) calcifications in the
achilles tendon; (d) gonarthrosis; (e) herniation of the discs
between sternal bones.

We may conclude, therefore, that as far as these two organ systems are concerned, whole-body X irradiation leads to
a dissociation in the time course of development of degenerative changes. This represents only one example of many differences found between naturally aging and irradiated mice.

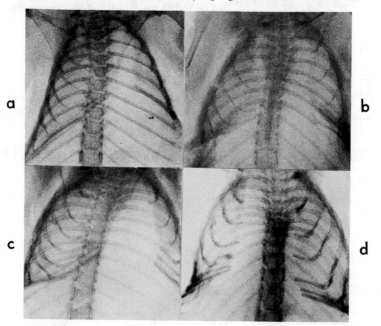

Fig. 80.—Various grades of calcification of rib cartilage

REFERENCES

1. Chvapil, M., and Z. Hruza. 1959. The influence of aging and under-
   nutrition on chemical contractility and relaxation of collagen fibres in
   rats. Gerontologia 3: 241-52.

2. Cottier, H. 1961. Strahlenbedingte Lebensverkürzung. Pathologische
   Anatomie somatischer Spätwirkungen der ionisierenden Ganzkörper-
   bestrahlung auf den erwachsenen Säugetierorganismus, p. 462. Berlin-Göttingen-Heidelberg: Springer Verlag.

3. Elden, H. R. 1962. Aging and the mechanical properties of rat tail
   tendons. J. Gerontol. 17: 452-53.

4. Glass, L. E., and T.-P. Lin. 1962. Irradiated and non-irradiated mouse oocytes transplanted to X-irradiated and non-irradiated recipient females, pp. 57-58. Abstr. Proc. 2d Internat. Congr. Rad. Res.

5. Gray, L. H., H. B. Chase, E. E. Deschner, J. W. Hunt, and O. C. A. Scott. 1959. The influence of oxygen and peroxides on the response of mammalian cells and tissues to ionizing radiations. Progr. in Nuclear Energy. Series VI 2: 69-81.

6. Haley, T. J., and R. S. Snider (eds.). 1962. A response of the central nervous system to ionizing radiation. New York: Academic Press.

7. Hamilton, K. F., G. A. Sacher, and D. Grahn. 1963. A sex difference in mouse survival under daily gamma irradiation and its modification by gonadectomy. Radiation Res. 18: 12-16.

8. Kaplan, H. S. 1948. Influence of age on susceptibility of mice to the development of lymphoid tumors after irradiation. J. Nat. Cancer Inst. 9: 55-56.

9. Kimeldorf, D. J. 1962. The progression of cataracts in neutron-exposed rat populations with respect to dose and age at exposure, p. 53. Abstr. Proc. 2d. Internat. Congr. Rad. Res.

10. Korenchevsky, V. 1961. Physiological and pathological ageing. New York: Hafner Publ. Co.

11. Lindop, P. J., and J. Rotblat. 1961. Long-term effects of a single whole-body exposure of mice to ionizing radiations. I. Life-shortening. Proc. Roy. Soc. (London) Ser. B. 154: 332-49.

12. Lindop, P. J., and J. Rotblat. 1961. Long-term effects of a single whole-body exposure of mice to ionizing radiations. II. Causes of death. Proc. Roy. Soc. (London) Ser. B. 154: 350-68.

13. Murray, D. H., W. R. Watts, and J. R. Ring. 1961. Hexosamine and hydroxyproline concentrations in skin and buccal mucosa of an aging rat population. J. Gerontol. 16: 17-19.

14. Peters, H., and E. Levy. 1962. The effect of radiation in infancy on the fertility of female mice, p. 59. Abstr. Proc. 2d Internat. Congr. Rad. Res.

15. Russell, W. L. 1957. Shortening of life in the offspring of male mice exposed to neutron radiation from an atomic bomb. Proc. Nat. Acad. Sci. U. S. 43: 324-29.

16. Sacher, G. A. 1959. (In discussion on paper by Furth et al.) Radiation Res. Suppl. 1: 263-64.

17. Upton, A. C. 1960. Ionizing radiation and aging. Gerontologia 4: 162-76.

18. Upton, A. C. 1961. The dose-response relation in radiation induced cancer. Cancer Res. 21: 717-29.

19. Upton, A. C., A. W. Kimball, J. Furth, K. W. Christenberry, and W. H. Benedict. 1960. Some delayed effects of atom bomb radiations in mice. Cancer Res. 20, No. 8, Pt. 2: 1-60.

20. Van Cleave, C. D. 1963. Irradiation and the nervous system. New York: Rowman and Littlefield.

21. Verzár, F. 1959. Influence of ionizing radiation on the age reaction of collagen fibres. Gerontologia 3: 163-70.

22. Verzár, F. 1963. Lectures in experimental gerontology. Springfield, Ill.: Charles C Thomas.

23. Wright, E. A., and J. M. Spink. 1959. A study of the loss of nerve cells in the central nervous system in relation to age. Gerontologia 3: 277-87.

Some Theoretical Approaches: Stochastic, System-Theoretic, and Molecular Models

Brues: Some essentially negative findings have been published on evidences of aging in exposed individuals at Hiroshima (33) and also on Rongelap Island (18), where many natives were exposed to one-third of the acute lethal radiation dose.

In Hiroshima, the examinations reports consisted in estimates of ages made by a nurse, compared with the chronological ages of individuals. These were divided into various groups, depending upon estimated radiation exposure.

None of the observations on the retractility and looseness of skin and graying of the hair showed any relation to the estimated exposure of individuals.

Fremont-Smith: There was no acceleration of aging?

Brues: That is the inference, yes. The study included a considerable number of persons who received doses up to the median lethal dose for man.

The Rongelap people were examined annually for a large number of characteristics, including those I mentioned in connection with Hiroshima—baldness, accommodation of the lens, arcus senilis, systolic and diastolic pressure, hand grip, and hematological examinations. Up to and including 7 years after exposure to fallout from the 1954 weapon test, there has been no significant difference between the exposed and unexposed groups.

Storer: There is some suggestion of an increased age-specific mortality rate in the Japanese, depending on how one chooses to do the analysis.

Brues: That is true. As far as I know, and you may be

263

more familiar with it, nothing has appeared that may be considered as absolutely definite.

Storer: That is my impression also.

Brues: The leukemia picture, as we all know, is a very definite one. There has been a considerable increase in leukemia in individuals exposed in areas where they would have received on the order of 100 rads or more, and non-significant changes below that, although further data have to be collected on this point (12, 20, 32).

Jarvik: It may be premature to make this comparison. In the mouse experiments, if leukemia is excluded, how long must one wait before delayed effects of radiation can be observed—the kind of effects that have been correlated with age changes? Would 7 years be a comparable period in man?

Cottier: Seven years may be too short a period of time to evaluate radiation-induced acceleration of degenerative changes in the human. In addition to the tests Dr. Conard's group (18) used to examine the fallout-exposed Rongelap people, it would be very desirable to have functional tests—for instance, for capillary flow rate.

Storer: The apparent completely silent period between radiation exposure of young animals and increased mortality rate is an artifact of sample size. In large samples of animals, at all times after radiation exposure, the irradiated population will show a higher mortality rate than the control population. Admittedly, for the first 2 or 3 months the differences are slight and then become exaggerated; but, at all time intervals, if the sample size is large enough there is a higher mortality rate in the irradiated population. Seventeen years, or whatever follow-up period has been completed in Japan, would perhaps not be long enough for the full difference in mortality rate to be expressed; but, because the samples are large, I think one would expect some difference in mortality rate between the lightly exposed and the heavily exposed.

Brues: In the case of leukemia—and this may be a partial answer—it appears that in man, after a single exposure to radiation, there is a limited length of time during which the disease developed. This appears to be the case in the data from Japan although leukemia has not subsided altogether. There is a peak between 5 and 8 or 10 years.

Lindop: There is another aspect to this, also. If the age distribution for different types of leukemia in the control population in Japan is studied, there is one type of leukemia that has increased with increasing risk up to 7 and 8 years after exposure. But if the population is followed for a longer period, there will be an increase in risk of incidence of the type of leukemia which comes later.

Cottier: In Japan, chronic lymphatic leukemia is apparently extremely rare as compared with the United States and Europe (32).

Lindop: Yes, I think one of the interesting things about the radiation-induced leukemia in Japan was that it was first analyzed against American and European incidences, and people said, "The shape of the induction of radiation does not parallel the control population." Now that comparisons have been made with the Japanese control group, the radiation-induced leukemia does correlate with the natural incidence (23).

Brues: It is a very extraordinary thing that chronic lymphatic leukemia is practically absent in Japan; yet it is about coequal with the chronic myeloid form in all other countries from which we have good data.

Atwood: I would like to comment on the question of whether radiation mimics natural aging. No matter how many radiation effects one can list that are different from natural aging, some component of the radiation effect must be identical with it. This statement is independent of any experimental evidence. It is based on the consideration that whatever individual microevents are summed to make natural aging, none of these are incapable of being produced by radiation. It follows from the physics of the situation: no biomolecules are exempt from radiation effects; hence, radiation should produce natural aging and, at the same time, many other effects.

Birren: How do you make that inference?

Atwood: If one considers the elementary processes involved in the interaction of radiation with matter, one concludes that anything that happens spontaneously would also happen to some extent as a result of radiation, although the reverse is not true. Radiation would then be expected to mimic natural aging to some extent no matter what our hypothesis of natural aging may be. A possible exception is the hypothesis of genetically programmed aging, in the generality of which I strongly disbelieve.

Quastler: Shouldn't one make an estimate of frequencies of those various events—the molecular changes due to thermal degradation or to radicals which occur spontaneously? They don't have the same frequency distribution.

Atwood: Not the same frequency distribution, surely, but it is certain to increase anything that already happens, as well as adding something to it.

Fremont-Smith: But I thought it could be limited to the molecular level. Since the frequency distribution could be quite different, its manifestations at a level more highly organized than molecular might always be different because it interacted with the other processes which were not identical.

Atwood: Yes. It will cause a lot of new processes.

Brues: I think this provides us with a suitable transition to the next topic. It seems to me the notion that the chronic action of radiation is equivalent to an acceleration of aging was derived largely from the first observations made on large numbers of small animals: specifically, the life tables were altered and the measured death rates for exposed animals were higher, resembling those of older animals. Certain other things, such as graying of hair, had been observed in dark-coated animals, although in several respects this is different from the graying of hair in aging humans.

Actuarial studies have been very useful, particularly with their bearing on several suggested theories of the aging process. Mr. Sacher is going to speak on that subject.

Sacher: My point of departure, Dr. Brues, will actually be far removed from the actuarial discussion of aging. I would like to start further back and put the problem into a broader perspective, the necessity for which has become obvious to me over the years.

I don't want to present this as a technical, mathematical analysis of a particular aspect of aging but, rather, as a framework within which a number of models can be assembled and unified. I shall try to indicate that for many of the problems presented there are two or more contrasting views. It is inherent in all research that it is a dialectic process. Each investigator approaches a problem from a particular viewpoint and works out the implications of that point of view. Only later are these special and partial points of view brought together and unified. To a greater extent in gerontology than in other fields (except perhaps cosmology), viewpoint is determined by one's philosophical position rather than by purely technical considerations. Thus it is important to have perspective and to realize that one is looking at just one side of a problem.

The first of these dialectical contrasts is between the view that aging is best understood in an evolutionary context and the view that aging can be most profitably approached in terms of the irreversibility characteristics of molecular structures.

A statement of the evolutionary point of view would be that aging is a time process in the organism, established by processes of natural selection. This process terminates life in such a fashion that the reproductive potential, subject to restrictions imposed by physical and organizational factors, is at a maximum. The problem then is to identify the restrictions and to discover how the maximization is achieved.

Simms: May I differ, in that I don't think it is exactly accurate to say that aging terminates life? The diseases terminate life.

Sacher: I certainly agree with that qualification. (Laughter) As you pointed out earlier, Dr. Simms, the diseases are not the aging process; they are consequences of it.

Simms: No, not consequences; their time of onset is influenced by aging.

Sacher: From the evolutionary viewpoint, one must ask: "In what way does aging become necessary in living nature?" It is characteristic of natural systems that they have a degree of irreversibility associated with any non-zero rate of reaction or any departure from thermodynamic equilibrium. The existence of such irreversibility sets a limit to how long any functioning physical system—whether it be a machine or an organism—can continue to live. From the standpoint of evolution, the one irreplaceable material that has to be conserved and which has to be maximized is the genetic potential of the species.

From this premise, the argument can be developed that the progressive degradation of the genetic information in the germ plasm during a typical individual life history is what ultimately determines the course of somatic aging. This is explicitly a Weissmannian view (63) of aging. But it was stated in various ways by Professor Dobzhansky at the beginning of this conference. In other words, Weissmannian thinking has been assimilated into present-day genetics and evolution.

Fremont-Smith: You are not referring to the aging of the species here, but to the aging of the individual as determined by the germ plasm?

Sacher: Yes.

Fremont-Smith: One could also pick up from the evolutionary point of view the aging of the species. That would be the aging of the germ plasm itself. This needs to be considered at some time if one approaches it from your point of view.

Sacher: Yes. I do not intend to discuss the nature of species aging. There is one important difference, however, between an organism and an interbreeding population. The organism inevitably, in consequence of its structure, has certain irreplaceable elements in it, whereas the gene pool of an interbreeding group does not really have any of these supporting members.

Fremont-Smith: Would you say there was nothing irreversible in the gene pool through time?

Sacher: There is irreversibility, but not of the structural kind.

Let us now consider two different patterns of reproduction. One is that of the mammal, with the formation of a placenta and the development to an advanced degree of several embryos, then birth and subsequent nursing and parental care. This can be contrasted to the pattern of Reptilia, in which the reproductive process is essentially the production of a large number of eggs which are small and simple in structure.

In effect, mammals have a declining fertility-versus-age function (Fig. 81). If that went on indefinitely, there would be a prolonged period of very inefficient reproduction. One could then infer that selective pressures would lead to the evolution of mechanisms for termination of the reproductive period, and for the subsequent termination of life, in a comparatively rectangular form.

In Reptilia, on the other hand, the relation of egg production to age looks more like B in Figure 81 (6). There is the additional consideration that as egg production increases and the animals increase in size, they move into somewhat different ecological niches. One might infer that in reptiles and other egg-layers there would be no strong selection pressures leading to the evolution of mechanisms for relatively abrupt truncation of the life table. This is of some importance in relation to the earlier theory of Ray Lankester (37) that animals that grow indefinitely do not age, where the inference is that continuation of growth is what retards the aging process.

One can turn this argument over and say that species that grow indefinitely and have a corresponding, even if not proportionate, increase in fertility with age, are not subject to strong selection toward rapidly accelerated somatic aging patterns.

Birren: How seriously should one take the fact that many animals continue to grow?

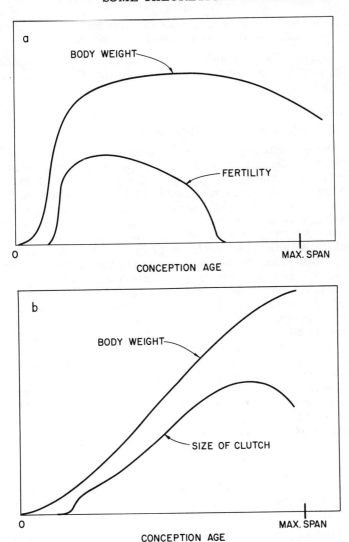

Fig. 81.—Schematic representation of the relation of fertility to age in different classes of vertebrates, in relation to growth pattern.
  a) Typical fertility and body-weight pattern for mammals.
  b) Typical fertility and body-weight pattern for reptiles.

<u>Sacher</u>: Many species of snakes and fish do (45).

<u>Birren</u>: Do they decelerate? Don't they approach some limit?

<u>Sacher</u>: Some of them seem to grow almost indefinitely,

as shown both by growth curves of individual animals and by the distribution of sizes of specimens taken in the wild.

Birren: Can you say with confidence there are species which continue to grow at an appreciable rate throughout their life span?

Sacher: Yes.

Atwood: Could you be specific?

Sacher: Sturgeon and many snakes are good instances (6). They might decelerate at some very advanced age, however. There is a conception in mammalian physiology of growth as a progression toward a steady state, in the mathematical sense, in which material balance is attained, so that body weight approaches asymptotically some constant value. We should not forget, however, the many possible—and plausible—kinds of unlimited or indefinite growth, which could be anything from linear to the logarithmic growth curve that seems to characterize some of these indefinitely growing species. There is a profound difference between any of these cases and the steady-state case. This, in turn, makes a great difference in our conceptions of the growth process: if a steady state clearly is not attained in certain growing forms, such as Reptilia and the others mentioned, one has to ask, in all seriousness, "Is there justification for the hypothesis of maturity as a steady state, even in the mammal?"

Let us take, for example, the rat or the mouse, as Dr. Lindop showed us earlier. At no period in the life of either of these species is there a perfectly stationary or constant body weight, much less body conformation. Since a great deal of the biochemical theory is based on the steady-state considerations, it is important to ask whether, indeed, there ever is a steady state of growth. The dichotomy between the steady-state and non-steady-state conceptions of the organism is therefore of great importance for our conceptions of the aging process.

Fremont-Smith: Is there any connection between this dichotomy and the dichotomy of a closed versus an open system?

Sacher: A steady-state system is an open one, in Bertalanffy's sense (5), and the non-steady-state systems are also open.

Fremont-Smith: The steady-state system is not completely open; it is partly closed and partly open. I thought the non-steady state had less constriction and, therefore, was more on the open side.

Sacher: They are both open in the sense that they are maintained by a dynamic interchange with the environment. The steady-state system, strictly, is subject to certain constraints; namely, it moves to a certain time-independent configuration wherein all material exchanges are balanced; the non-steady-state system is not subject to such constraints. In that sense it is indeed more open.

Another kind of dichotomy was called to our attention quite vividly by the writings of Medawar (40) and Comfort (17). It concerns whether the senescence process is primarily under control of the genetic apparatus, subject to positive forces of natural selection, or whether it is an adventitious thing, a "running out of program," in Medawar's apt phrase.

If the latter hypothesis is accepted, it leads to different inferences in the minds of different people. One is that aging is a nondescript process, just an accumulation within the organism of all kinds of errors in the program. If that is the case, there would hardly be any rational approach to it. From the same sort of premise—that aging is just due to the unfortunate occurrence of a gene mutation which is not operated on by natural selection—a number of people have thought: "Well, let's look for the gene. Let's try to select against aging or look for some enzyme system that has a late action." If this were the model, there would be no reason why the aging process should be subject to very heavy selection pressures. There wouldn't be the kind of polygenic systems Dr. Dobzhansky discussed, and one might hope to alter the nature of the aging process rapidly by a very modest program of genetic selection.

Lansing: With a fixed reproductive period, it would follow that any gene that expresses itself after cessation of the reproductive period would fall in the category of what we call senescent change. It would not be subject to natural selection, particularly if this were an unfavorable change. This, in essence, is the argument. Wouldn't it follow that in those species with no fixed reproductive period there would be no senescence? If we look back phylogenetically, the majority of species don't have fixed reproductive periods. In the human population, of course, the female has a clean-cut, three-decade reproductive period. If we were to discuss senescence in the human population, this would be fine. But there are many, many species to which this doesn't apply. Where there is no fixed reproductive period, then this selective factor we have been talking about really isn't pertinent.

Sacher: I dwelt on this earlier but inadequately, and that was, in effect, what I said.

Atwood: Is it pertinent to ask whether the reproductive span is determined secondarily, by senescent changes cutting it off, or whether it initiates the senescent change?

Sacher: I think both of these things are true; it is a chicken-or-egg situation.

Atwood: Organisms with fixed numbers of oocytes don't live long enough to use them all up. I wondered whether the reproductive span is cut off consequent to other changes.

Fremont-Smith: Prematurely cut off.

Atwood: Yes. Russell's back-transplantation of mouse ovaries, which have a fixed number of unused oocytes, shows that the ovary can function for much longer than the normal reproductive period if back-transplanted to a young mouse.

Sacher: The question is: "What rate of accumulation of deleterious mutant genes in the gene pool would become too much to bear?" The dependence of mutation rate on parental age is the significant factor there, rather than fecundity.

Atwood: Nobody knows whether this dependence is autonomous in the ovary. If the ovary were always kept in a young animal, as by back-transplantation, maybe there wouldn't be any of these age-correlated defects.

If it is possible for any metazoan to be so constructed that it is immortal, it seems remarkable that none of them have made use of this particular adaptation. We decided at the beginning of this conference that natural selection for longevity would depend on how the postreproductive individuals are related to the rest of the population. There must be some species in which the postreproductives are related to the rest of the population in such a way that it would be better if they all lived indefinitely. Possibly the need for recombination would select against indefinite life span. But recombination has been discarded in some species—for instance, in those that are parthenogenetic.

Sacher: The existence of some selective advantage for some postreproductive individuals would be part of the contribution to the total reproductive potential. On an evolutionary basis, according to Haldane's theory (31) which Dr. Dobzhansky discussed earlier, such individuals would not have negative adaptive value. Hence, postreproductively, there would still be positive evolutionary forces leading to the maintenance of a certain degree of superannuation, and the elders of the tribe would have satisfactory life tables.

Atwood: I meant to suggest that it is not possible to con-struct a metazoan in such a way that it will last forever.

Jarvik: Could I have a clarification of some experimental observations? The Russells transplanted ovaries from old animals into young ones. If I understood Dr. Lindop correctly, opposite has been observed by other investigators.

Atwood: The Russells had stocks that were isogenic ex-cept for one coat-color marker. This served to identify the transplant. So you can judge what the experiment amounts to.

Lindop: Dr. D. M. V. Parrott (41) has transplanted ova-ries which were showing decreasing function toward the end of life back into isogenic young animals and tested their func-tion again.

Atwood: The Russells transplanted the ovary while it was not declining.

Lindop: The age at which they make the transplantation might be important. One might not be able to reverse some-thing that has already taken place.

Atwood: That is true.

Fremont-Smith: So the results are not contradictory be-cause the experiments were not the same.

Lindop: That is why I didn't want to bring it up.

Sacher: The point is, the actual selection process oper-ates on ovaries that have to live within a single host.

Programed aging can be easily seen and understood in terms of life tables of parts of organisms. The leaf ages and falls off the tree when the time comes. The red cell ages and dies in an extraordinarily precise fashion. These aren't really cognate because these processes are controlled by the geno-type of the organism at large. But the instance I brought up earlier (7, 8) (of the procryptic and aposematic moths) is a clear-cut illustration of selection acting in an adaptive man-ner to produce in the postreproductive period the kind of life table that confers the greatest survival advantage on the par-ticular genotype. The procryptic moths lay eggs and die very shortly thereafter; the aposematic moths, brilliantly colored and nasty tasting, lay eggs and then survive for a longer time. So the signal value of this aposematic character could be im-printed vividly on birds or other enemies. There is the addi-tional, beautiful property that, here, aging is clearly not a "running out of program" but a single specific mechanism, namely, the escape from inhibition of a pattern of rest after flight. It is this particular process that governs the survival characteristics of these two species of moths.

Birren: Markert, the embryologist, at a recent meeting of the Gerontological Society, cited instances of early-life-programed necrosis, which is necessary for successful survival.[*] His example was that in the development of a fowl the separation of the wing from the body depends upon the successful dying of cells.

Atwood: That is a very common thing in embryos. Many structures are formed and then die.

Birren: So the concept, at least, of programed necrosis is admissable.

Storer: Dr. Atwood, did I understand you to say it is not possible to select for longevity?

Atwood: For indefinite longevity.

Storer: That is a very important qualification.

Sacher: Let us turn from the evolutionary to the structural side of the aging problem. The question commonly regarded as the essence of the aging problem is: "What are the changes in the material structure of organisms?" The usual approach is to study aging in the rat, or in some other single species of choice. But there is a possibility of studying these structural aspects in an interspecies way, by regarding a group of related species as so many different realizations of a single structural plan and examining the relation of life span, rate of aging, etc., to various linear and mass dimensions.
The question is: "Do the Mammalia constitute a similarity group, in which one species can be mapped onto another by the continuous transformations introduced by D'Arcy Thompson (61)?" It is worthwhile seeing how far one can go in that direction. I have approached this by way of the allometric relations, which are relations of the dimension of homologous parts of organisms. One interesting outcome is that a quantitative statement can be given to the widely recognized fact that the larger mammals live longer (28).

Lansing: Again, that is a generalization we had best look at carefully because, while it is true that men live much longer than rats and mice, there are many, many exceptions to the rule—about as many exceptions as there are species.

Sacher: That is precisely what I want to discuss. The relation of life span to logarithm of body size (Fig. 82) does

---

[*] Unpublished observations.

BODY WEIGHT, GRAMS

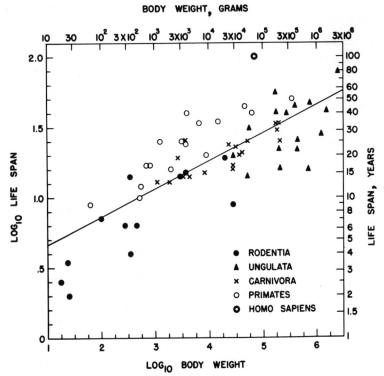

Fig. 82.—Relation of life span to body size in mammals. Life span as ordinate and body weight as abscissa, both plotted on logarithmic scales. Reprinted by permission from G. E. W. Wolstenholme and M. O'Connor (eds.), CIBA Colloquia on Ageing (Boston: Little, Brown, 1959).

indeed show exceptions, but the correlation of 0.6 is highly significant.

Ehret: What do you get if you plot body size versus maturation time?

Sacher: The relation of life span to body weight would be matched by similar plots for maturation period versus body weight. However, I don't think the two things are a single factor—that maturation time, in other words, is always strictly proportional to life span.

As we know from Brody's extensive investigations (13), body weight is about 0.99+ with basal metabolic rate. The relation of life span to body weight is necessarily a relationship of life span to metabolic rate.

Keys: You have a correlation surface and you put down a

point for each species in order to get some information, is that right?

Sacher: Yes.

Keys: You say this occurs within one class of animal, the mammal?

Sacher: This is a relation for terrestrial placental mammals. It excludes bats, seals, whales, and marsupials.

Keys: Isn't it true that the majority of species larger than man have shorter life spans?

Sacher: That is quite true.

Keys: That is a rather large exception, isn't it?

Sacher: The existence of that exception is why I am interested. Man exceeds by a factor of 3 the life span expected in terms of his body size. This raises one of our major problems: If we are to gain our knowledge about aging in man by using small mammals as homunculi, we have to find out whether it is possible, on any basis whatever, to relate the life span of man quantitatively to the life spans of the lower mammals.

This discrepancy in the body-weight–life-span relation for man tells us that when we have done the best we can in terms of the mechanisms by which life span is related to the integrated lifetime energy dissipation, we are still far short of accounting for the length of the human life span. So it becomes urgent to determine what additional factor is operative and whether this factor can be identified and studied experimentally in the lower mammals.

Fortunately, there is in the literature a large amount of data on brain weight in relation to body weight, because the so-called index of cephalization was, in times past, of great interest to anatomists and evolutionists (9). Therefore, it was possible to look at the relationship of life span and brain weight.

The outcome was that brain weight is a better predictor of life span than body weight. If one takes the two variables together in a multiple regression relation, the prediction is better still. Brain weight is correlated about 0.9 with body weight; but one can use a quantity called the index of cephalization, a measure of relative brain size that is orthogonal to body size (9). Therefore, any dependence of life span on index of cephalization is a relation completely independent of body weight. It turns out that there is a significant dependence of life span on the two, of the form

$$x = 0.636w + 0.198y + 0.471 \qquad (1)$$

where x is log life span, y is log body weight, and w is index of cephalization given by

$$w = \log [(\text{brain weight})/(\text{body weight})^{2/3}]. \qquad (2)$$

With this multiple-regression prediction function (Fig. 83), one gets a much tighter cluster. It does not account for everything perfectly, but the big exceptions have now been removed. Most important, man has now found his place in nature. He is right on the over-all multivariate regression relationship. The primates and the other orders are now almost superimposed on one another.

To return to your question, Dr. Lansing, this means that body weight alone is not sufficient to account for the human life span but that, when we introduce a measure of cephalization, we greatly improve the over-all predictability of life span and, what is more important for us, we find that this prediction works quite well indeed for the human species.

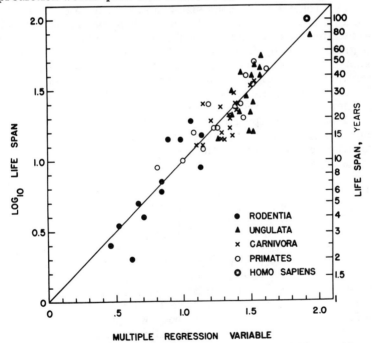

MULTIPLE REGRESSION VARIABLE

Fig. 83.—The dependence of life span on a linear combination of logarithm of body weight and logarithm of brain weight, given by the right-hand side of Equation 1, above. The coefficients of this relationship were estimated by least squares. Reprinted by permission from G. E. W. Wolstenholme and M. O'Connor (eds.), CIBA Colloquia on Ageing (Boston: Little, Brown, 1959).

Lansing: One could do the same using heart beats rather than index of cephalization. One could have lots of games with the general correlation.

Atwood: The elephant would be way off. It has bradycardia.

Lansing: It has about the same number of total heartbeats as the mouse.

Atwood: Its heart rate is much slower than man's; yet it lives about the same length of time as man.

Lansing: The figures comparing heartbeats of the mouse and the elephant are amazing: both come out to about one billion beats per lifetime.

Sacher: There is a group of variables, all related to energy metabolism and cardiovascular function, that have high intercorrelations and high correlation with body size. Heart rate is one; heart weight, stroke volume, oxygen pulse, are others. Together with body size and metabolic rate, they constitute a single factor, so that a relation that holds for one holds almost as well for any of the others. This is discussed in great detail by Brody (13). Rubner (48) was the first to point out that the energy expenditure per gram of body tissue per lifetime is approximately constant for a number of domestic animals. He also noted that man had about threefold greater lifetime energy expenditure.

I would add, Dr. Lansing, that although we have greatly increased our knowledge about the dimensional attributes that govern life span in mammals, we probably have not yet got the full story. There is every possibility that relationships between organs, and other second-order relations, may yet enable us to account for life span more precisely, perhaps not in terms of correlation over all the Mammalia, but by more detailed study within single orders.

I will give you one instance: I had always considered rodents to be small-brained, short-lived animals, but the fact finally forced itself above threshold that this isn't true for all rodents. The gray squirrel can live for 15 years, for example. A few months ago, I compiled newly available data on brain weights (46) and life spans of rodents. One finds a picture for the relation of brain weight to body weight as in Figure 84. The astonishing thing is that the allometric relations for the Sciuridae (members of the squirrel family) and Muridae (members of the mouse family) are parallel and non-overlapping. No squirrel has a brain as small as a like-sized mouse or rat.

If one looks at the assembled life spans for all of these small rodents, one finds just as complete a disjunction. I don't know of any member of the mouse family that lives more than 6 years or so. I have no records on the squirrel family of less than a 6-year life span.

Here is a case where, within a single order, there is a strong stratification in the brain-size factor. It might be possible, because of the similarities of body structure, to make much more detailed comparisons within this order than could be made, say, between any rodent and a small primate.

Lansing: Has anyone worked up an index on the shrew?

Sacher: The index of the shrew is not greatly different from that of the small murids.

Birren: Do you think this should hold within a species also? What puzzles me, for example, is that if we took data on rats in the wild state, we would likely find that about 1 year was the maximum life span. If we put them in artificial laboratory circumstances, the life span goes up to 2-1/2 years, and if we put them in Dr. Simms's laboratory, it goes up to 5 years. That is a huge variance. Furthermore, when Dr. Simms's rats live longer, they are lower in body weight. From this I am led to think that if a condition leads to improved longevity, it would also lead to an increase in body weight.

Sacher: Very few of the data included here are taken from life spans in the wild because of heavy mortality from disease, starvation, and predation. The data are almost entirely from zoo records. These records are of course fallible, but I should say that few, if any, of them are in error by so much as a factor of 2.

Fremont-Smith: You said earlier that the bat was an exception. Where do the bats fall in?

Sacher: I left out bats because they are hibernators. Bats are more like birds; small ones can live 15 years. Flying birds have a strong diurnal temperature cycle and have entirely different brain-weight–life-span relations from mammals.

Brues: If the body weight is reduced, the cerebral index is increased.

Sacher: That is the second point, that there are two opposed actions here. When one gets a high index of cephalization within a species, it is usually for a small breed of that species, such as small breeds of dogs versus large, or ponies

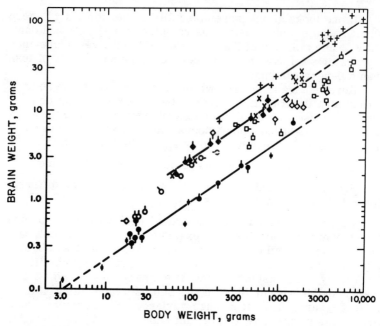

Fig. 84A.—The allometric relation of brain weight to body weight for rodents, insectivores, and small primates. Brain weight and body weight plotted on logarithmic scales.

versus horses. In this case, the short-lived breed is almost always the larger one. It is true for horses and for dogs. Dogs, in particular, have been discussed by Comfort (17). So between these two actions increase in index of cephalization more than compensates for decreased body size (51). This is a matter for empirical investigation. We will have to gather a great deal more data.

Birren: Has anyone done an experiment on small organisms in which the investigator deliberately selected for longevity? If one were successful in producing an increasingly longer-lived species or strain, then, according to earlier statements made here, one would predict that with increasing longevity there should be increasing brain size and body weight. I believe the point was also brought up that there is an analog here in the experiments on resistance to radiation.

Storer: Dr. T. H. Roderick (47) in our laboratory has successfully selected mice for radiation resistance and radiation sensitivity. The divergence was rather rapid after a few generations. He now has a resistant line and a sensitive line. Some of these animals have been set aside for longevity stud-

	CLASSIFICATION	SYMBOL	SIZE OF SAMPLE
Order	RODENTIA		
Suborder	MYOMORPHA		19
Superfamily	Muroidea		
Family	Muridae	● }	11
Family	Cricetidae, exc. Microtini	● }	
Tribe	Microtini	○̇	3
Family	Spalacidae	○-	1
Superfamily	Dipodoidea	-○	3
Superfamily	Gliroidea	○	1
Suborder	SCIUROMORPHA		18
Superfamily	Sciuroidea >1 kg	◇	5
Superfamily	Sciuroidea <1 kg	◆	10
Superfamily	Aplodontoidea	◇	2
Superfamily	Geomyoidea	-◇	1
Suborder	HYSTRICOMORPHA		16
Superfamily	Cavioidea	☐	8
Superfamily	Chinchilloidea	☐-	4
Superfamily	Hystricoidea	-☐	2
Superfamily	Octodontoidea	☐	2
Order	PRIMATES		22
Suborder	PROSIMII	×	9
Suborder	ANTHROPOIDEA	+	13
Order	INSECTIVORA	✚	6	6
		Total	81

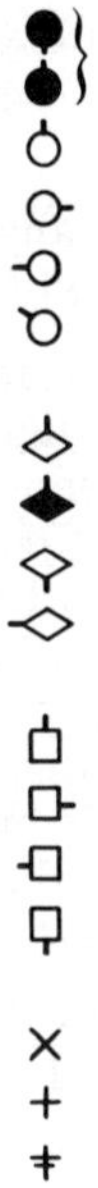

Fig. 84B.—Key to Figure 84A. Filled symbols indicate data points used to fit allometric relations. Classification according to Simpson, 1945.

ies. Again, the data are not complete, but it appears that the radiation-resistant line may be longer lived than the sensitive line. Interestingly enough, the resistant line is also considerably larger than the sensitive line. This could be a chance fixation of these genes, but I doubt it. I think the larger body size may very well have some bearing on the longevity problem. We plan to measure oxygen consumption in these lines and also do some measurements of brain size. Just as a matter of interest, we are currently selecting for brain size in mice and also for brain–body-weight ratios. On theoretical grounds we are sure we will be able to select relatively easily. Once we get a good separation of lines, we plan to study longevity and make associated measurements. If there is a cause-and-effect relationship by selecting for favorable brain–body-weight ratios, we should select a long-lived line of animals. Perhaps we will have the answer in 5 years.

Brues: What sort of factor of difference are you getting so far?

Storer: The resistant line is nearly twice as resistant as the sensitive line. It is really premature to say much about longevity, but it appears that it may be increased considerably.

Birren: Is anybody aware of any study in which longevity has been selected for?

Sacher: The instances I know of don't contribute anything to the brain-weight–body-weight issue. Pearl (43) selected for long- and short-lived strains in Drosophila and studied life tables. It is possible to achieve quite a large factor of increase in survival of Drosophila.

Maynard Smith has long- and short-lived lines of Drosophila subobscura. He also did an experiment that Pearl had done earlier, which is to hybridize long- and short-lived lines. Pearl observed intermediate length of life in the hybrid, whereas Maynard Smith observed marked increase in longevity, hybrid vigor (16).

Fremont-Smith: Has radiation in Drosophila ever led to increased longevity?

Sacher: Yes, several investigators have found an increased survival of irradiated Drosophila and irradiated flour beetles. I did one such experiment (52). Strehler (55, 58) has reported a similar result on fruit flies. Cork (19) recently repeated a classic study that Wheeler Davey (21) did in 1919 on the effects of radiation on flour beetles. The best condition for bringing about an improvement in longevity is that of a daily exposure throughout life, or quite highly fractionated exposure.

Lansing: Baily* has done a similar experiment on favorable effects on longevity of exposure to radiation.

Fremont-Smith: All species throughout evolution have been exposed to background irradiation. Therefore, it would not be an unnatural assumption that background radiation has been taken advantage of by evolution. One could raise the question of whether, for some species, current background radiation is optimum.

---

*Baily, N. A., Roswell Park Memorial Institute: personal communication.

There has been a certain kind of assumption that all radiation is a life-shortening process. Had this been the case, one would expect that evolution would have led to shorter and shorter living and, eventually, the elimination of life. It has worked the other way. Therefore, the fact that it is possible to increase longevity experimentally by increasing radiation over background suggests that this deserves further consideration.

Sacher: In answer to your first question, the best thing to do is to discuss the dose rates involved. Drosophila has an LD_{50} dose for 50% acute kill, on the order of 10^5 r. The flour beetle has an LD_{50} on the order of 10 kr.

When I produced about a 33% increase in the survival of Drosophila melanogaster, starting irradiation shortly after emergence, the most efficacious dosages were on the order of 2 kr/day. On this regime, the control survival was close to slightly less than 30 days, and the survival of some of the irradiated population went up over 40 days.

Atwood: They must have been fairly sterile males.

Sacher: They were males. I didn't attempt to breed them.

Atwood: They would be sterile after a few days. The only dividing tissues in the adult Drosophila are the gonads and a few divisions in the brain.

Sacher: For flour beetles, the optimal dosage level is on the order of a couple of hundred roentgens per day. In each case the optimal accumulated dose is approximately one LD_{50} spread over the lifetime.

The exposed groups of flies, at doses up to 20 kr/day, show a virtual cessation of mortality for a number of days after the beginning of exposure. When the death process begins, it accelerates rapidly, so that even at treatment levels of 2-5 kr/day, which yield a 20 to 30% increase of mean after-survival, the maximum life span is not as great as that of the controls. The same thing happens in the flour beetle: the increased expectation of life is due to a lower mortality at early ages. There is a like phenomenon in the mouse and rat also.

Lorenz et al. (39), using mice and guinea pigs, and Carlson et al. (14, 15), using rats, found that daily gamma-ray exposures at levels from about 0.1 to 2.0 r/day produced small but significant increases in after-expectation of life. Grahn and I (53) have found a similar phenomenon. In the rodent, we know that the mortality is due to infectious disease. In different animal colonies, these can be different diseases. Because there was mortality in the control groups from these causes, it became possible to observe that in the irradiated groups this mortality pressure had been lifted.

Brues: Is there any evidence at all that the species life spans of mammals are quantized–that they cluster around certain times? I am thinking of one of the models for cancer development worked out by Fisher (27)—based on an analogy with crystallization in metals—whereby the rate of development of various types of cancer in different species might be quantized in this way. The basic hypothesis was that a certain limited number of events take place randomly, at the end of which the tumor develops.

Sacher: Fisher's hypothesis was the stimulus to a number of publications about target theories of carcinogenesis and aging. They all assert that the age dependence of cancer incidence can be accounted for by the statistics of occurrence of a small number of events—four, for example—within a cell or in contiguous cells (2, 26, 27).

I don't think that such target models imply a quantization or clustering of species life-span values. Even if the target number could only take on integral values such as 3, 4, or 5, the remaining continuously distributed parameters, not to mention external random influences and error, would probably obliterate the quantization. To my knowledge, nobody has noted the occurrence of modal values of life spans. If the target number took on only integer values, the best way to discover it would be by examining the life tables for a number of species. Plots of logarithm of age-specific mortality rate versus age for various species should then tend to be straight lines with slopes differing by integer values. Such an analysis has not yet been done.

It is certainly true that after examining maximum longevity the next thing to look at is the slope parameter, that having to do with the steepness of the plot of logarithm of death rate versus age, the K of Dr. Simms's equation (55), on page 104. I know Dr. Simms has been interested in doing that. I intend to get back to it when I have more data.

Atwood: When you look at various species, is the difference in the position of the curve or in its slope?

Sacher: You want to know about the relationship between the mean survival time and the slope parameter?

Atwood: Yes.

Sacher: In the mouse and rat the slope is smaller relative to the mean than it is in man.

Let's turn to aging in populations. In the laboratory, we

really don't look at the general case of interbreeding populations; rather we look at cohorts of animals. We produce
simultaneously many animals of almost identical genotype,
start them all out, and follow them. On the other hand, the
other major source of actuarial data is that for human populations, where one has an outbreeding population and a considerable degree of genetic heterogeneity. I believe the existence
of these two very different pools of data may be partly responsible for the two kinds of theories that are most appropriate
in each instance.

Earlier, Dr. Kallmann and Dr. Jarvik presented data on
the survival of fraternal and identical twins and on their performance of various psychological tests. These data could be
used to calculate a quantity which the geneticists call the heritability of a trait. In particular, it appeared from the data
that the heritability of length of life in man was quite high, in
the sense that the identical twins had a much smaller mean
difference in ages at death than the fraternals. The presence
of a high coefficient of heritability would lead one to conclude
that the appropriate model to account for the observed spread
of the survival curve in man is one in which the major source
of variance is genetic.

This is, in effect, the conclusion reached by Szilard (60)
in consideration of the Kallmann data (34). His position was
that the environmental or non-genetic term is negligible, so
that a theory of the human life table is essentially a theory of
the genetic inheritances of the individuals making it up.

Szilard then constructed a specific model. Accepting the
hypothesis of a genetic model, he then had to produce a genetic
mechanism that would give the proper kind of life table statistics. He pointed out that it is very hard to understand this
in terms of independent inheritance of genes, because the statistics of random assortment of tens of thousands of genes in
genetic segregation would give a very narrow spread of ages
at death. So he turned his attention to the chromosome as the
unit of inheritance of the survival character. In effect, he said
that chromosomes are not only inherited as units, as indeed
they are, but that, in regard to the transmission of vitality,
length of life, and the subsequent aging process, whole chromosomes behave as units. So there is something like 50 independent units instead of 10,000.

In effect, Szilard said that an ideal genetic type is one in
which all of the chromosomes are present and intact. He
didn't mean that a chromosome is physically lost, but rather,
that it becomes inactive or inert as a whole. And if all chromosomes were transmitted intact, the bearer of such a perfect set would have the maximum life span attainable by the

species. This follows from his further assumption that the rate of inactivation of chromosomes is constant throughout life, for all cells in the body and for all members of the population. Then the aging process, in terms of the number of intact chromosomes left per cell, would, in effect, be a straight line which would finally intersect some critical value, a fraction of denatured or inactivated chromosomes corresponding to a lethal state.

Since this slope is immutable and is given, there is such a thing, to his way of thinking, as a maximum life span. In the U. S. female life table he used, that was about 115 years. If there was a defective inheritance, for example, whereby one inactive chromosome was transmitted, that would be replicated in every cell in the body of the offspring. Such an individual starts at a disadvantage, and that disadvantage is preserved throughout life, and so he dies earlier. So what happens is that a frequency distribution of number of faults transmitted to the zygotes in a population is mapped into a distribution of ages at death.

Beard (3), an actuary in London, used the same sort of model with a good deal less theoretical genetic consideration. He used a Chi-square distribution, which can be related to the distribution function for a multiple-hit killing process and in which the variable is the number of years deficit from a maximum survival age. This, he showed, does succeed in fitting the human life table, for the reason that the human life table is negatively skewed and, as I remarked earlier, seems to go to what one would almost consider a maximum terminal age. Target curves are positively skewed. If one fits a target curve from a maximum age backwards, one can actually fit, with a relatively small number of parameters, a good piece of the typical life table.

Although this is a model of aging that employs random distribution, namely, the distribution of inherited chromosome faults, it is, from the standpoint of the organism or the population, a theory of predetermination. Everything about the survival and the pattern of disease in a given individual, according to theories of this class, is determined completely at conception.

Birren: Isn't there a qualification necessary? It is not theoretical how the limit itself is set; it is only theoretical why a person lives less than the limit or optimum.

Sacher: Yes, I said it was a theory to account for the shape of the life table on purely genetic grounds—a working-out of implications of the assumption that chromosomes are lost at some uniform rate.

Birren: It is a theory about aging in a very qualified sense, because it doesn't tell us why life spans have characteristic limits.

Atwood: I want to say something good about Szilard's theory (60). It leads to certain predictions that can be tested experimentally, and this alone is enough to make it far superior to most theories of aging. The "faults," as Szilard calls them, correspond in genetic terms to recessive cell lethals. The elementary aging event is a functional blockade of a chromosome or chromosome arm such that the homolog behaves in effect as though it were hemizygous. Thus, if the homolog carries a "fault," the cell dies. Senescence is then a depletion of some unspecified cell population, the probability of death becoming essentially unity when the population is depleted to a certain level. I believe one-sixth was the value chosen.

Such a specification is, of course, rather arbitrary. One prediction is that inbreeding would get rid of the cell lethals, so that inbred strains would reach maximum longevity. This is not exactly true, because inbreeding may have other effects that are deleterious. The hybrid between the inbred strains, however, may be free of such other effects and also carry no faults; hence it may show maximum longevity. Another prediction is that the F_1 of irradiated parents should show life-shortening because of radiation-induced faults. Russell's preliminary results (49) on this point seem not to be holding up, in view of what Dr. Lindop has said. So the theory, even though erroneous, is basically sound. (Laughter)

Fremont-Smith: This illustrates beautifully the great virtue of a concept or a theory or a speculation—it leads to predictions that can be tested. It leads to experiments that might not otherwise be done and which will show either the erroneousness of the theory or the degree of its limitations.

Atwood: I think the theory is basically right. The theory that will turn out to be right will have very much the same structure as this, but the particular, specified elements in it will be different from the ones that Szilard shows.

Brues: Does this theory predict that chromosome number would be an important factor, or, in other words, that the Chinese hamster should have a very odd survival function?

Atwood: It depends not only on chromosome number but on what Szilard calls the probability of inactivation of chromosomes, as well as on frequency of these faults in the population.

Sacher: One could also point out that where it leaves genetics and goes into the somatic life of the chromosomes, the theory is very reminiscent of many observations that the genetic defects of somatic cells are, to a considerable extent, chromosome aberrations.

Atwood: Actually, there are so many other reasons why longevity should be highly heritable that that starting point is still a pretty good one. After all, maybe the brain sizes of twins are more alike, or something like that.

Birren: Could I go back to my previous point? Perhaps I am being a little bit dull at the moment. My impression is that these considerations deal only with conditions which lead to a less-than-optimum life span for the animal but do not relate to mechanisms involved in setting the optimum life span for species.

Sacher: No, that is taken as given. In different species one has to introduce a parameter, quite unexplained by the theory, specifying the rate of accumulation of faults. Thus, if one wanted to compare man and mouse and fruit fly, as Failla (25) has done in his own approach to a genetic theory of aging, one has to introduce an assumption that there is an invariant mutation rate per generation for different species. Once one accepts that as a starting point, a genetic model of aging follows quite naturally, because now mutations will occur at such a rate that, at some particular stage of life, such as the time of 50% survival in fruit fly and man alike, there would have been approximately the same number of somatic mutations accumulated per locus. But these theories don't account for the existence of this wide interspecies variation in the somatic mutation rate, or in the germinal mutation rate that is actually used to infer the somatic mutation rates.

Ehret: But Szilard's theory included a footnote (60) in which he qualified his target determinants to be the chromosomal genes and/or gene products. In the current sense of messenger RNA's, one might consider populations of messenger RNA receiving the aging hits. How does that fit? Is it possible to save the theory by saying that the target is not always or only the gene, but is sometimes the gene product?

Atwood: That doesn't save it because it is essential in the theory that the heritable fault is a recessive cell lethal, regardless of whether the somatic change resulting from that cell lethal is something wrong with the RNA or not. Still, it is just a regular recessive cell lethal that makes the heritability of longevity. That is the point at which the theory is disproved by facts.

Brues: Any genetic theory, it seems to me, has to take into account the possibility that it may predict a widely different somatic cell mutation rate between species of different life span. I wonder whether there is any evidence as to whether, although germinal mutation rates seem to be about the same in these species, somatic cell mutation rates might be as different as that.

Atwood: No information.

Cottier: Is there any indication that somatic mutations do occur at a constant rate? I don't know how good that assumption is.

Sacher: Isn't it true that in some plants and microorganisms the mutation rate is quite low in the young organism and shoots up very rapidly when it reaches a "senescent" state?

Atwood: Yes.

Sacher: The mutation rate is not a constant over all ages in all organisms. But perhaps one could say that for man or the other mammals with an essentially constant internal milieu, the assumption of constancy would be plausible.

Keys: What is the critical level? What evidence is there for that?

Sacher: It is an adjustable parameter in Szilard's theory (60). I don't think it has any physical justification at present.

Lansing: Dr. Brues raised a question concerning variations in somatic mutation rate, as against the known low level of variability in the germinal mutation rate. His question is basic to this whole scheme of things.

Atwood: The inactivation constant for the elements involved is one thing that must be known, but in making comparative studies of different species the multiplicity factors must be known as well. One has to know how many elements there are in one species as opposed to another, and what proportion of them must still remain for viability, which might be different among various species. The elements will have to be identified in order to construct an entirely successful theory. That is what is lacking in Szilard's theory, and necessarily so, because we do not yet have the required information.

Brues: I quite agree with you. I wanted to indicate that this has to be considered in the evaluation of any theory.

Atwood: It is vaguely suggested that it is a cell population that is dying off, or something similar, but exactly what cells is not clear.

Quastler: Does anybody know how far we are from finding out the mutation rate in tissue culture?

Atwood: I think that the Kleins' experiment (36) on the loss of histocompatibility alleles in ascites tumors is the most precise measurement of this. I think the rates were something like 10^{-5} per cell division.

Quastler: Do they have mouse-cell cultures and man-cell cultures that would begin to answer this question?

Sacher: Of course, the pertinent mutation rate is that in the normal environment.

Atwood: These rates are in tumor cells growing in the peritoneal cavity of a mouse.

Fremont-Smith: It has no normal environment.

Sacher: What is, in fact, the heritability of longevity in human populations? As I said earlier, Szilard's assumption was that longevity is about 90% heritable. On this basis, all one's effort in developing models of aging should be devoted to the genetic aspect of the problem. However, I believe the combined evidence indicates a heritability of longevity in man on the order of 50%. This means that one is in the worst possible case: if we are to have an adequate theory of the human life table, we must give equal attention to two aspects—the genetic, as well as the non-genetic determiners, including environment, nurture, etc.

With laboratory-animal populations, the situation is almost at the other extreme. With very few exceptions, the major laboratories use inbred populations showing a very high degree of homozygosity resulting from 100 generations or so of brother-sister mating.

On the basis of the theories of a wholly genetic origin of the dispersion of survival, we would expect virtually a step-function survivorship curve for laboratory populations if the genes were the only significant determinants.

Atwood: It wouldn't be quite that good. The individual microevents are matters of chance, and the role of chance in the effect of a given level of depletion on the organism would introduce further variance.

Sacher: There would be a variance of genotype of somatic cells within and between animals. This could be estimated from the mutation rate and the replication of mutations as a function of the stage of embryonic development at which they had occurred. One would, nevertheless, expect a very sharp curve indeed, even taking all these things into consideration. There should, perhaps, be a long tail for a very small mutant fraction of the population. If one looks at survival curves of inbred populations, one sees instead the same familiar sigmoid survivorship curve. Since I am laboratory-oriented, that was what I focused my attention on. There was also the consideration that even in man, if one uses all available evidence, including the studies of heritability conducted earlier by Beeton and Pearson (4) and Pearl (44), the heritability values for longevity are seemingly close to 50%. Both these things led me to conclude that it would be important to look at the non-heritable fraction. What aspects of the organism, structural or functional, should one look to in seeking to account for this non-genetic variability?

My point of departure was the postulate that organisms in general exist in a dynamic steady state: this state is maintained by constant adjustments or corrections the organism makes to compensate for the displacements produced by environmental disturbances or by the deficiencies of function of the organism itself. The concept of malfunctions arising without environmental causation is a natural consequence of the view that the organism is, after all, a finite self-regulatory system, with only finite capabilities for discriminating its own states and for responding to them.

My major assumption is that the physiological state of an organism can be adequately described by specifying the instantaneous values of a set of major physiological variables, each averaged over the body volume. These would be such things as the composition of the blood in terms of cells, nutrients, enzymes, antibodies, etc., and the performances of the major organs—very much the same kind of information a physician would wish to have about his patients. A specification of the physiological state by a string of such numbers is appropriately called a macroscopic description. I make no gesture toward a theory based on a complete microscopic description of the state of an organism because I am convinced that such a complete description of a living organism is neither operationally meaningful nor physically possible. A physiological state so specified by a list of numbers would then be engaged in a random walk around a mean value whose existence can be inferred from the fact that the deviations are bounded and kept confined within a certain region.

The next intuitive postulate is a restatement of the principle of homeostasis in negative terms. The positive statement given by Claude Bernard is that homeostasis maintains the stability of the milieu intérieur. For our purposes it is better to invert the emphasis and say that the capability of a given homeostatic mechanism can be specified by the degree to which it fails to maintain constancy of the internal milieu. This degree of failure is measured in units of variance or equivocation.

Then there is another fundamental postulate of physiology, namely, that there is some maximum deviation; there can only be a certain amount of displacement of blood potassium, or hormone levels, or oxygen, or any other physical or biochemical or cellular variable one can name, compatible with life.

Now the question is: "Can we specify the nature of this fluctuation process, and can we proceed to calculate the probability that by random concatenations of events the trajectory of the point representing the mean physiological state crosses the boundary between viable and non-viable states?" We will define this to be a lethal event in a formal sense. It implies strictly that diseases have infinitesimal duration.

This is shown diagrammatically in Figure 85, which conceptualizes physiological regulation and stability in terms of a potential well. The physiological state (here represented in one dimension) of an organism in a steady state fluctuates in a small region centered on the bottom of the well. If the fluctuation exceeds distance Λ from the mean, the state will no longer tend to return to the point 0. This is an "escape" or "death." If such events occur, at a rate at least an order of magnitude lower than the recovery rate of the system, then this can be treated as a quasi-stationary process, and an asymptotic time-independent death rate can be calculated. If V, the height of the well, varies as the square of the distance from the mean,

$$V = \beta y^2 / 2 \qquad \infty < y < \Lambda \qquad (3)$$

$$\rho = \frac{1}{\sqrt{2\mu}} \; \frac{\beta \Lambda}{\sigma} \; e^{-(\Lambda^2/2\sigma^2)} \qquad (4)$$

where β is the recovery rate constant of the system, σ is the standard deviation of the distribution of instantaneous values of $y(t)$, and Λ is the value of y at the edge of the well.

We know one more thing about regulatory processes, namely, that the strength of the restoring tendency begins to decrease when the system is displaced too far from normal. The restoring force, instead of increasing linearly, proportionally to the displacement, becomes a curved line as in Figure 86. There is, then, a magnitude of displacement at which restoring forces are essentially nil. In a turning-over cell

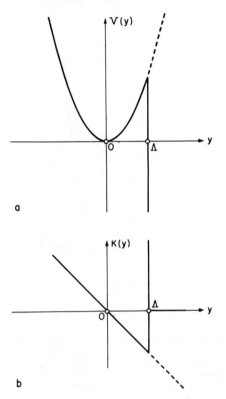

Fig. 85.—Illustration of a homeostatic mechanism with linear recovery, K (y), if to a point, Λ, at which recovery fails. The corresponding quadratic potential function, V (y), is shown also, with stationary point at 0, and discontinuous decrease at Λ.

population, for example, this limit would be reached at zero cells left in the proliferative pool. That system is never going to come back at all. In point of fact, it is not necessary for the proliferative pool to reach zero cells. If the system is driven down to a very small number of proliferative cells, by X irradiation or benzol poisoning, for example, there would be a very low rate of increase initially, until the surviving cells multiplied themselves to the point where restoration becomes rapid. However, the time involved in getting to that state might be incompatible with life, since anemia or infection or hemorrhage could supervene.

I have tried to show that in consequence of the accepted facts of homeostatic regulation there has to be a mechanism of this sort generating randomness or uncertainty in the fates of stressed animals. The problem is to establish, by calcula-

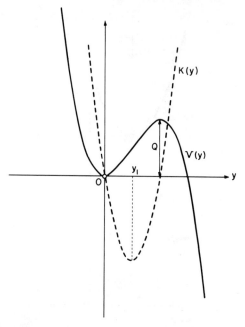

Fig. 86.—Illustration of the case of a quadratic restoring force, K (y), which is the negative gradient of a cubic potential function, V (y). The recovery force diminishes beyond $y = y_1$, and the maximum of V (y) is here in a region of finite curvature. This model is in better accord with the properties of real physiological mechanisms than the model of Figure 85.

tion, the magnitude of the uncertainty in terms of acceptable values for the parameters of the physiological restoring forces, and the parameters of the observed physiological fluctuations. The latter terms are the variances and relaxation times computed from time-series observations of specific physiological performances of individual subjects. The techniques of lag-correlation analysis and spectral analysis must be brought into play here.

In summary, then, I am confident that in the organisms we are most interested in, the Mammalia, a considerable part, perhaps half, of the observed variance of the life table can be accounted for in terms of the known facts of systemic physiology, homeostatic regulation, and its limitations.

Fremont-Smith: Does this imply that the restoration will be a direct reversal of the displacement? Physiological processes, for instance, in Henderson's nomograms of the blood, would indicate that the restorations are, rather, compensatory forces that come in great variety one after another, in sequence, to protect, for instance, the pH of the blood.

Sacher: Yes. That is more than I can discuss at the moment. If one wrote deterministic models, such a model would describe a multivariate system in terms of a set of continuous differential equations and one would say the organism is going to solve these equations in a simultaneous and continuous fashion. So from some initial point there would be a determinate trajectory back to the equilibrium point.

Fremont-Smith: Not along the same line; it could be a different trajectory, couldn't it?

Sacher: It would almost always be different.

I hasten to say I have not the slightest evidence that living systems do obey simple equations of this kind. It is possible that the recovery process consists of steps taken sequentially by a central integrative mechanism: reading the whole state of affairs and not being able to do everything at once, the mechanism says:"What should we do next?" This has some resemblances to computational algorithms developed by G. P. E. Box (10, 11) and other statisticians (30), which are used to solve problems such as we have when the yield of a reaction vessel must be maximized and there are a number of reactants and physical factors such as temperature, pressure, etc. The question there is: "What is the mix that will give the maximum return for our investment?" This became a serious problem in the culture of penicillin and other antibiotics, because a large number of factors had to be adjusted.

Fremont-Smith: This is the first time I have heard anyone but a Soviet use the word "algorithm."

Sacher: An algorithm is a stepwise computational procedure. We use simple ones such as long division all the time. In the case of chemical engineering, yield as a function of the controlled variables is presumed to be a surface with a maximum. The problem is to find the top of that hill by the most economical procedure; so the method is also referred to as "hill climbing." Since the physiological problem is formally similar, it is not impossible that the brain tackles the physiological problem in a similar way. That would mean that the kind of potential well models shown in Figures 85 and 86 would be convenient crutches for the present, to get us to the point of thinking about a random process and its implications for disease and death; they need not have any close relation to the actual process as accomplished in organisms.

It should be noted, however, that the only real difference between the model I presented earlier and the algorithmic hill-climbing model is that the former is continuous and the latter discrete. The idea of a potential function is also essential to the discrete process. The value in moving to an algorithmic conception of physiological regulation is that it prompts us to ask how maturation and learning contribute to the ontogeny of regulatory patterns.

Atwood: What experiment does this suggest?

Sacher: If one looks at mortality rates in almost any of the metazoan populations, one finds that age-specific mortality rate versus time is a rapidly accelerated function, approximately exponential. So, in regard to the problem of accounting for aging actuarially, that is, in terms of increased probability of disease, the question is: "How do we account for risk of death increasing by a factor of 10^3 to 10^4 during a lifetime?"

Atwood: What is the experiment?

Sacher: Be patient. If one examines the constitutive physiological variables, one sees that the description of the state of the organism as a function of age can be comprised by the statement that mean levels of physiological variables only occasionally change by so much as a factor of 2 over the life span.

One must ask, then, what kind of statistical process can relate this slow, linear age change with the rapidly increasing mortality process? My answer is that a fluctuation process of the kind I described, utilizing values of the fluctuation parameters, will give the required relation.

A statistical model resembling this in some respects was proposed by Dr. Simms (54) in a paper on hemorrhage as a cause of death. He bled a number of animals and found that the volume of blood that could be delivered from the decapitated rat decreased as a function of age more or less linearly.

Storer: That isn't exactly right. He bled them with a controlled hemorrhage and determined how much blood loss is necessary to kill the animal as a function of age.

Sacher: That is true. Next he noted that there was a sigmoid distribution of number of animals with bleeding volumes less than or equal to a given value. Then he said in effect: "Suppose there were some disease condition in which loss of blood was a critical event? It would follow that, in the young animal, it is far less probable that this critical depression of the blood level would be attained. The variation of blood level between animals is small compared to the total distance and, as age increased, this probability would increase rapidly."

In effect, he got a relation of the death rate to the cumulative probability, P, that a blood volume would lie below this critical value. He then showed that if one plotted the log of P versus age for the hypothetical case of an aging process in which the population median diminishes in linear fashion while the standard deviation is constant, such a plot would approximate fairly well to an exponential relation to age. I understand that Dr. Simms no longer holds with this model, and that his presentation here represents his current views. I cannot say I ever completely accepted it because the details of the statistical model are somewhat contradictory. But I did accept the basic conception of a statistical relation between the distribution of values of physiological variables and the probability of mortality, and I hold it today.

The point is that when one develops a consistent statistical model, albeit oversimplified, it does give, with these same assumptions, the observed exponential relation of death rate to age. Moreover, experimentally, this exponential relation holds for genetically uniform populations maintained in constant (including aseptic) environments, so that genetic and environmental variance terms are minimal. That is about as close as I can get to answering your question, Dr. Atwood.

Atwood: A number of different models could be used which would give excellent fits.

Sacher: You have to recall that the model here includes the parameters of the physiological systems involved. The real test, then, is to find a system in which there is a disease or death process that can be uniquely characterized and that arises from a particular physiological variable that can be adequately measured: then tie the two together.

This is the kind of experiment I think would be quite determinative, because this is a phenomenological model. If one did it and could make the necessary physiological measurements, there would be no parameters left over to be adjusted.

In the same sense that the Szilard type of theory (60) is testable, I would maintain this one is testable also. The difficulty is that it is hard to isolate a system adequately to permit a measurement of both the parameters of the continuous fluctuation process and the mortality process.

Atwood: I don't understand. Could you give a sample protocol of an experiment?

Sacher: The writing of a protocol is a matter of first finding and isolating the physiological system that has the properties.

Atwood: Just think of one.

Sacher: Some few years ago, Dr. Quastler and I discussed the possibility of comparing theory and experiment in regard to the estimation of the probability of bacterial infection as a function of a leakage rate of bacteria into the system, and of the number of white cells circulating in it. However, one still needs some mediating assumptions and therefore adjustable variables. We don't know what kind of search pattern white cells use, or what the capture cross-sections of bacteria are, for example. Given these parameters, however, an expectation-of-disease probability would be a function of controllable parameters, such as mean white-cell level. By definition, then, a disease would be the growth of a bacterial clone beyond a critical size.

Atwood: For example, take a group of animals of different ages.

Sacher: Age has nothing to do with it.

Atwood: This is analogous to the Simms experiment, but instead of bleeding the animals are injected with graded numbers of bacteria.

Sacher: Age is not the crux of the testing of this hypothesis. The hypothesis is really one about the nature of the death process in its relation to a physiological fluctuation process. That the parameters of this process have a dependence on age is merely an empirical fact.

Atwood: It is of interest to us.

Sacher: If one could, for any state of affairs, test the relation of death rates to physiological states, the further application to the aging problem would be merely an exercise. Let's go back to the bacteria and white cells. If we wanted to study this problem meaningfully, it would be desirable to set up a condition in which we could control the mean circulating white-cell level at will instead of sitting around and waiting for the animals to get so old that the white cells decrease, granting they do—which they don't. (Laughter) In other words, the major part of the hypothesis is better testable within a circumscribed laboratory situation than it is by employing age to generate the change in a physiological parameter, since aging changes all parameters, many of them in still unknown degree.

I am also hopeful that erythrocyte lysis in vitro will have all the essential properties necessary to permit a test of this stochastic model, because erythrocytes are very uniform, lack genetic apparatus, live in a remarkably constant environment, and present a sharp, unequivocal death process. They also undergo an aging process that can be characterized biochemically, and can be lysed by a variety of simple, precisely controllable physical and chemical agents.

Quastler: I have a feeling your model suggests certain things to check. However, I don't see why you call it phenomenological; it does not look very phenomenological to me.

Sacher: It is phenomenological in that it presents a relation between two classes of phenomena, continuous physiological variation and probabilistic death events. The phenomena have been left unmeasured, but that does not mean that their nature is undetermined.

Quastler: All right, but the model, of course, is not vulnerable.

Sacher: I wouldn't say that is right.

Quastler: Any time one gets the wrong results, one can adjust the shape of the potential variables or the restoring functions.

Sacher: Not if the case is one in which these things are physically and independently calculable.

Quastler: Suppose one takes, say, leukocyte count as the critical variable, and one gets only wrong relations. No matter, it was just the wrong variable; it must be some other variable or combination of variables. Indeed, one might easily suspect that some combination of six variables is involved— and for six variables with four parameters each, one can really construct a variety of potential wells that will accommodate almost any kind of available data.

Sacher: You express very well the difficulties I see in trying to establish critical experiments.

Quastler: It just suggests places to go. It would help one to know when one had reached a wrong place.

Sacher: One can find two kinds of consistencies, I should say. One is to measure the continuous physiological parameter and the mortality-rate parameter and show that one of them is enough to account for the other in a sufficiently well-isolated system. I am not much closer to doing this experiment today than I was 10 years ago. The other is to look at the shapes of the curves obtained and consider the formal consistency between the predictions of the model and observation. In other words, to ask what would happen if we observed the system and looked at the actuarial outcome.

One cardinal fact is, and here I am subject to correction from those here present, the aging of the major constituent

variables of organisms—not trace elements or clinker sub-
stances such as age pigments, but such things as metabolic
rate, various critical cell population sizes, and so on—is one
of gradual linear decrease with age, and the picture of mortality rate is of a rapidly accelerated kind. Introducing the
model of a statistical fluctuation process as the intermediary,
one gets back the proper relation between these. This, I agree,
is not unique. What other way is there to go from the observed
physiological picture to the observed mortality picture while
still getting the same kind of mathematical relationship? I
don't know any alternative way of deriving this exponential relationship from different considerations that I can give credence to. But that is perhaps a matter of the limitations in the
exhaustiveness of my examination of alternative hypotheses.

Suppose we were to produce some sort of insult to the
organism, such as by radiation, for example. Let us accept
the various lines of evidence, the genetic in particular, that
radiation will leave a residue of damage such as point mutations, chromosome aberrations, denaturations of information-
bearing macromolecules, etc. Then consider the case where
one gives a single radiation exposure in early adult life. Let
us assume that the exposure is such that the transient acute
injury and mortality can be ignored. By this model, we would
expect the permanent radiation injury to combine with the
aging injury already present or accumulated subsequently; we
should then get a displacement in that irradiated population
such that the rate of mortality in it would be increased above
the control rate by a constant factor at subsequent ages.

Figure 87 shows what happens when we take empirical
data. This is one of the first tests I made of radiation mortality data (50). The data came from a study by Furth et al.
(29, 62) on the late effects of weapon-quality radiations. We
looked at about a dozen experiments from our own and other
laboratories, and the general outcome is as shown. By Chi-
square test there is no deviation from parallelism. I don't say
these were all straight lines; that is not a necessary part of
the theory. As you will recall, the theory states that if the
physiological aging process consists of a linear decrement,
the rate of mortality will go up exponentially; but it doesn't
state that the physiological decrements with age must be
linear.

I think other people are dissatisfied with the Gompertz
equation as a way of fitting data. For example, Lindop and
Rotblat (38) used the probit of survival versus the square of
time. Others use other transforming functions. These may
linearize the curves better, but I would point out that (a) lin-
earization of the curve of log death rates is not essential to

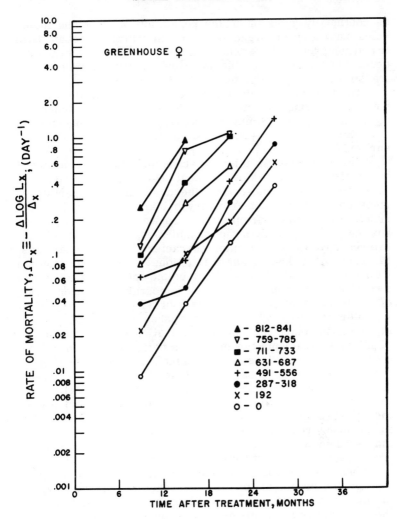

Fig. 87.—An example of the effect of a single exposure to ionizing radiations on the subsequent death rates of populations of mice. Death rates plotted on a logarithmic scale versus time after irradiation in days. Data of Furth et al. (29). Reprinted by permission from Radiology 67: 250-57, 1956.

the correctness of the stochastic theory and (b) the transformations chosen have no theoretical support; they just, by random search, turned out to be things that worked.

Carrying this same stochastic concept downward, one can say that as a consequence of fluctuation and as a function of the magnitude of fluctuations, a number of little deaths would be continually going on in the population of cells and molecules making up an organism. The same kind of probabilistic transition process I described for death of the whole organism occurs in the irreplaceable macromolecules that store and transmit the information that is needed for continued survival. The latter part of the theory leads to the consideration of how major aging parameters, such as the $\underline{k}$ in the Gompertz equation, which Dr. Simms evaluated for several species, can be related to the physiological parameters we discussed earlier.

The basic idea is this: an organism would be considered to consist of a network of chemical reactions whose rates are determined by enzymes. The thermodynamic properties of these enzymes are not arbitrary but are established as the result of an evolutionary process. So we can say an organism has certain thermodynamic capabilities, in terms of the evolved specificity and other characteristics of the enzymes, to carry out a desired set of reactions of the living organism with what one might consider to be the optimum efficiency in a particular environment, that is, temperature, concentration of electrolytes, etc. The organism provides this for itself by its internal milieu which is established by various homeostatic mechanisms. In some ideal situation, one could conceive of all these reactants flowing in at a perfectly uniform rate; a steady state might thus be maintained at as near the physiological optimum as possible, in terms of the genetically determined thermodynamic properties of the set of enzymes. Then by intuition and by resort to the concepts of information theory, one could state that the probability of an error—that is, an undesired side reaction per unit of time in the steady state—would be proportional to the number of molecular transactions per unit of time.

Such a term would thus depend on the flux of material through the organism, the rate of reaction, and the measure of this in the metabolic rate. Therefore, one could say that the life spans of organisms depend on metabolic rate, in inverse fashion to the way the information transaction per unit of time would depend on metabolic rate, if the organism could be maintained in a physiologically or biochemically ideal state. In fact it cannot; it is constantly being disturbed. Every displacement from the ideal means that the efficiency of the desired reaction is diminished and, quite probably, that the yield of undesired reactions increases. Therefore, one would say there would be a term for an additional contribution to the degradation of molecules in the organism—and therefore to aging—arising from a term in the form of a weighted sum of the mean square fluctuations of all the physiological variables from the biochemical ideal.

Just as the mean state is presumably established upon thermodynamic considerations, the degree to which the mean can be approximated is determined by the competence of the integrative mechanisms. I consider the latter term—the one arising from the fluctuations from the biochemical ideal—to be primarily influenced by the nervous system, and by this I mean all of the integrative mechanisms. If an organism has a large nervous system, it necessarily has more information in its genetic complement, which, I am sure, indicates greater enzyme specificity and more integrated cellular machinery, etc. The only extractable measure I know of today is this incredibly gross quantity, the weight of all the nervous system inside the skull.

Atwood: What do you mean by more enzyme specificity? Bacteria have wonderful enzymes, for example.

Sacher: Maybe enzyme specificity won't increase. As I see it, every species alive has had exactly the same length of time to evolve fundamental metabolic systems. However, the characters that make a mammal what it is are of more recent origin than those that make oxidative metabolism what it is; those that make a man a man are of even more recent origin. These latter factors are still susceptible to evolutionary improvement. They wouldn't be the basic enzymes but the kinds of things involved in polygenic control of development, where a lot of genetic determiners make small contributions to a number of different systems.

Atwood: So this is the "sackful-of-enzymes" theory?

Sacher: If you want to call it that. I haven't found any way of meaningfully introducing the concept of structure, and I don't want to give mere lip service to it. This is established by the information contained in the genotype. How, I don't know.

Atwood: I want to make a comment about the wearing out of the template. We have done an experiment on this, and I think a number of other people have done a similar one.
Some excellent bacterial systems are available in which the rate of use of a template can be changed at will. One is the induction of β-galactosidase by external inducers. In the uninduced cell the amount of β-galactosidase formed is about 1 molecule/cell division, and in the induced cell it is about one thousand times greater than that.

Fremont-Smith: What is the induced cell?

Atwood: A cell in the presence of an inducer substance such as β-methyl-thiogalactoside.

Fremont-Smith: Put in the environment?

Atwood: Yes. The enzyme is then formed in large quantities, whereas otherwise it is formed in small quantities. The mechanism of induction operates at the level of gene transcription; it can be shown that when inducer is given to the cell, the cell makes a polyribonucleotide which is a copy of the β-galactosidase gene locus and is exactly complementary to it. The gene is a template for the copying of this RNA. This then goes out to the ribosome and sits there, and the molecules of amino-acid-charged transfer RNA line up on this RNA messenger and the polypeptide is formed, which is the enzyme. If the template is worn out by use, one would expect that the mutation rate at the structural locus for β-galactosidase would be much higher when the cells are kept induced than when they are not induced. The fact is that the mutation rate is the same under the two conditions. Thus we do not see any evidence that the gene template is worn out by use.

Quastler: What you said implies that bacteria have a superbly efficient machine for making enzymes. As my colleague Zubay has pointed out, they also have much more evolutionary experience, in terms of generations passed, than we have.

Atwood: I should point out these mechanisms of protein synthesis have very great generality in all forms of life. In fact, we extremists would say there are no other mechanisms but those. The process is essentially the same in all organisms although the stability of messages may vary and some of the components may show more or less species specificity.

In my opinion the wearing out of templates by use is a very unlikely basis for senescence. Of course, "wearing out" goes on without use. The point is that these bits of matter are not indestructible; they have lifetimes of their own on which use may have little or no influence.

Sacher: Only the opposite inference is open to me when I consider the near invariance of energy expenditure per lifetime over a wide range of homologous homeothermic species. The value of 250,000 cal/g for typical mammals is a fact staring us in the face.

Atwood: I should judge this is just as likely to be a coincidence as to be a significant starting point. For example, is a hypothyroid individual whose metabolic rate is much lower going to live correspondingly longer?

Sacher: That is not a fair question because he is an abnormal individual.

<u>Atwood</u>: He is not abnormal enough to die right away.

<u>Sacher</u>: He is not normal, in the sense that his physiological function has to go on in rather an unfavorable set of circumstances.

<u>Atwood</u>: Then, in that case, one should always be able to assign his cause of death to the pathology. I don't think that is true. I think people have significant individual differences in metabolic rate that cannot be traced to any obvious pathology. I doubt that such differences, if carefully studied, would show the expected correlation with longevity.

<u>Brues</u>: In the course of this discussion, I continue to be reminded of certain more naive approaches to theory of aging. Specifically, I have been led to reflect on what Bernard Strehler (57) has called the "clinker" theory. This theory equates aging with the accumulation of some undesirable matter that cannot be disposed of. The hypothyroid individual accumulates a very specific "clinker," namely, cholesterol, which places a limitation on his life span.

<u>Atwood</u>: You're right.

<u>Brues</u>: Which is probably why we would not have adjusted in that direction in evolution.

<u>Atwood</u>: As to the clinker theory, the pigment in heart muscle that Strehler (59) measured looked promising because it increases with age. But his graph shows a lot of scatter. Certain young individuals have more pigment than is average for the very old, and vice versa. Since the variance of the age-specific pigment content seems greater than that of the age at death, this particular clinker does not seem to be an important cause of death.

<u>Ehret</u>: Returning to the wearing out through use, how does it go? Is it a direct function of time? You mentioned the two circumstances of use and non-use, Dr. Atwood.

<u>Atwood</u>: The cells were dividing at about the same rate under the conditions of use and non-use.

<u>Ehret</u>: But there is another use to which the template is put, and that is replication.

<u>Atwood</u>: Copy errors would affect the strand being newly synthesized, rather than the template strand. We can probably dismiss copy errors in non-dividing cells, since they would not affect the DNA, and a faulty message can be replaced. In dividing cells, they may contribute to the mutation rate.

Tyler: Were you postulating wearing out of the enzymes, and also instability of messenger RNA?

Atwood: The factors affecting the stability of RNA message are incompletely known. In cell-free systems such as Nirenberg's, message can be unstable without use.

Tyler: In the cell there probably is continued production of more messenger RNA.

Atwood: Right. As to other kinds of molecules wearing out, I think the evidence on enzymes would be generally against it. That is, enzyme molecules on standing in solution inactivate spontaneously and, if anything, faster when there is no substrate there than when there is. If enzymes wear out in cells, it wouldn't make much difference because they can always replace them. So I can't see that the wearing out of enzymes is a likely basis for senescence.

Tyler: Even in the non-mitotic cell there might still have to be a reasonably intact complement of DNA molecules.

Atwood: That is certainly true.

Tyler: Because they are read presumably from one end.

Atwood: Right.

Tyler: If there are breaks or interruptions, then the proper messenger RNA just won't be produced.

Atwood: Absolutely.

Tyler: So, there is no need to make a basic distinction between the dividing and non-dividing tissues.

Atwood: That is an inevitable cause of senescence in non-dividing cells. Our only problem in evaluating it is whether we live long enough to die of that rather than something else. But if we didn't have any other processes, that one would suffice and would be inevitable.

Brues: I wonder if you have any general thoughts, Dr. Keys.

Keys: I am reminded of the New Yorker cartoon showing a professor at a cocktail party who was left alone because he always insisted on talking about facts.
Mention was made earlier of exponential functions and how one could arrive at situations in which exponential functions would describe some of the conditions involved in aging and in senescence.
Let us consider one condition we know a bit about now,

which greatly affects our own longevity because it currently threatens to result, eventually, in the death of 50% of American men, and perhaps 40% of the women, such as are gathered at this conference. I am referring to myocardial infarction and other complications of coronary heart disease.

We said many years ago, and it is generally agreed now, that there is a relationship between the risk of this disease and the concentration of cholesterol in the blood (1). We now have enough follow-up material from large-scale studies at Framingham (22), Albany (24), Minnesota (35), and very recently from Chicago (42), to look critically into the situation and see what kind of a relationship we have to deal with.

In all of these studies, the picture of the risk of dying of this disease or developing myocardial infarction proves to be much the same. Let us say that the total risk, R, of future infarction is the sum of the effects of all influences unrelated to serum cholesterol plus a function of the pre-disease cholesterol concentration. For the moment we know nothing about all these influences unrelated to serum cholesterol and we simply put down their total effect as A. So we write the equation: $R = A + $ function of Chol.

We have tried to apply many mathematical models to the data from Framingham, Albany, and Minnesota, but the simplest and most promising are exponential or logarithmic equations of the forms

$$R = A + B \, (\text{Chol.})^k \tag{5}$$

or

$$\log R = A' + B' \log (\text{Chol.}). \tag{6}$$

To solve these equations and test their effectiveness in predicting the risk, R, we have data from several studies in which over 6,000 initially "healthy" men were followed for from 6 to 15 years during which time 251 of these men had infarcts or died from coronary heart disease. We began by classifying all of the men according to their pre-disease serum cholesterol concentration, under 200 mg/100 ml, 200-219, etc. Then for each such cholesterol class we write: $R_1 = A + B \, (\text{Chol.}_1)^k$, where R_1 is the incidence rate of infarction of men in a particular cholesterol class with average serum cholesterol, before disease, of Chol._1. Then with these numerical equations the constants A, B, and k may be found by least squares.

The result of these manipulations was that a good fit was found with values of k of the order of 2.5 to 3.0. For these data the average "predicted" values for the risk of infarction associated with the serum-cholesterol average were correlated with the observed risk with $r = 0.9$. Further, it appeared that about three-fourths of the total risk was accounted for by the serum-cholesterol level alone. The logarithmic equation (6), above, gave much the same good fit to the observed data.

It should be noted that the relationship between risk and serum-cholesterol level was substantially the same in all of the follow-up series. In other words, the relationship was not significantly different for businessmen in Minnesota, state employees in Albany, or men in the general population of Framingham, Massachusetts. In general, men with cholesterol levels less than 200 mg/100 ml proved to have less than one third the susceptibility to myocardial infarction of men with cholesterol levels of 260 or more. And there is no critical level; the risk simply rises roughly as the cube of the serum cholesterol concentration.

The high correlation found between observed risk and that predicted from cholesterol applies to the averages of groups of men who represent particular cholesterol classes. The risk for the individual, of course, is a matter of statistical probabilities.

It can be shown that the high correlation found is actually an underestimate of the true correlation between serum cholesterol and risk of infarction. This follows from the fact that the men were classed according to the serum-cholesterol value found in a single sample of blood, but we know that a single sample is far from a perfect representation of the true average serum-cholesterol level of the individual over all the time of atherogenesis preceding the infarction, that is, over all the time when, presumably, the cholesterol concentration in the blood is influencing atherogenesis and thrombogenesis.

A single blood sample is not even a very reliable indicator of the average serum cholesterol of the individual over a short period of time. When we take repeated blood samples from the same individuals over a few days or weeks, we find that the average intra-individual standard deviation around the individual's mean value is of the order of 20 to 25 mg cholesterol/100 ml serum. This means that about one-third of the samples will have cholesterol values that are 20 to 25 mg/100 ml or more above or below the true mean for the individual. Larger variations occur if the mode of life and other variables are not constant, if there are dietary changes, alterations in physical activity, minor illnesses, etc.

This intra-individual variation is a considerable fraction of the total inter-individual variation. For all the groups we have studied, the inter-individual standard deviation is of the order of 40 to 45 mg cholesterol/100 ml. A part of the intra-individual variation can be explained by spontaneous, unnoticed variations in the diet. When men are kept in a metabolic ward with the diet absolutely constant from day to day, the average intra-individual variation in serum cholesterol is only about 12 mg/100 ml. But even this residual variation is appreciable and we have no explanation for it at all.

Nor, for that matter, do we have much explanation for the differences among individuals in regard to serum cholesterol. A few cases with habitually very high cholesterol levels are explained by genetic factors and a few others by thyroid hypofunction. A major influence of the habitual diet is seen when we compare men whose diets are greatly dissimilar in regard to fats. But within populations with relatively homogeneous dietary customs there is still much inter-individual difference and this is not explained.

For our present purposes, the upshot is that if we had better representations of the true long-time average serum cholesterol levels of individuals we should undoubtedly find a closer relationship to the risk of infarction than observed so far.

Fremont-Smith: That is, if you trace the trend over a period of years?

Keys: Yes.

Fremont-Smith: Does this mean if the cholesterol is going up?

Keys: No, this is simply random variation. We pick out one blood sample and say that the analysis labels the fellow. We find this a poor label because it doesn't differentiate him well enough to allow us to take full advantage of whatever the underlying relationship may be.

Sacher: Dr. Keys, is this individual standard deviation essentially the error of measurement?

Keys: No, the error of measurement for serum cholesterol is rather small with proper methods. The variance attributable to measurement error is less than 20% of the total intra-individual variance in cholesterol.

Sacher: Has the heritability of blood cholesterol level been measured in an experimental animal, such as the chicken?

Keys: There has been quite a bit of work done on this in man, as you know.
    It depends on the population. If we take a population of Japanese and Finns and mix them up, we get very large cholesterol variation between individuals. If we take a population of garment workers in New York, the variation is much less.

It was in the latter situation that Adlersberg (1) did his work. As I recall, the estimated genetic component of the variation was something of the order of 30 or 40% in Adlersberg's material. The differences between individuals beyond genetic explanation are, of course, fascinating and very important. But we haven't the foggiest idea as to why and how they exist.

Brues: I think this would be a good time to have Dr. Quastler embark on the summation.

Atwood: I don't want to have the last word, so if the summation is about to begin, this is the time to issue the molecular manifesto. (Laughter)

Fremont-Smith: Molecules, unite! (Laughter)

Atwood: Aging is a summation of individual microevents at the molecular level, and the explanation we want of the phenomenon is the identification and characterization of these events. This will involve a knowledge of the nature of the events themselves and, in particular, of the biomolecules that are subject to them in any important sense. I just want to give some hunches about what this may involve.

One thing is this. If we consider any replaceable component of the organism, it should be replaced in response to depletion if the homeostatic mechanisms operate—and we are often much impressed by how well they operate, for a while at least. So I take the view that the replaceable constituents are unlikely to be involved in the process as I described it. They will, of course, show changes secondary to the process in which we are really interested. These will confuse investigators. Indeed, such secondary changes probably constitute the bulk of our present information.

Now the principle that what is replaceable is unimportant can be carried down through all levels. If a cell is replaceable and we believe that the daughter cells are usually accurate copies of the mother cell, then we can dismiss such cell populations as primary sites of aging. If a wrong copy is made it too can be replaced. Similarly, inside a cell that is not itself normally replaceable, we can dispense with the replaceable intracellular components as primary aging sites. Proceeding in this manner, we end up with the DNA of non-replicating cells as the primary site.

Another source of confusion for the problem of localization is the presence of entities (for example, the crystalline lens) that seem to age autonomously, and yet in so doing contribute little or nothing to the probability of death. Whenever such an entity is recognized, it should be steadfastly ignored.

Still another canard is the roster of organisms that die

in some specialized manner, such as moths with flight-release hormone, or salmon with Cushing's syndrome. These make interesting topics of conversation, but the tendency to regard them as relevant is a palpable hindrance to progress.

Now, what kinds of experiments could be undertaken to pursue the foregoing ideas? One approach is seriously to attempt anatomical localization of the process. This must be carefully distinguished from the search for pathology, which has, in my opinion, already been carried to its inherent limits. The techniques that suggest themselves at present are back-transplantation and radiation shielding. To make use of the latter technique, we must temporarily adopt the hypothesis that whatever the process is, it is sure to be mimicked by radiation. The difficulty is the profusion of side effects which will confound the investigator who does not, for the time being, hold fast to his assumptions. Shielding experiments have been done in many previous contexts. In the present context, their purpose would be to localize the long-term effect on longevity, independent of recognized pathology. By "recognized" I mean recognized as radiation sequelae: tumors, and so on. Even if the detailed molecular lesions with radiation are different from the spontaneous, such experiments would tell us where in the organism truly irreplaceable biomolecules reside. I hold the prejudice that these locations will be different from those that are most significant for the acute syndrome at moderate doses.

Another approach is to devise experiments based on some plausible conjecture concerning the nature of the quanta of aging. The free-radical trapping agents you spoke of, Dr. Lindop, and the inconclusive result there should be pushed with this idea in mind.

Simms: I am not sure I understood you correctly. First you brought out a hypothesis that aging must take place at a molecular level.

Atwood: Yes, obviously.

Simms: I don't think we know enough about aging to draw that conclusion. Second, if I understood you correctly, you said that aging is affected by radiation. I don't think that has been proved.

Atwood: I should say not, but I think that to make radiation a useful tool we have to make the assumption for a while that that is true.

Simms: Since it has been presented at this meeting, I take it that radiation has been shown to affect the time of onset of one or two diseases but not all of them. My own feeling is that unless radiation can be shown to produce a similar effect to the one I discussed earlier, that of a reduced diet in which all major lesions are affected, I don't think the effect is necessarily on the aging process.

Quastler: I would like to see incidence curves of the major lesions in all the irradiated animals, not only those that are presumed to have died from each specific disease. Lesion incidence curves tell us much more than survival curves.

Lindop: I think there is a slight misinterpretation of what I was trying to say earlier. Radiation, in fact, does affect all diseases, but it affects some more than others. I like your suggestion, Dr. Atwood. That is the hypothesis we have been working on up to now. The only part I find puzzling is your statement that one should, when studying the results, exclude what is known to be specific radiation damage such as tumor induction. From our data and from many other people's, one can't differentiate what is a specific radiation-induced lesion.

Atwood: In order to understand a process it is often helpful to exclude others temporarily from consideration. In a sense, tumors are relevant since their age incidence is proportionate in animals of widely disparate longevity. In a more important sense, they are irrelevant since the tumor-free animal ages, even so.

Birren: I wonder why you put the question on the level of the cell rather than, say, the extracellular space in the mammal.

Keys: Or the organization of the cells.

Birren: Don't collagen fibers age somewhat autonomously in the extracellular space?

Atwood: Yes, but is that what we die of? If collagen did not age would we be immortal?

Birren: Let me display my naivete. I thought some people had developed a theory of mammalian aging in terms of changing permeability of extracellular space.

Atwood: They have developed it. (Laughter)

REFERENCES

1. Adlersberg, D., L. E. Schaeffer, and A. G. Steinberg. 1957. Studies on genetic and environmental control of serum cholesterol level. Circulation 16: 487-88.

2. Armitage, P., and R. Doll. 1957. A two-stage theory of carcinogenesis in relation to the age distribution of human cancer. Brit. J. Cancer 11: 161-69.

3. Beard, R. E. 1959. Notes on some mathematical mortality models. In G. E. W. Wolstenholme and M. O'Connor (eds.), Ciba Foundation Colloquia on Ageing. 5. The lifespan of animals, pp. 302-11. Boston: Little, Brown.

4. Beeton, M., and K. Pearson. 1901. On the inheritance of the duration of life and on the intensity of natural selection in man. Biometrika 1: 50-89.

5. Bertalanffy, L. von. 1951. Theoretische Biologie (2d ed.). Berne: A. Francke.

6. Binet, L., and F. Bourlière. 1955. Précis de gérontologie. Chap. 1. Paris: Masson et Cie.

7. Blest, A. D. 1960. The evolution, ontogeny, and quantitative control of the settling movements of some New World Saturniid moths, with some comments on distance communication by honey-bees. Behaviour 16: 188-253.

8. Blest, A. D. 1963. Longevity, palatability, and natural selection in five species of New World Saturniid moth. Nature 197: 1183-86.

9. Bonin, G. von. 1937. Brain weight and body weight in mammals. J. Gen. Psychol. 16: 379-89.

10. Box, G. E. P. 1954. The exploration and exploitation of response surfaces: some general considerations and examples. Biometrics 10: 16-60.

11. Box, G. E. P., and J. S. Hunter. 1957. Multi-factor experimental designs for exploring response surfaces. Ann. Math. Stat. 28: 195-241.

12. Brill, A. B., M. Tomonaga, and R. M. Heyssel. 1962. Leukemia in man following exposure to ionizing radiation. Ann. Int. Med. 56: 590-609.

13. Brody, S. 1945. Bioenergetics and growth. New York: Reinhold.

14. Carlson, L. D., and B. H. Jackson. 1959. The combined effects of ionizing radiation and high temperature on the longevity of the Sprague-Dawley rat. Radiation Res. 11: 509-19.

15. Carlson, L. D., W. J. Scheyer, and B. H. Jackson. 1957. The combined effects of ionizing radiation and low temperature on the metabolism longevity and soft tissues of the white rat. I. Metabolism and longevity. Radiation Res. 7: 190-98.

16. Clarke, J. M., and J. Maynard Smith. 1955. The genetics and cytology of Drosophila subobscura. XI. Hybrid vigour and longevity. J. Genetics 53: 172-80.

17. Comfort, A. 1956. The biology of senescence. New York: Rinehart.

18. Conard, R. A., H. E. MacDonald, L. M. Meyer, S. Cohn, W. W. Sutow, D. A. Karnofsky, A. A. Joffee, and E. Riklon. 1962. Medical survey of Rongelap people seven years after exposure to fallout. Brookhaven Nat. Lab. Report BNL-727.

19. Cork, J. M. 1957. Gamma-irradiation and longevity of the flour-beetle. Radiation Res. 7: 551-57.

20. Cronkite, E. P., W. Moloney, and V. P. Bond. 1960. Radiation leukemogenesis: an analysis of the problem. Am. J. Med. 28: 673-82.

21. Davey, W. P. 1919. Prolongation of life of Tribolium confusum apparently due to small doses of X-rays. J. Exp. Zool. 28: 447-58.

22. Dawber, T. R., and W. B. Kannel. 1961. Susceptibility to coronary heart disease. Mod. Conc. Cardiovasc. Dis. 30: 671-76.

23. Doll, R. 1962. Age difference in susceptibility to carcinogenesis in man. Brit. J. Radiol. 35: 31-36.

24. Doyle, J. T., A. S. Heslin, H. E. Hilleboe, P. F. Formel, and R. F. Korns. 1957. A prospective study of degenerative cardiovascular disease in Albany; report of three years' experience. I. Ischemic heart disease. Am. J. Publ. Health 47, No. 4, Suppl.: 25-32.

25. Failla, G. 1958. The aging process and carcinogenesis. Ann. N. Y. Acad. Sci. 71: 1124-40.

26. Fisher, J. 1958. Multiple-mutation theory of carcinogenesis. Nature 181: 651-52.

27. Fisher, J. C., and J. H. Hollomon. 1951. A hypothesis for the origin of cancer foci. Cancer 4: 916-18.

28. Flower, S. S. 1931. Contributions to our knowledge of the duration of life in vertebrate animals. Vertebrate mammals. Proc. Zool. Soc. London: 145-234.

29. Furth, J., A. C. Upton, K. W. Christenberry, W. H. Benedict, and J. Moshman. 1954. Some late effects in mice of ionizing radiation from experimental nuclear detonation. Radiology 63: 562-70.

30. Gel'Fand, I. M., and M. L. Tsetlin. 1962. Some control methods for complicated systems. Uspekhi Mathematicheskikh Nauk 17: 3-25. (Available as JPRS translation No. 13707, U. S. Dept. of Commerce, Office of Technical Science.)

31. Haldane, J. B. S. 1932. The causes of evolution. London: Longmans Green.

32. Heyssel, R., A. B. Brill, L. A. Woodbury, E. T. Nishimura, T. Ghose, T. Hoshino, and M. Yamasake. 1960. Leukemia in Hiroshima atomic bomb survivors. Blood 15: 313-31.

33. Hollingsworth, J. W., G. Ishii, and R. A. Conrad. 1961. Skin aging and hair graying in Hiroshima. Geriatrics 16: 27-36.

34. Jarvik, L. F., A. Falek, F. J. Kallmann, and I. Lorge. 1960. Survival trends in a senescent twin population. Am. J. Human Genetics 12: 170-79.

35. Keys, A., H. L. Taylor, H. W. Blackburn, J. Brozek, J. T. Anderson, and E. Simonson. 1963. Coronary heart disease among Minnesota business and professional men followed fifteen years. Circulation 28: 381-95.

36. Klein, G., and E. Klein. 1958. Histocompatability changes in tumors. J. Cell. Comp. Physiol. 52, Suppl. 1: 125-68.

37. Lankester, E. R. 1870. On comparative longevity in man and the lower animals. London: Macmillan.

38. Lindop, P. J., and J. Rotblat. 1961. Long-term effects of a single whole-body exposure of mice to ionizing radiations. I. Life-shortening. Proc. Roy. Soc. (London) Ser. B. 154: 332-49.

39. Lorenz, E., L. O. Jacobson, W. E. Heston, M. Shimkin, A. B. Eschenbrenner, M. K. Deringer, J. Doniger, and R. Schweisthal. 1954. Effects of long-continued total-body gamma irradiation in mice, guinea pigs and rabbits. III. Effects on lifespan, weight, blood picture and carcinogenesis and the role of the intensity of radiation. In R. E. Firkle (ed.), Biological effects of external X- and gamma radiation, part I, pp. 24-148. New York: McGraw-Hill.

40. Medawar, P. B. 1957. The uniqueness of the individual. London: Methuen.

41. Parrott, D. M. V. 1959. Ovarian grafting as a method for research into ageing. Gerontologia 3: 91-96.

42. Paul, O., M. H. Lepper, W. H. Phelan, G. W. Dupertuis, A. MacMillan, H. McKean, and H. Park. 1963. A longitudinal study of coronary heart disease. Circulation 28: 20-31.

43. Pearl, R., S. L. Parker, and B. M. Gonzalez. 1923. Experimental studies on the duration of life. VII. The Mendelian inheritance of duration of life in crosses of wild type and quintuple stocks of Drosophila melanogaster. Am. Nat. 57: 153-92.

44. Pearl, R., and R. DeW. Pearl. 1934. The ancestry of the long-lived. Baltimore: Johns Hopkins Press.

45. Petter-Rousseaux, A. 1955. Recherches sur la croissance et le cycle d'activité testiculaire de Natrix natrix helvetica. Terre et Vie 100: 175. (Summary in L. Binet and F. Bourlière. 1955. Précis de Gérontologie. Paris: Masson et Cie.)

46. Pilleri, G. 1959. Beiträge zur vergleichenden Morphologie des Nagetiergehirns. Acta Anat. 39, Suppl. 38: 1-124. 1960. 42, Suppl. 40: 1-188. 1961. 44, Suppl. 42: 1-84.

47. Roderick, T. H. 1963. Selection for radiation resistance in mice. Genetics 48: 205-16.

316 AGING AND LEVELS OF BIOLOGICAL ORGANIZATION

48. Rubner, M. 1908. Das Problem der Lebensdauer und seine Beziehungen zur Wachstum und Ernährung. Munich: Oldenbourg.

49. Russell, W. L. 1957. Shortening of life in the offspring of male mice exposed to neutron radiation from an atomic bomb. Proc. Nat. Acad. Sci. U.S. 43: 324-29.

50. Sacher, G. A. 1956. On the statistical nature of mortality, with especial reference to chronic radiation mortality. Radiology 67: 250-57.

51. Sacher, G. A. 1959. Relation of lifespan to brain weight and body weight in mammals. In G. E. W. Wolstenholme and M. O'Connor (eds.), Ciba Foundation Colloquia on Ageing. 5. The lifespan of animals. Boston: Little, Brown.

52. Sacher, G. A. 1963. Effects of X-rays on the survival of Drosophila imagoes. Physiol. Zool. 36: 295-311.

53. Sacher, G. A., and D. Grahn. 1963. Survival of mice under duration-of-life exposure to gamma rays. I. The dosage-survival relation and the lethality function. J. Nat. Canc. Inst. 32: 277-319.

54. Simms, H. S. 1942. The use of a measurable cause of death (hemorrhage) for evaluation of aging. J. Gen. Physiol. 26: 169-78.

55. Simms, H. S. 1946. Logarithmic increase in mortality as a manifestation of aging. J. Gerontol. 1: 13-26.

56. Strehler, B. L. 1959. Origin and comparison of the effects of time and high energy radiations on living systems. Quart. Rev. Biol. 34: 117-42.

57. Strehler, B. L. 1960. Dynamic theories of aging. In N. W. Shock (ed.), Aging: some social and biological aspects. AAAS Publ. No. 65.

58. Strehler, B. L. 1962. Further studies on the thermally induced aging of Drosophila melanogaster. J. Gerontol. 17: 347-52.

59. Strehler, B. L., D. D. Mark, A. S. Midvan, and M. V. Gee. 1959. Rate and magnitude of age pigment accumulation in the human myocardium. J. Gerontol. 14: 430-39.

60. Szilard, L. 1959. On the nature of the aging process. Proc. Nat. Acad. Sci. 45: 30-45.

61. Thompson, D. W. 1952. On growth and form. Cambridge: Cambridge Univ. Press.

62. Upton, A. C., A. W. Kimball, J. Furth, K. W. Christenberry, and W. H. Benedict. 1960. Some delayed effects of atom-bomb radiations in mice. Canc. Res. 20: 1-62.

63. Weissmann, A. Ueber die Dauer des Lebens. 1882. Jena: G. Fischer.

Summation of the Conference

Quastler: I feel diffident about summarizing this conference since I see a number of people around this table who have written a good deal more about aging than I have read—but I'll try. I'll put some large chips on my shoulder which I expect will be knocked off. My summary will be restricted to those parts of the proceedings which touched directly on the specific topic of "concepts of aging and biological organization."

The topic of "levels of biological organization" was put before this conference at the very beginning when Dr. Fremont-Smith asked: "Are we troubled because we have fewer cells or because we have cells that are not so good?" For the present purpose, I'd like to reduce the complex hierarchy of biological organization to just three levels: individuals, including populations of individuals, and organs; cells and cell populations; and macromolecules, including cell organelles. At each level, different problems are encountered. As this conference unfolded, it was very noticeable that for each biological entity different sets of facts were discussed. With each set of facts went a set of theories—often many theories. Since aging is a field where experimental data are very hard to come by, it has been blessed or plagued (whatever you want to call it) with an unusual amount of theorizing. This is the unavoidable consequence of having to make the most out of limited data.

The theories show an interesting range in the number of causative factors involved. There are examples of the single-factor theory, the classical type of theory which tries to single out one critical factor; there are plurifactorial theories, probably most important biologically and, unfortunately, exceedingly difficult to treat mathematically; there are many-factor theories, assuming factors too numerous to be dealt with individually and calling for statistical treatment. Some theories make explicit use of random elements. These were put before the conference in the opening remarks, when Dr. Brues spoke about cellular information being shuffled and reshuffled more or less randomly until it loses validity—one of the ways of looking at the aging process. It was interesting to note that to some of us (myself included), a role of random events seemed quite natural although others obviously found it repugnant. At any rate, there is no technical difference between effects due to random events and effects due to unknown (preferably numerous) factors; both are treated by the same statistical approach.

A population of individuals is the result of a gene pool acted upon by a particular surrounding. The gene pool came to be what it is by selection, and selection depends on gene action. In discussing gene action, Dr. Dobzhansky brought out the difference between single-factor and multiple-factor mechanisms: there are "good" genes, classical genes in the Mendel-Morgan tradition, genes responsible for the "one-gene–one-trait" situations; and there are genes connected with plurifactorial mechanisms—polygenes where several genes affect one trait, pleomorphic genes where one gene affects several traits. For very good reasons, in the early stage of a science, scientists select for single-factor mechanisms, "good" genes in this case. For equally good or better reasons, nature selects for plurifactor mechanisms. Important features of the aging process may well be dominated by pleomorphic polygenes.

The plurifactorial approach helps to mitigate a problem which is still very much up for discussion, the selection for limited spans of reproductive activity and of life itself. As Dr. Lansing pointed out, termination of reproductive activity is not a necessary consequence of biological organization; death seems to be. Since both are genetically determined, they have presumably been arrived at as the result of natural selection, and the question arises as to how something as negative as death or the cessation of reproductive activity can be selected for. One answer is in plurifactorial determination: genes which now tend to limit the life span may have conferred advantages at the time they were selected for. Sickle-cell anemia is a good example of this. Others may simply be linked to advantageous genes. To some of us here, however, it seemed easy to see that limitation of life span itself could confer an advantage to the species and thus be selected for. To others, this thought was difficult to accept. Mr. Sacher brought up a beautiful example: one species of moth looks inconspicuous, seems to be acceptable food to birds, and dies soon after reproduction; another species looks conspicuous, tastes very bad, and is longer-lived. In the latter case, the advantage to the species is clear. Each non-reproductive surviving moth may teach some bird, at no cost to the species, to leave this kind of thing alone. The advantage of early death in the former case is less clear. While each non-reproductive survivor may help some bird form a dangerous habit, that particular moth may also be taken instead of a reproductive member of the tribe. The application of selection principles to the determination of the human life span is not easy to see. In some populations old individuals are of great value as teachers and leaders; in others they are an intolerable burden. Could selection have taken place in the very limited lifetime of the human species?

One of the most frequently studied features of a population is the life table. As everyone here pointed out at one time or another, death is a miserable end point because there are so many ways of dying. Still it is a reasonably objective end point and one about which a great deal is known. How much does genetic constitution, and how much does environment contribute to shaping the life table? In some species, death is strictly and simply programed. A good example of a single-factor programed death was given by Dr. Tyler: the Pacific salmon after spawning develops Cushing's syndrome and dies. Such strict reliance on a particular mode of death seems to be exceptional. A less strict relation between reproduction and death can be seen in female mice of a strain with high incidence of breast cancer, where each pregnancy increases the probability of developing a lethal cancer. In many cases, death is not tied up with any particular function.

Let us leave the attempts to identify the mechanisms underlying the life table, and turn to the shape of the life table in general. This problem is treated by statistical methods. With most higher organisms, a curve of fraction surviving versus time shows a definite S-shape, usually skewed to the left. The logarithmic derivative of this curve can be described by the Gompertz function or some similar expression. All these curves have essentially two parameters. One is a scale factor, converting something like "speed of living" into units of absolute time. (Dr. Ehret brought up the interesting question of whether time should be measured appropriately in terms of revolutions of the earth, or in terms of circadian rhythms.) The other is related to the width of the shoulder of the S-curve, and is some kind of expression of stability of the biological system. There are half a dozen or so mathematical models which will result in S-curves of survivors or Gompertz curves of mortality rate, and in each of these models the two parameters acquire a distinct and very precise meaning. Unfortunately, all these models result in curves which are quite indistinguishable between 10 and 90% survival. Since, in higher organism, one does not put much credence in the results based on the first few decedents or the last few survivors, it follows that the analysis of the mortality curve gives very little insight into the underlying mechanisms.

This does not mean that the statistical parameters extracted from the life table are useless. If one accepts—and not everybody does—Hardin Jones's contention that all human mortality data share a common time-scale parameter, then a whole life-table characteristic of a given situation can be described reasonably adequately in a single number. Dr. Lindop gave another example: by plotting probit of survival versus the square of time elapsed, she obtained parallel straight lines. This again is a very useful descriptive device. However, if the one parameter thus extracted from a life table is treated as a function of some variable, and then a parameter is extracted from this function and again studied for dependence on something else, one risks getting into deep water through distortions due to accretion of empirical approximations.

Some of the participants stated that if one had a truly homogeneous population, kept under truly homogeneous conditions, the survival curve should then be rectangular, with all individuals dying at the same age. Real curves are not rectangular, but this, to some of us here, including myself, does not imply heterogeneity of the population or the conditions but simply the working of random elements. After all, if one takes a perfectly homogeneous collection of atoms and watches the result of, say, three successive transformations (disregarding the first two), the resulting curve will be sigmoid, just like a typical life table. The deviation from "rectangularity" is due to randomness. Now, random events may very well enter into the determination of the life span. Mr. Sacher discussed models of this type. There is, for instance, Szilard's model (and several others) where differences in survival time are ascribed to randomly distributed amounts of damage accumulated before birth. Mr. Sacher is concerned with the effects of randomness at the other end of the life span: a given physiologic state is associated with a certain probability of dying, which does not jump from 0 to 1 but shows a slow transition. In addition, random events may well affect the density of "aging events" along the life span. This sounds like a very realistic model which embodies all the likely features of a survival function, but it has one critical weakness. To determine a life table in terms of this model, at least four free parameters are available. The statistical analysis of the life table yields only two good parameters; hence, a model of the type described can be neither disproved nor proved through analysis of the life table. In other words, any number of models can be proposed that will be invulnerable to anything that may be extracted from a life table.

One can attempt to add to the stochastic models more detail and, implicitly, more vulnerability, by specifying what particular mechanisms are involved in the progress toward death. Mr. Sacher is trying to do just that but—old friendship will permit a harsh criticism—his physiological model with its potential wells, force functions, and restoring functions, has so many undefined variables as to be quite invulnerable. Now, I came to this conference believing that a model that was not vulnerable by any facts was not worth anything. I've changed my mind. While I still prefer a vulnerable model to an invulnerable one, I can realize the great value of invulnerable models in suggesting avenues of approach.

A simple life table can be used to achieve great progress if one registers not just the time of death but the time of various changes, including onset of various diseases. An example of this approach was given by Dr. Simms. Or one can go even further, as Dr. Lindop did, and discuss the inducibility of pathological conditions as a function of age.

A pattern of appearance of changes in time is a sophisticated way to define aging. The pattern certainly depends on genetic factors as well as on surroundings. Dr. Keys talked about human populations which are genetically poorly defined but, in some cases at least, live in well-defined surroundings; the pattern of disease incidence is very much affected. The question of surrounding comes up whenever the details of the aging process are discussed, and particularly when one tries to identify the normal, or natural, aging process. But what is natural surrounding? Is Dr. Simms's rat palace a natural surrounding? Is the condition of the underfed rat a natural or unnatural one?—a wild rat will seldom eat to satiation. Dr. Storer mentioned that when control mice are caged together with irradiated mice they experience a shortening of the life span. There are many factors which affect the life table as a whole and the detailed patterns of incidence of pathological changes. It is difficult if not impossible to pick out one set of conditions and label it as the normal situation that will reveal the normal course of aging. Dr. Barrows pointed out that some enzymes change in the underfed rat while others don't. This certainly does not mean that these enzyme changes should be excluded in a study of aging.

This brings us to the irradiation studies. It is well known that in many ways an irradiated individual resembles an unirradiated but older individual of the same kind. Certain effects of irradiation on the life table discovered by Dr. Brues and Mr. Sacher (1) suggested that in some ways irradiation can be equated to a normal lapse of time. By causing accelerated or premature aging, radiation would then be an invaluable method of studying normal aging. As experience with late effects of irradiation accumulated, more and more differences between irradiated and aged individuals became known, and any lingering belief in the nice, simple idea of equating late effects of irradiation to aging was destroyed by the sledge-hammer treatment applied by Drs. Cottier and Lindop. It seems to me, however, that this is the right moment to rehabilitate radiation studies as a legitimate method in aging research. Certainly, the time pattern of changes in the irradiated animal has some specific features; so does the time pattern characteristic of the underfed animal; so does the time pattern of the pampered rat in Dr. Simms's palace; so, presumably, does the time pattern for any well-defined set of conditions. All we have to do is free ourselves of the idea that some particular set of conditions has more inherent virtue than any other, and a whole host of conditions become equally legitimate foundations for research in aging.

Related to variations in time pattern of aging changes is the question of an objective criterion of aging. The quest for criteria has been going on as long as research in aging, and it has been going on during this conference too. There still does not seem to be a better criterion than that furnished by the calendar.

The most widely respected criteria of aging are still those furnished by the pathologist. One event that made me very thoughtful in this context was the violent attack Drs. Lansing and Keys delivered on the kind of qualitative judgment that goes into the findings of pathologists. They don't want to believe any statements not based on measurements, and they are not willing to accept the experienced pathologist as a fairly good digitalized disease meter. I had bad visions of simple statements such as "stomach cancer," "gall stones," and "atherosclerosis" being replaced by some formidable array of numbers which had to be fed into a computer since no human could deal with them. Having recovered from the first shock, however, I admit that it might be a very good idea to break with a great deal of medical tradition and start thinking along such lines as Drs. Lansing and Keys suggest. When I was still practicing medicine I might have found it a bit more difficult to consider such a thorough revolution in medical thinking.

Since the "naive," largely qualitative criteria of aging are of doubtful value, one tends to define aging changes in terms of measurable responses in test situations. Drs. Birren and Jarvik presented results obtained with beautiful batteries of tests. Incidentally, I enjoyed hearing at last of tests in which people get better between 68 and 80. My guess is that we might find more such tests if we looked for them; we are much too preoccupied with the detrimental changes associating with aging. This brings out one weakness inherent in the use of batteries of tests: they tend to reveal what one is looking for and no more.

The question of genetic and environmental determination of the aging process has been approached in a very interesting way through the study of twins, as reported by Drs. Kallmann and Jarvik. I'd like to refer to one small part of their study—the account of the twin sisters who were just about indistinguishable in every way, except that one was a missionary and the other a farmer's wife. I'd like to submit that this illustrates the play of random events on the level of the individual, rather than plasticity in the sense of reacting to environment in an adaptive way.

We now proceed to the cellular level of organization. Dr. Atwood made the case for the non-dividing cells as the chief actors in the aging process. Dr. Jarvik argued that dividing cells may play a larger role than suspected. To be sure, nobody dies of old age because a system of dividing cells gives out. One does not die in old age from aplastic anemia, or from denudation of the intestinal lining, or from loss of the epidermis. Yet there are a number of things that change in dividing cells as an individual grows old.

Dr. Court-Brown talked about the loss of the X and Y chromosomes which occurs with progressive frequency as age increases. One rarely observes loss of other chromosomes. It may well be that any chromosome can get lost but that cells which have lost large chromosomes are selected against. Perhaps related to the loss of sex chromosomes is Dr. Fry's finding that duration of the phase during which DNA is replicated varies increasingly with age. Since the chromosomes that tend to get lost are those which double last in DNA synthesis, it could be that they sometimes fail to accomplish their duplication before the synthesis phase ends.

The increasing frequency of chromosome losses with age may well be correlated with the increasing frequency of anomalies in children as the parents grow older. This, however, contrasts strikingly with the integrity of the germ line. What keeps the germ line intact? Is it selection pressure on the cellular or subcellular level?

An interesting aspect of aging changes was discussed, too briefly, by Dr. Storer. It appears that in a number of instances tested, the mean value of some feature showed little or no change with age, but the variance increased with age. Of particular interest in this context is the increase in variance of red-cell size with age, which is evidence of an age-related change in a cell-renewal system. Dr. Brues and some of us agreed at lunch that it would be fun to find out whether variance goes up at different rates in long- and short-lived animals; if the variance in man goes up as fast as it does in the mouse then by the time he has reached 80 his red-blood cell sizes should be scattered all over the map. There must, therefore, be some factor controlling the rate at which variability changes with age.

Very much in this context belongs Dr. Tyler's unifying hypothesis of carcinogenesis. His theory, a plurifactorial one, is based on the idea that cells in older persons tend to lose some of their genetic material. That makes them different from other cells, and immunological differences, among others, will result. Immunological difficulties between cells can result in rapid and uncontrolled growth. This is a very attractive hypothesis but, I'm afraid, invulnerable.

Tyler: It is very vulnerable.

Quastler: Can you name one experiment whose outcome would make you drop the hypothesis forever? I doubt it. It seems invulnerable, together with all the auxiliary hypotheses. At any rate, it is very useful in suggesting approaches for further experimentation.

Dr. Lindop reported that radiosensitivity increases steeply in very old mice. Under the conditions used, radiosensitivity depends on the reproductive capabilities of the stem cells which form platelets and granulocytes. The increased sensitivity may well mean decadence of the stem cells.

With all these indications that everything is not right with cell-renewal systems in aging individuals, one may wonder about the range of validity of the statement that people don't die from depletion of cell-renewal systems. Suppose we do conquer the degenerative vascular diseases; won't the life span then be terminated by breakdown of cell-renewal systems?

An observation concerning a conditional renewal system was not brought up during the conference, but it is so relevant that I want to mention it here. This is work done by H. J. Curtis on liver cells in mice (3). In the normal adult mouse, liver cells divide about once a month. If a good fraction of the liver is removed, however, the remaining cells proliferate rapidly until the organ size is restituted. During this period, chromosomal anomalies are easily detected. In normal young mice the frequency of such anomalies is low. As the mice age, however, the frequency increases until in old mice there is hardly a cell which has not some anomaly. The increase of frequency with age was followed in two strains, a short-lived and a long-lived one, and the rise was significantly steeper in the short-lived strain. It seems that the accumulation of chromosomal anomalies does not keep a liver cell from living reasonably well, unless it tries to divide.

The liver is the only system I know of where changes with age in the genetic apparatus have been tested directly in a slowly dividing cell population. As to other slowly dividing or non-dividing cell populations, particularly those of the central nervous system, we know that they dwindle in number and tend to accumulate abnormal components. What this means functionally we really do not know.

I don't want to leave the cells without reminding you that Dr. Tyler has developed a case of a cell endowed with a very specifically programed mode of death: the sea urchin sperm, if given sufficient time, commits suicide by ingesting metals.

There is not much to say about the molecular aspect of aging after the molecular manifesto Dr. Atwood delivered. Considering the tremendous vogue of molecular biology, there really was very little talk about molecules at this conference. The aging pigment has not shown up, probably by accident. Dr. Barrows produced some very interesting data on enzyme levels which clearly showed that there is no simple correlation between aging and levels of enzymatic activities, as tested so far. Only cathepsins seemed to go up regularly, and there may be good reasons for this. DNA does not change much; it decreases in total amount in accordance with the loss of cells. RNA does not change much either; but tracer uptake into RNA is greatly increased in some cells, and this may have something to do with decaying templates.

I should not leave the molecules without reminding you of a warning Dr. Dobzhansky sounded at the beginning of this conference. The Mendel-Morgan kind of genetics went through a "one-gene–one-trait" stage which was dominated by an unrealistically simple model of gene properties and gene action, but this was probably necessary in the development of the discipline. Could it be that molecular genetics, or "DNology" as Dr. Dobzhansky calls it, with its nice, clean "one-gene–one-messenger–one-enzyme" scheme is in a similar stage of adolescence?

Tyler: I think it is up to Mr. Sacher and me to defend ourselves briefly with respect to invulnerable hypotheses. I thought mine was quite vulnerable. In fact, I presented a general concept and then a very special derivation, a simple form of the concept. I thought I had presented data to prove that the simple form of the hypothesis was wrong but that the general form remained. I don't consider the general concept invulnerable; I think we can attack it. I can see at least one other general concept in opposition to it, namely, that the neoplastic cell possesses something intrinsically that determines its special properties. This could be a mutated gene or a virus affecting directly the phenotype of the cell. Such a concept is a distinct alternative to ours, which supposes that the neoplastic property results from an effect of materials from other tissues of the body to which the gene-loss cell has a new relation. I think experiments will soon permit us to decide between these general concepts.

Sacher: I certainly am concerned with the comparative invulnerability of the stochastic model. That is why I say as often as possible that one finds evidence of consistency with the model and not proof of it, and so I continue to look for a satisfactory test situation.

[(Afterthought) Meanwhile, it has been fruitful to me because, in Dr. Quastler's phrase, "it suggests a way of going about finding things." The role of brain size in longevity is one thing the theory set me to looking for. Above all—and here I must disagree with Dr. Quastler—it is a phenomenological theory in intent, if not yet in fact. The theory has a great avidity for data and this keeps me running in the effort to find enough to satisfy it.]

Tyler: In our experiment, as Dr. Keys pointed out, we had three tumors out of 48 F_1 animals, and we expected 48 out of 48 on the basis of the special form of the theory that used the minimum number of ad hoc assumptions.

Quastler: You could account for 45.

Tyler: Then we begin to add that hypothesis. This, of course, is exactly where we get into the danger that you mentioned, namely, of becoming invulnerable. But I think we have so far avoided this in that our added assumptions are based on experimental evidence and the modified special hypotheses remain experimentally testable.

Quastler: I really think I should state the attitude about invulnerable hypotheses which I have developed during these last three days. Clearly, every idea goes through an invulnerable stage. In principle, I don't see why one should be in a great hurry to get it into the vulnerable stage. It may be very profitable just to develop the picture and see where it leads without trying to test it severely, for a while at least. I consider both Mr. Sacher's and Dr. Tyler's hypotheses as very fertile in guiding exploration. I may also be persuaded that Dr. Tyler's has indeed reached the stage of test.

Sacher: I might call attention to another model that could be considered invulnerable because it seems so absolutely right. This model, one form of which was espoused by Dr. Atwood in his ringing manifesto, states that aging ultimately is a molecular degradation. There could equally well be intact molecules and degradation of order. This could happen, particularly in our favorite noble-cell system, the nervous system. With enough cross-connections made or enough overwriting done, it gets progressively less useful as a logic or memory unit, as Dr. Atwood pointed out earlier. I think one might be able to produce other models of degradation of order and not leave the molecular-denaturation model arraigned as the only one.

Fremont-Smith: We wouldn't have to start at the macromolecular; we can go to the atomic and subatomic. Certainly there will be reflections all along the line. What we need is not to try to find a final solution but to try to look at the same phenomenon on many different conceptual levels simultaneously—on the levels of the social group, the individual, the organ system, the organ, the cells, the macromolecular, and further down if possible. It seems to me the picture will only be a whole one when we relate these different levels to one another rather than select one and say: "This is it."

Atwood: We can safely assume that most of our atoms are stable.

Tyler: Don't we really complete the cycle when we reach the point where we are dealing with elementary particles that are mathematical concepts?

Atwood: As to the dividing-cell problem, I felt much less sure that non-dividing cells were the only possible candidates at the cell level after I became convinced that the tissue-culture people had found a time limit of about 2 years for the propagation of normal diploid cells. If the culture has not converted to an aneuploid strain by then, the stock is lost. This could still be because the medium is wrong. Maybe they haven't tried Versene. (Laughter)

Tyler: I'm afraid they have, Dr. Atwood.

Brues: I might mention that we have had some lines that have remained stable for the past 2 years, even after a dose of X ray; however, this seems to be unusual (5).

Atwood: Have they converted?

Brues: No.

Atwood: You are doing it very well.

Lansing: Two hours ago I would not have believed our conference could have been summarized as brilliantly as it has been. I mean that! I am impressed with the quality of the summary, and I think Dr. Quastler has made a very important point. The study of senescence is one that is characterized by speculation and too seldom subject to experimentation. The data in this field are shockingly scarce. We have very few pegs on which to hang our hats. One thing is certain: I think we all agree that practically all living things die. I say "practically all" because there is always that rare exception that eludes careful analysis. But this is a fact, and I think one should pay attention to it rather than accept it uncritically.

It is also a fact that senescence has escaped the process of natural selection as a presumably unfavorable trait for the individual. Natural selection has failed to eliminate it from the vital series over millions of years, or however long it is that life has existed.

There is more than one possible explanation of this failure of natural selection. One possibility is that unfavorable genes that express themselves after the reproductive phase and that cannot be eliminated produce senescence—I don't believe it, but it is a possibility. Another is that senescence is desirable to the species. Perhaps the moth analogy gives us an idea here. Again it is quite possible that in the animal kingdom, which survives by way of predation and only by way of predation, it is desirable for the species to have a useless component in its population—useless because it has already reproduced—a component that can serve as ready prey for the predators, leaving those who have yet to do a breeding job free of predators. I say that with tongue in cheek; I don't believe it, but it is a possibility. I think the important thing is that data are very scarce. We come up with all sorts of models based on permeability or lack of permeability, age pigments—or "clinkers." All of these are entertaining to us, but they only add value if they lead to experiments. I think it is incumbent upon us to seize on the few facts we have in this field and to ask nature the right questions. I beg a question when I say "the right questions." What constitutes a right question? It is one that will lead to useful data. It is painful that we have so few facts with which to work, for this further encourages the speculative.

One last point. I am not sorry I shocked Dr. Quastler; I don't know about Dr. Keys. But, again, we have a very important problem. Unless we as scientists are working for our own amusement and collecting data for ourselves, it is very important that we communicate. In order to communicate, then, the recipient of the communication must understand the language that is used. When one deals with analytical material it is very simple to communicate. Once I know what a millimole is we have a common basis for exchange. But when one has to use descriptive procedures that depend to a large extent on art and undocumented observation, it is very important to describe carefully the process or phenomenon the communicator wishes to get over to the recipient. That was the basis of my protest.

I am reminded of Bacon, four hundred years ago, with his four stumbling blocks to truth. I have an atrocious memory, but one of the stumbling blocks, I think, is custom—the use of custom to dignify an approach. This has been done for so many years, and we continue to do it, and it inhibits the evolution of truth. Another one is the use of authority. "I have been a professor for twenty years and I have seen so many thousand cases. On the basis of my experience, there is no question that I am right." We are all familiar with this. The third one, if I remember correctly, is concealment of ignorance by ostentation of seeming wisdom; and the fourth, use of inaccurate senses.

I think this is what is being protested, not the method of the morphologist, whether he be anatomist or pathologist.

Brues: I like your point about asking questions. It is easy to give good answers but it takes much more to formulate and ask the right questions.

I imagine that if we were to look at the proceedings of this conference from the standpoint of a practicing geriatrist reading the record, we would see that he is expected to go on doing the same things he has always done. He will help to minimize the fluctuations in the internal environment. He will help to protect his patients against the insults of the external environment. He will try to avert the accumulation of the "clinkers." These things he has done all along, but perhaps he will ask better questions and thus advance the state of the art and extend the scope of our understanding.

Atwood: Dr. Quastler, I would like to raise a minor question about your interpretation of the increased sensitivity of older animals to an acute radiation dose—one producing bone-marrow death. This was taken to mean that the dividing stem cells had suffered an effect over time.

Suppose the sensitivities of young and old were compared as before, except that in each case an injection of bone-marrow cells of standard viability from a young animal was given after the challenge dose. If an age effect is still produced (and

I suspect it would be), it would indicate that the ability of the animal to tolerate bone-marrow depletion—rather than the resistance of the bone-marrow cells themselves—has decreased with age.

Lindop: I am not quite sure I agree with your interpretation, Dr. Quastler, that the increasing sensitivity of old age was the result of the dividing cells, or stem cells, being less resistant. We get exactly the same quantitative relationship for the long-term effect. This is an expression of result occurring many weeks after the dose and therefore isn't bone-marrow failure as such. The stage has been passed at which the bone marrow is replicating dividing cells or bone-marrow cells, which are the important ones. There is still a quantitative, increasing sensitivity with old age.

Quastler: Yes, you are both right. Death is due to a failure of the stem cells to produce enough platelets or granulocytes before fatal dysfunction occurs. The failure may indeed be due to the ambient as well as to the cells themselves. The experiment Dr. Atwood suggested—irradiating an old mouse to see whether it can be protected with young bone marrow—is a very simple one and would be decisive.

Atwood: The predicted result is well in line with Dr. Simms's bleeding experiment.

This kind of experiment actually bears on the problem of localization, as a variant of the back-transplant approach.

Transplantation from old to young is more direct; if an organ could be maintained for, say, one and one-half times the life span of the whole animal, this would permit one to exclude that organ from consideration as a primary site of aging.

Jarvik: I have some difficulty in visualizing any such precise localization of aging. At least, judging from Lashley's experience, we should not be too optimistic. Lashley (4) started out trying to specify the anatomic sites for certain brain functions and ended up with the concept of equipotentiality, which we are just beginning to get away from (2). It took almost a quarter of a century.

Atwood: It is simply a matter of technical feasibility. There is nothing obscure or difficult about the concept. One transplants a kidney from an 8-month rat back into a 2-month rat. One takes out the other kidney too so one knows that is the one. Then, when the rat gets to be 8 months old, one transplants it back into another 2-month-old rat.

Jarvik: It isn't the technical aspect that is difficult to understand but the concept of localizing within any one organ something as complex as the initiation or maintenance of aging processes. Thus we may be able to ascribe certain age changes to alterations in a given organ such as the kidney, but there will undoubtedly be other phenomena of aging that must be described at different levels of organization, be they molecular, submolecular, or organismic. As Dr. Fremont-Smith said earlier, we have to talk of aging at different levels. We can't hope to explain solely at the molecular level, for instance, what we mean by psychological aging.

Tyler: I would like to comment on Dr. Court-Brown's work on the sex chromosomes to which Dr. Quastler referred. Before I do so let me also express my admiration for the summation. It was not just a brilliant performance but also another bit of evidence concerning what goes on and what doesn't go on during aging. I think you have proved to all of us, Dr. Quastler, that there is at least one faculty which need not be impaired with age. I can't imagine anyone processing information, mostly new information, better than you have done. I can't even imagine you, at an earlier age, doing it any better.

There was, however, one little slip about sex. The sex chromosomes are not inactive in mammals. There are many genes present in the X chromosome and some have recently been found in the Y chromosome in addition to those for maleness. Dr. Court-Brown reported on increased losses of X chromosomes and Y chromosomes with aging.

Fremont-Smith: I am grateful to every one of you for participating. I speak on behalf of A. I. B. S., and naturally we don't have any unkind feelings toward the National Heart Institute, which made this conference possible.

REFERENCES

1. Brues, A. M., and G. A. Sacher. 1952. Analysis of mammalian radiation injury and lethality. In J. J. Nickson (ed.), Symposium on radiobiology, pp. 441-65. New York: John Wiley.

2. Chow, K. L., and P. F. Hutt. 1953. The association cortex of Macaca mulatta; a review of recent contributions to its anatomy and functions. Brain 76: 625-77.

3. Curtis, H. J. 1963. Biological mechanisms underlying the aging process. Science 141: 686-94.

4. Lashley, K. S. 1929. Brain mechanisms and intelligence. Chicago: Univ. of Chicago Press.

5. Stroud, A. N., B. R. Svoboda, and A. M. Brues. 1962. Characteristics of long-term variant clones of pig kidney cells. Rad. Res. 16: 589.

Aging and Space Travel

Quimby: If a conference can be said to switch gears, this one is now doing so. The title of my presentation is "Aging in the Space Age."

There is probably little that the exploration of space, as I see it, can contribute directly to solving the problem of aging, except the remote possibility that, if man can approach the velocity of light in space flight, he may not age so rapidly. That is, at such velocities, the formulas of normal physics must be replaced by those of the relativity theory.

The relativistic time dilatation, as it is characteristically called, is a theoretically effective gain over real time on earth, if the crew members can spend more than 10 years of their lives on a voyage at the speeds near the utmost limit of velocity. Von Hoerner (1) has made calculations to show that the time dilatation accumulates so rapidly that it is nearly incredible, like money at a very high rate of compound interest.

Table 31 shows the immense contrast we would have, according to the theory. You will notice that the crew in space for 1 year would be spending essentially the equivalent of 1 year on earth; after 2 years in space they will have spent slightly more time than that on earth. And, as one proceeds, there is an exponential effect so that, after 60 years in flight, one passes the fantastic figure of 5 million years on earth. This is because of the time dilatation that takes place at velocities near the velocity of light.

Atwood: Is this travel at uniform velocity or uniform acceleration?

Quimby: It is acceleration and deceleration at 1 g.

Fremont-Smith: I am not sure I understand the implication. Does this mean that when the crew has been in space for 10 years, they will have aged 24 years, or that they will only age 10 years in 24 years of earth time?

TABLE 31

Total Duration and Distance Reached with Constant Acceleration and Deceleration at 1 G (1)

Time for crew in space (Years)	Time for people on earth (Years)	Distance reached (Parsecs)*
1	1.0	0.018
2	2.1	0.075
5	6.5	0.52
10	24	3.0
15	80	11.4
20	270	42
25	910	140
30	3,100	480
40	36,000	5,400
50	420,000	64,000
60	5,000,000	760,000

*One parsec equals 3.26 light years. A light year is slightly less than 6 trillion miles.

Quimby: These men would age 10 years, and their brothers on earth would age 24 years. That is what it means.

Fremont-Smith: If they come back!

Quimby: I will come to that in a moment.

Let us apply these numbers to a hypothetical case. A crew could spend 30 years on a voyage to the Orion nebula and back and, upon their return, find that 3,000 years have elapsed on earth. When they returned, earth civilization could be as strange, perhaps, as any they visited in space; or the earth might be uninhabited as a result of one or more thermonuclear wars. In fact they might find they should have stayed where they were.

Perhaps Orion is a poor destination. Let us think of a more interesting journey. Let us think of the nearest 10 star systems which might have one or more planets with an environment similar to our own and, perhaps, intelligent beings. These are, on the average, 18.6 light years away. The distance the crew would travel, incidentally, is 2×10^{14} miles. A trip there and back would consume 12.3 years in flight and 42 years on earth. Thus, any child 10 years old at the time of the rocket's departure from earth could hear or read the report from the crew if he lived to be 52 years old. He would theoretically see a crew of his own age, if the crewmen were 40 years old at the time of takeoff.

These calculations are not wild. They simply assume very

large spacecraft and a constant acceleration and deceleration at 1 g, which is what we are subject to here on earth. With a closed ecological system and with a crew society geared to life in a large-rocket environment, the venture is not impossible, if aging is indeed decreased by a relativistic time dilatation. The limits are not set by biological considerations. The constraints for interplanetary space travel are, instead, exactly where they are in space advancements today—energy!

It appears that the requisite acceleration and velocities cannot be achieved by uranium reactors, controlled fusion of hydrogen to helium, or ion propulsion, in part because these systems are all so massive. The power-to-mass ratio required for relativistic velocities must be achieved by a technology which we cannot at present foresee. The alternative would be to render man ageless, or nearly so; then the unattainable relativistic velocities would not be required. By "ageless" I mean possessing a life span of at least 380 years. That is the time we should need to reach and return from the nearest stars, using the most efficient possible nuclear propulsion.

Perhaps only hypothermia or hibernation of the crew is the solution. But it would be difficult to communicate a growing terrestrial technology to men with frozen or inactive brains. In fact communication with any crew at distances measured in light years is a severe problem, because radio waves travel at the speed of light, which is 3×10^9 cm/sec.

Since intergalactic trips remain for the next generation, let us look at some closer celestial bodies for our destination in space. Voyages to planets in our own solar system are possible within the limits of modern spacecraft technology and of man's natural life span. This is apparent from Table 32, which gives the one-way time of flight to these planets, calculated for minimum energy paths from the earth. Some astronomers may disagree with the exact numbers listed here. I did not list Pluto because it is not a real planet. I think it is regarded as a satellite of Saturn that moved out of its original moonlike orbit.

By taking advantage of the periodic proximity of the planets, using the gravity of the sun and target bodies, and planning trajectories and times of departure, it seems that we could eventually orbit the planets in manned spacecraft. Temperature would have to be controlled in the spacecraft while it is near the sun or far away from it.

Mars seems to be the most habitable planet, whether for life of indigenous origin or for the crew of a spacecraft. Mercury and Venus are too hot and the rest of the planets are all regarded as too cold. Even if these planets were merely orbited, the vehicle would be in the same solar-temperature in-

TABLE 32

One-Way Time of Flight to the Planets
(Minimum-energy paths from earth)

Planet	Time to planet (Approximate)	Sidereal period (Revolution in years)
Mercury	106 days	.24
Venus	146 days	.62
Mars	259 days	1.88
Jupiter	2.7 years	11.86
Saturn	6.1 years	29.46
Uranus	16 years	84.01
Neptune	30.7 years	248.4

fluence as the planet itself. It would take propulsion energy to keep from hitting the major planets and more energy to escape from them. It would take energy to keep us warm, and with respect to Mercury and Venus we might need energy for a little refrigeration.

Mars then appears to be the most definite possibility within our lifetime. A trip to Mars and back will require more than double the time needed to reach Mars at opposition, because return would require a wait for proper orbital opportunity between the earth and Mars. Also the distances at different oppositions vary. In February of 1963, which is the next opposition, Mars will be about 62 million miles from us. In 1971, it will be 34.6 million miles away from us.

Fremont-Smith: How long would it take to go back and forth at the shortest opposition?

Quimby: If you mean during the same opposition, that is now impossible.

Fremont-Smith: Roughly speaking, what is it in years?

Quimby: With current propulsion technology, around 3 years. Round-trip trajectories for manned voyages to Mars have been calculated by Von Braun and Ley (2). I remember it as 900 days, but I am not sure. I can also give you Glenn Seaborg's recent calculation: he has indicated that by using some form of nuclear propulsion, he could get us there and back in 11 months. The time schedule for this voyage is not mentioned by Dr. Seaborg.

Fremont-Smith: That gives the range.

Quimby: Even available spacecraft technology can do this job, if an adequate and reliable life-support system can be developed and if the metabolic requirement of the crew can be met for a 2-1/2- to 3-year period of time. For three men, assuming a 900-day voyage, something like 8 million calories would be required. I allow 3,000 cal/man-day. That would be a little over 1-1/2 tons of completely dehydrated food. They would also need about 10 tons of water. (Of course, we might recycle the latter, especially the urine, and perhaps some of the moisture which accumulates in the cabin atmosphere.) Oxygen requirement runs a little over 2 lb/man-day or 3 tons for the entire voyage. This weight would be greatly reduced, of course, if we could reliably recycle the respiratory gases. Such a system would also eliminate the weight of equipment for the absorption of carbon dioxide.

The biologists at NASA are not exclusively interested in or dedicated to manned space flight, or the origin of life on earth, or to proving the cosmic principle of life by detecting it on Mars, although we are of course trying to do all three of these. We are mindful of and concerned with terrestrial biological and medical problems, such as the one which inspired this conference. We are prepared, politically and scientifically, to contribute to the resolution of this and other biological problems. After all, the earth is a planet and, like all others, it is in space too. We simply know more about the planet earth and its biology because we have more convenient access to it—we are on it. While conquering space, with its other planets and celestial bodies, we shall also conquer this little terrestrial sphere to which we are temporarily restricted. We shall somehow prolong the life span of man, who altogether too often succumbs to death at his most productive age: that, I think, is the most serious aspect of the aging problem.

Fremont-Smith: How about siphoning a little energy from the sun for the long-range flights? There may not be any lying around on the earth, but there is quite a lot up there.

Quimby: Energy could be tapped from the sun with solar cells. This is done on all of our satellites and deep space probes. It is being done now on Mariner II for the Venus flight. If we didn't recharge those batteries with solar energy, we wouldn't get any information back from the planet when we pass it ten or eleven days from now.

Fremont-Smith: I was being slightly fantastic in suggesting going up and grabbing a good chunk of that energy and taking it along with us—I haven't got the metallurgy worked out for it.

Quastler: The energy requirement depends very much on

just how closely the speed of light is to be approximated. How much energy is needed to get up to, say, 90%?

Quimby: If 90% or better of the speed of light can be reached, the time dilatation effect of relativity apparently comes into effect. If we could completely annihilate matter, 98% of the velocity of light could be achieved.

Fenn: When an astronaut is coming back at nearly the speed of light, does he get a similar contraction?

Quimby: It wouldn't make any difference whether he is going or coming; as long as he is traveling near the speed of light, time is theoretically "shortened."

Fremont-Smith: Would he stay young?

Quimby: He would not stay young, but he would not manifest the usual signs of terrestrial age as rapidly. You see, in order to make a long space voyage, the velocity of light must be approached very slowly. Otherwise the crew could not stand the acceleration. The calculations have been based upon 1 g. It would take a certain amount of time before one approached the speed of light at an acceleration of 1 g.

Then, as he reached his destination which, shall we say, would be Jupiter, he would have to slow down, also at a rate of 1 g. During the early acceleration and later deceleration, he would not be so near the speed of light and would not be getting the relativistic time dilatation.

Fremont-Smith: I have a formal suggestion to make to NASA, and I am very happy to make it in the presence of Dr. Kallmann. That is that only one member of identical twins be selected for space astronauts. Then we will really have an experiment!

Quimby: I am a little more serious, but there are theoretical limits to this entire matter; it may never happen.

Fremont-Smith: You mean hardly ever.

Quimby: "Impossible" is a word I hate to use. However, according to the mass-energy physicists, we cannot get the necessary energy out of any known material. A series of booster stages might optimize the capability of hydrogen fusion engines to achieve velocities approximating those of this discussion.

REFERENCES

1. Hoerner, S. von. 1962. The general limits of space travel. Science
   137: 18-23.

2. Ley, W., and W. von Braun. 1956. The exploration of Mars. New
   York: Viking Press.

PARTICIPANTS

Dr. Kimball C. Atwood
Department of Genetics
University of Illinois
  School of Medicine
Urbana, Illinois

Dr. C. H. Barrows
Gerontology Branch
National Heart Institute
Baltimore City Hospitals
Baltimore, Maryland

Dr. James E. Birren
Section on Aging
National Institute of Mental
  Health
Bethesda, Maryland

Dr. Austin M. Brues
Division of Biological and
  Medical Research
Argonne National Laboratory
Argonne, Illinois

Dr. Hans Cottier
Medical Research Center
Brookhaven National
  Laboratory
Upton, Long Island, New York

Dr. W. M. Court-Brown
Medical Research Council
Western General Hospital
Edinburgh, Scotland

Dr. Th. Dobzhansky
Department of Zoology
Columbia University
New York, New York

Dr. Charles F. Ehret
Division of Biological and
  Medical Research
Argonne National Laboratory
Argonne, Illinois

Dr. Wallace O. Fenn
Department of Physiology
University of Rochester
  School of Medicine and
  Dentistry
Rochester, New York

Dr. Frank Fremont-Smith
Interdisciplinary Conference
  Program
American Institute of Biologi-
  cal Sciences
New York, New York

Dr. R. J. Michael Fry
Department of Physiology
Trinity College
University of Dublin
Dublin, Ireland

Dr. Lissy Jarvik
Department of Psychiatry
New York State Psychiatric
  Institute
Columbia University
New York, New York

Dr. Franz J. Kallmann
Department of Mental Hygiene
New York State Psychiatric
  Institute
Columbia University
New York, New York

Dr. Ancel Keys
Laboratory of Physiological
    Hygiene
University of Minnesota
Minneapolis, Minnesota

Dr. Albert I. Lansing
Department of Anatomy
University of Pittsburgh
    School of Medicine
Pittsburgh, Pennsylvania

Dr. Patricia J. Lindop
Radiobiology Unit
St. Bartholomew's Hospital
    Medical College
London, England

Dr. Henry Quastler
Department of Biology
Brookhaven National
    Laboratory
Upton, Long Island, New York

Dr. Freeman H. Quimby
Division of Biosciences
National Aeronautics and
    Space Administration
Washington, D. C.

Mr. George A. Sacher
Division of Biological and
    Medical Research
Argonne National Laboratory
Argonne, Illinois

Dr. Henry S. Simms
Department of Pathology
Columbia University College of
    Physicians and Surgeons
New York, New York

Dr. H. Burr Steinbach
Department of Zoology
University of Chicago
Chicago, Illinois

Dr. John B. Storer
Roscoe B. Jackson Memorial
    Laboratory
Bar Harbor, Maine

Dr. Albert Tyler
Department of Biology
California Institute of
    Technology
Pasadena, California

Index of Names

Adlersberg, D., 310
Alexander, P., 236
Alpatov, W. W., 185
Anderson, E. C., 118
Andrew, W., 111, 112, 153
Aschoff, J., 210
Ashley, W. R., 146
Atwood, K., 66, 67, 68, 69, 70, 72,
74, 75, 76, 79, 80, 81, 82, 101,
102, 103, 107, 116, 118, 120,
121, 142, 143, 144, 146, 147,
170, 171, 174, 182-85, 187, 212,
213, 242-46, 250, 265, 266, 270,
272, 273, 274, 278, 283, 284,
287, 288, 289, 290, 296, 297,
298, 303, 304, 305, 306, 310-12,
323, 325, 327, 328, 329, 330,
332

Bacon, France, 329
Baily, N. A., 282
Banga, I., 236
Barnes, D. W H., 68
Barrows, C. H., Jr., 40, 102, 103,
104, 105, 106, 107, 110, 111,
112, 121, 152-86, 187, 190, 193,
233, 235, 236, 321, 325
Beard, R. E., 286
Beeton, M., 291
Berg, B. N., 89, 90, 96, 110, 111,
112, 116, 117, 118, 119, 175,
232, 324
Bernard, C., 291
Billingham, R. E., 58
Birren, J. E., 7, 13, 21, 27, 80,
103, 111, 122-38, 142, 144, 145,
146, 184, 188, 208, 209, 212,
236, 255, 265, 268, 269, 270,
274, 279, 280, 282, 286, 288,
312, 322

Blest, A. D., 18
Bond, V. P., 191
Botwinick, J., 132
Box, G P. E., 295
Boyse, E. A., 61, 71, 77
Brandt, K. F , 112
Braun, S. von, 332
Brent, L., 58
Brody, S., 275, 278
Brown, M. B., 68
Brues, A., 16, 29, 33, 35, 38, 39,
44, 45, 46, 50, 61, 65, 66, 67,
71, 72, 73, 74, 75, 76, 77, 78,
79, 81, 82, 117, 126, 141, 142,
144, 152, 154, 161, 162, 174,
188, 189, 192, 203, 204, 209,
218, 220, 221, 247, 263, 264,
265, 266, 279, 282, 284, 287,
289, 305, 306, 310, 317, 321,
324, 327, 328, 329

Calhoun, J. B., 153
Calloway, E., 132
Carlson, A., 103
Carlson, L., 187
Carlson, L. D., 283
Clark, L. C., Jr., 158
Comfort, A., 14, 271, 280
Conard, R. A., 264
Cork, J M., 282
Cottier, H., 76, 92, 113, 114, 116,
118, 119, 121, 122, 126, 154,
155, 161, 162, 191, 234, 255-60,
264, 265, 289, 322
Court-Brown, W. M., 19, 28, 29,
31, 65, 70, 78, 79, 80-82, 323,
331
Cross, R. J., 169
Curtis, H. J., 324

344 INDEX OF NAMES

Verzar, F., 111, 235, 236
Vos, O., 68

Waksman, S. A., 51
Weissmann, A., 267
Welch, G., 31
Whipple, G. H., 120
Williams, G. C., 14

Wolf, A., 116
Wright, E. A., 255
Wulff, V. J., 187, 210

Yiengst, M. J., 112

Zorzoli, A., 157, 158
Zubay, 304

Index of Subjects

Adaptedness, meaning of, 13
Age: and alerting reaction, 132;
and behavior in communication,
137; creativity as function of,
146; and digit-symbol test performance, 134; and mental test
performance, 134, 136; and
recognition speed, 134; and
speed of performance, 129; and
stored information, 136, 137;
and vocabulary test, 139
Aging: actuarial approach to, 296;
and aneuploidy, 31; biochemical
processes in, 152; blood pressure and age of parental death,
205-7; and blood pressure in
different populations, 206; and
body weight, 194, 197, 232-33;
and cancer, 74; and cell loss,
152; chromosomal hypothesis
of, 25; criteria for, 122, 322;
crucial question of, 7; definition of, 220; as disease, 87-
120; and disease, semantics of,
111; distinct from senescence,
25; in extracellular space, 312;
genetic control of, 14, 19; and
homeostasis, 204, 291; immunogenetic theory of, 56; localization of, 310-11, 330; and loss
of chromosomes, 79, 285-86,
323; and loss of nerve tissue,
143; at molecular level, 267,
310, 327; and neoplastic disease, 55; and nerve conduction,
34-35; and nervous system,
122-38; non-lethal diseases in,
114; and physical activity, 103;
programed, 14, 18, 271, 273;

radiation exposure in Hiroshima, in Rongelap Island, 263;
radiation-induced, 218, 264-65,
311-12; and replication of DNA,
79, 323; and reproductive period, 268, 271; of sea-urchin
eggs, 53; and sensitivity to
acute radiation, 237-39, 248;
of space crews, 332, 334; and
species-specific factors, 186;
spontaneous, and free radicals,
188; and target model of carcinogenesis, 284; in unicellular
organisms, 27; uniformity of,
32; a universal process, 208;
and variability of performance,
192-201; and X-ray toxicity,
194; see also Senescence, Theories of aging
Aging process: and non-dividing
cells, 323; theories of, 208
Algorithms, computational, 295-
96
Allergic death, basis for tumor
therapy, 71
Alzheimer's disease, 13, 15
American Negroes, and sickle-
cell anemia, 16
Amino acids, and life of sea-
urchin sperm, 53, 54
Amyloidosis, in mice, 113
Anencephaly, and developmental
stability, 5
Aneuploidy, and aging, 31, 80
Animal behavior, circadian as-
pects of, and aging, 209
Antibiotic patulin, 8
Antigens, methods for identifying
loss of, 72

age, 202; and environmental
variance, 193; and hormonal
system, 204; individual and genetic, 6
Homeostatic mechanisms, 193,
292–94, 302
Homeostatic regulation, and mammalian life-table, 294
Homosexual behavior, genetic determinants of, 14
Hormonal system, and homeostasis, 204
Human life-table: Szilard's theory
of, 285–87; theory of, 290
Huntington's chorea, and lethal
gene, 22
Hypertension: and age, 206; and
genetic differences, 209; in
rats, 92, 111–12; and reaction
time, 144
Hypertrophy, of muscle in swimming rats, 127
Hypodiploidy: and age constancy,
81; and sex differences, 80
Hypotheses, invulnerable and vulnerable, 325-26
Hypoxia, and radiation sensitivity,
245

"Incidence," meaning of, 97
Industrial mechanism, 17
Information theory, 302
Infradian rhythm, 212
Inheritance: concept of, 1; distinguished from heredity, 1; semantics of, 1; see also Heredity
Intelligence, and life span, 141–42
Ionizing radiation, and leukemia,
65
Irradiation: of Drosophila, and
longevity, 282–83; effects on
life table, 218–26, 300–301, 321;
and incidence of leukemia, 239;
late effects on aging, 322; and
longevity in mice, 198

Japan: leukemia in, 264-65; mortality rate and radiation exposure, 264

Kidney: cell change, in rats, 153,
171; regeneration of, by rats,
110

Learning ability, and genetic fixity, 9
Lens opacities: chromosomal damage and, 32; radiation-induced,
250–51
Lesions, onset of, 93–97
Lethal gene: definition of, 23; in
mice, 22; in Pacific salmon,
23; and termination of life, 22
Leukemia: age-dependent, 241;
and Down's disease, 65; hormone dependent, 241; incidence
of, and age at irradiation, 239;
and ionizing radiation, 65; in
irradiated mice, 225; and Philadelphia chromosome, 82; and
radiation exposure in Japan,
264–65; radiation-induced, and
age, 241
Life expectancy, for rats, 93
Life span: and autopsies, 117; and
body size, 274–77; and brain
weight, 276–77; and enzymes,
157–58; extension of, 108, 109;
and heart beats, 278; in irradiated mice, 253; in mammals,
278; relation to brain and body
age, 275–80; of rodents, 278,
279; and space research, 336;
and stress, 109; and use of
thyroxin, 109; ways of altering,
108, 109
Life table: mechanisms underlying,
319; statistical models of, 319,
320
Life termination: in Huntington's
chorea, 22; and lethal gene, 22;
in moths, 18; in Pacific salmon, 23
Liver, cell changes in rats, 154
Liver weight, in mice, 161
Longevity: and brain size, 202,
276–77; and enzyme activity,
179; gene control of, 20, 21;
and homeostasis, 202; human
heritability of, 290, 291; in irradiated Drosophila, 282, 283;
in irradiated mice, 198; and
metabolic rate, 189; and motor
activity, 103, 104; and mutation
rate, 21; and natural selection,
18; of Old Testament patriarchs,
45; and oxygen consumption,
186, 187; of prehistoric man,